Principles of Clinical Cancer Genetics: A Handbook from the Massachusetts General Hospital

Daniel C. Chung · Daniel A. Haber
Editors

Principles of Clinical Cancer Genetics: A Handbook from the Massachusetts General Hospital

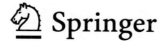 Springer

Editors
Daniel C. Chung
Massachusetts General Hospital Cancer Center
and Gastrointestinal Unit
Harvard Medical School
Boston, MA
USA
dchung@partners.org

Daniel A. Haber
Massachusetts General Hospital Cancer Center
Harvard Medical School and Howard Hughes
Medical Institute
Boston, MA
USA
dhaber@partners.org

ISBN 978-0-387-93844-8   e-ISBN 978-0-387-93846-2
DOI 10.1007/978-0-387-93846-2
Springer New York Dordrecht Heidelberg London

Library of Congress Control Number: 2010926039

Printed on acid-free paper

Springer is part of Springer Science+Business Media (www.springer.com)

Preface

Cancer is fundamentally a genetic disorder, and the rapid accumulation of insights into the broad spectrum of genetic alterations that underlie human cancers has been staggering. Equally exciting has been the translation of many of these insights into the clinical management of patients with cancer or at high risk of developing cancer. Over the past decade, the field of "clinical cancer genetics" has entered a renaissance that has thrust it into an integral position in modern cancer care.

Our goal with this textbook is to provide a comprehensive reference on current topics in cancer genetics for the clinician. At the Massachusetts General Hospital Cancer Center, our multidisciplinary group of clinicians, basic scientists, translational scientists, and geneticists strive to seamlessly integrate cancer genetics into the care of our patients and their families. The basic principles of cancer genetics (Chapter 1) and genetic testing (Chapter 2) are first reviewed. In Chapters 3–13, we highlight the hereditary cancer syndromes most commonly encountered in the clinic, focusing on the underlying genetics, clinical presentations, screening and surveillance strategies, genetic testing algorithms, risk-reducing surgical approaches, and management of cancer. These syndromes encompass a broad range of hereditary tumors of the breast, colon, pancreas, stomach, kidney, skin, and endocrine organs, as well as Wilms, retinoblastoma, and neurofibromatosis syndromes. Finally, Chapters 14 and 15 explore new directions in cancer genetics: the role of low penetrance cancer susceptibility alleles as well as the impact of molecularly targeted cancer therapies.

The number of genes that contribute to both hereditary and sporadic cancers continues to grow. As a consequence, the impact of genetics on strategies for cancer prevention and therapy is increasing at a similar pace. The care of the cancer patient is continually being transformed by genetics, and we hope to share with the reader the excitement, importance, and potential of clinical cancer genetics.

Boston, MA

Daniel C. Chung
Daniel A. Haber

Contents

1 **Basic Principles of Cancer Genetics**... 1
  Leif W. Ellisen and Daniel A. Haber

2 **Principles of Cancer Genetic Counseling and Genetic Testing**......................... 23
  Kristen M. Shannon and Devanshi Patel

3 **Genetics of Hereditary Breast Cancer** 41
  Paula D. Ryan

4 **Surgical Management of Hereditary Breast and Ovarian Cancer**...................... 53
  Michelle C. Specht, Marcela G. del Carmen, and Barbara L. Smith

5 **Hereditary Colon Cancer: Colonic Polyposis Syndromes**................................. 63
  Andrew T. Chan and Daniel C. Chung

6 **Hereditary Colon Cancer: Lynch Syndrome**... 77
  Eunice L. Kwak and Daniel C. Chung

7 **Hereditary Pancreatic Cancer** 89
  Janivette Alsina and Sarah P. Thayer

8 **Hereditary Diffuse Gastric Cancer** 97
  Prakash K. Pandalai and Sam S. Yoon

9 **Familial Renal Cell Cancers and Pheochromocytomas**.................................... 109
  Gayun Chan-Smutko and Othon Iliopoulos

10 **Familial Atypical Mole Melanoma (FAMM) Syndrome** 129
   Elizabeth D. Chao, Michele J. Gabree, and Hensin Tsao

11 **Multiple Endocrine Neoplasia** 145
   Yariv J. Houvras and Gilbert H. Daniels

12 **Pediatric Malignancies: Retinoblastoma and Wilms' Tumor**........................... 163
   David A. Sweetser and Eric F. Grabowski

13 **Neurofibromatosis and Schwannomatosis** 181
   Miriam J. Smith and Scott R. Plotkin

14 **The HapMap Project and Low-Penetrance Cancer
   Susceptibility Alleles**... 195
   Edwin Choy and David Altshuler

**15   Somatic Genetic Alterations and Implications for Targeted
       Therapies in Cancer (GIST, CML, Lung Cancer)**.................................... 205
       Alice T. Shaw, Eyal C. Attar, Edwin Choy, and Jeffrey Engelman

Index... 221

Contributors

Janivette Alsina, MD, PhD
Resident in General Surgery, Department of Surgery, Massachusetts General Hospital, Boston, MA

David Altshuler, MD, PhD
Professor of Medicine, Harvard Medical School, Boston, MA;
Department of Molecular Biology, Massachusetts General Hospital, Boston, MA

Eyal C. Attar, MD
Instructor in Medicine, Harvard Medical School, Boston, MA;
Director, Translational Leukemia Research, Massachusetts General Hospital Cancer Center, Boston, MA

Andrew T. Chan, MD, MPH
Assistant Professor of Medicine, Department of Gastroenterology, Massachusetts General Hospital, Boston, MA

Gayun Chan-Smutko, MS, CGC
Senior Genetic Counselor, Center for Cancer Risk Assessment, Massachusetts General Hospital, Boston, MA

Elizabeth D. Chao, PhD
Harvard Medical School, Boston, MA

Edwin Choy, MD, PhD
Instructor in Medicine, Department of Medicine, Massachusetts General Hospital, Boston, MA

Daniel C. Chung, MD
Director, GI Cancer Genetics Program, Gastrointestinal Unit and Cancer Center, Massachusetts General Hospital, Boston, MA;
Associate Professor of Medicine, Harvard Medical School, Boston, MA

Gilbert H. Daniels, MD
Professor of Medicine, Harvard Medical School, Boston, MA;
Co-Director, Thyroid Clinic, Massachusetts General Hospital, Boston, MA;
Co-Director, Endocrine Tumor Genetics Clinic, Massachusetts General Hospital, Boston, MA

Marcela G. del Carmen, MD
Assistant Professor, Harvard Medical School, Boston, MA;
Department of Obstetrics and Gynecology Service, Massachusetts General Hospital, Boston, MA

Leif W. Ellisen, MD, PhD
Associate Professor of Medicine, Harvard Medical School, Boston, MA;
Massachusetts General Hospital Cancer Center, Boston, MA

Jeffrey Engelman, MD, PhD
Chief, Thoracic Oncology, Massachusetts General Hospital Cancer Center,
Boston, MA

Michele Jacobs Gabree, MS, CGC
Certified Genetic Counselor, Center for Cancer Risk Assessment,
Massachusetts General Hospital, Boston, MA

Eric F. Grabowski, MD, D Sci
Associate Professor of Pediatrics, Harvard Medical School, Boston, MA;
Department of Pediatric Hematology/Oncology, Massachusetts General Hospital,
Boston, MA

Daniel A. Haber, MD, PhD
Director, Massachusetts General Hospital Cancer Center; Kurt J. Isselbacher /
Peter D. Schwartz Professor of Medicine, Harvard Medical School;
Investigator, Howard Hughes Medical Institute,
Boston, MA

Yariv J. Houvras, MD, PhD
Instructor in Medicine, Massachusetts General Hospital Cancer Center,
Boston, MA

Othon Iliopoulos, MD
Assistant Professor of Medicine, Harvard Medical School, Boston, MA;
Director, Familial Renal Carcinoma Clinic, Massachusetts General Hospital Cancer Center,
Boston, MA

Eunice L. Kwak, MD, PhD
Assistant in Medicine, Department of Hematology and Oncology,
Massachusetts General Hospital Cancer Center, Boston, MA

Prakash K. Pandalai, MD
Fellow, Surgical Oncology, Massachusetts General Hospital,
Harvard Medical School, Boston, MA

Devanshi Patel, MS, CGC
Senior Genetic Counselor, Center for Cancer Risk Assessment, Massachusetts General
Hospital, Boston, MA

Scott R. Plotkin, MD, PhD
Assistant Professor of Neurology, Harvard Medical School, Boston, MA;
Department of Neurology, Massachusetts General Hospital, Boston, MA

Paula D. Ryan, MD, PhD
Medical Director, Breast and Ovarian Cancer Genetics and Risk Assessment Clinic,
Massachusetts General Hospital, Boston, MA

Kristen Mahoney Shannon, MS, CGC
Program Manager/Senior Genetic Counselor, Center for Cancer Risk Assessment,
Massachusetts General Hospital, Boston, MA

Alice T. Shaw, MD, PhD
Assistant Professor of Medicine, Harvard Medical School, Massachusetts General Hospital
Cancer Center, Boston, MA

Barbara L. Smith, MD, PhD
Associate Professor of Surgery, Harvard Medical School, Boston, MA;
Director, Breast Program, Massachusetts General Hospital Cancer Center,
Boston, MA

Miriam J. Smith, PhD
Postdoctoral Research Fellow, Department of Neurology, Massachusetts General Hospital, Boston, MA

Michelle C. Specht, MD
Assistant Professor of Surgery, Harvard Medical School, Boston, MA;
Department of Surgical Oncology, Massachusetts General Hospital, Boston, MA

David A. Sweetser, MD, PhD
Associate Pediatrician, Department of Pediatric Hematology/Oncology, Massachusetts General Hospital, Boston, MA

Sarah P. Thayer, MD, PhD
Assistant Professor of Surgery, Harvard Medical School, Boston, MA;
Director, Pancreatic Biology Laboratory, Massachusetts General Hospital, Boston, MA

Hensin Tsao, MD, PhD
Director, MGH Melanoma and Pigmented Lesion Center, Massachusetts General Hospital, Boston, MA;
Director, MGH Melanoma Genetics Program, Wellman Center for Photomedicine, Massachusetts General Hospital, Boston, MA

Sam S. Yoon, MD
Assistant Professor of Surgery, Harvard Medical School, Boston, MA;
Department of Surgery, Massachusetts General Hospital, Boston, MA

Chapter 1
Basic Principles of Cancer Genetics

Leif W. Ellisen and Daniel A. Haber

Keywords Oncogene • Tumor suppressor gene • DNA repair • Cell cycle • Apoptosis • Telomerase • Genetic instability • Epigenetics • MicroRNA

Introduction

Cancer results from the stepwise accumulation of genetic alterations within a cell. These alterations lead to abnormal proliferation and clonal expansion, and ultimately to invasion of surrounding tissues and metastasis to distant sites. Genetic abnormalities providing a selective advantage are maintained and ultimately become dominant within the population. The accumulation of genetic abnormalities, which in most cases occurs over a period of years, underlies both the process of tumorigenesis (the transition from normal cells to invasive cancer) and tumor progression (the transition to a metastatic and often treatment-resistant cancer). Histologic correlates of the process of tumorigenesis are recognized in a subset of cancers (e.g., colon and bladder cancers), whereas for others such cancer-precursor lesions have not been identified. Dozens of genes involved in tumorigenesis and tumor progression have now been identified. The products of these genes regulate key cellular processes including cell proliferation and survival, cellular motility and differentiation, and the establishment of cellular immortality.

Environmental factors influence the genetic evolution that occurs during tumorigenesis. In some cases, an environmental carcinogen exposure (e.g., tobacco) leads directly to mutation in a key tumor-promoting gene such as the K-Ras oncogene or inactivation of a tumor suppressor gene,

e.g., p53 (also known as TP53). In other cases, more subtle alterations occur following long-term exposure to carcinogenic agents such as asbestos or ultraviolet radiation. Cancer incidence following exposure to ionizing radiation also clearly demonstrates the link between genetic damage and tumorigenesis. Thus, survivors of the atomic bomb exhibited a dose-dependent incidence of leukemia and other solid tumors. The same spectrum of cancers can also be observed in some patients who have undergone treatment for an initial tumor with genotoxic agents including radiation and chemotherapy. The probability that such environmental exposures will lead to cancer development for any given individual is governed by both tumor-cell intrinsic factors (that is, which genetic abnormalities occur and whether they provide a growth advantage) and host factors (subtle germline genetic variations that govern cancer sensitivity through a variety of mechanisms) [1].

Additional causes of environmental carcinogenesis are infectious agents including certain tumor viruses and, less commonly, bacteria. Cancer-virus linkages include cervical carcinoma with specific subtypes of human papillomavirus; hepatocellular carcinoma with chronic hepatitis B and C virus infection; nasopharyngeal carcinoma and lymphomas with Epstein-Barr virus in immunosuppressed hosts; the rare acute T cell leukemia with acute transforming human T cell lymphotrophic virus type I; and Kaposi sarcoma with human herpesvirus 8. A specific subtype of gastric lymphoma has been linked to infection with the H. Pylori bacterium. Most cancers, however, do not have a known link to infectious agents. Nevertheless, much of our initial understanding of cancer genes and their functions was the product of studies focusing on the mechanisms by which tumor viruses cause cancer in rodents and birds. Thus, the first tumor-promoting genes or "oncogenes" were identified within such tumor viruses [2]. Only later was it recognized that these viral genes were actually normal cellular genes that had been taken up by these viruses in a slightly altered or activated form.

L.W. Ellisen (✉)
Harvard Medical School, Massachusetts General Hospital Cancer
Center, Boston, MA, USA
e-mail: ellisen@helix.mgh.harvard.edu

Germline Versus Somatic Genetic Alterations in Cancer

For most common cancers, the genetic lesions that promote tumorigenesis are acquired somatically and do not involve germline alterations. In some cases, however, inherited germline abnormalities contribute to cancer pathogenesis. In the latter case, a single defective copy of a gene is typically inherited, and transformation requires somatic loss of the second (non-mutant) allele. Because the rate of somatic loss of a single allele is exponentially higher than the independent mutation of two alleles, the incidence of specific cancers in mutation carriers is dramatically elevated over that of the general population. For inherited cancer predisposition, it is typically (but not always) loss, rather than gain of function of these genes that promotes carcinogenesis. These genes are therefore by definition tumor suppressors. In contrast, somatic genetic alterations in cancer are associated with both activation-of-function (of oncogenes) and loss-of-function (of tumor suppressors).

Different cancers are associated with both overlapping and distinct patterns of genetic alterations. Thus, some genetic events, particularly specific somatic chromosomal translocations, are associated exclusively with one type of cancer. In these cases, the genetic abnormality (for example, the EWS-FLI 1 translocation in Ewing's sarcoma) serves as a useful diagnostic hallmark for this tumor [3]. Other somatic abnormalities, such as mutational activation of the K-Ras oncogene or inactivation of the p53 tumor suppressor, are associated with numerous different cancers. In the case of germline genetic defects, inheritance of a specific tumor suppressor gene abnormality most commonly results in a tissue-specific pattern of cancer predisposition. Perhaps surprisingly, such tissue-specificity is observed even for genes whose functions appear to be required across tissues and cell types. For example, the BRCA1 gene is required for genomic stability and DNA repair in all cell types. However, inherited mutations in BRCA1 are associated almost exclusively with predisposition to breast and ovarian cancer. We have only a limited understanding of the basis for this observation, although many different hypotheses have been proposed. A related finding is that genes associated with inherited cancer predisposition may also be targeted for somatic inactivation – but in a distinct subset of tumors. Thus, 90% of small cell lung carcinomas (SCLC) demonstrate somatic mutational inactivation of the retinoblastoma tumor suppressor (RB1) [4]. Nevertheless, germline mutation of RB1 is associated with a high incidence of retinoblastoma and osteosarcoma, but not with SCLC. It has been proposed that this paradox reflects different roles of the RB1 gene in different cellular contexts, such that its inactivation can be sufficient by itself to drive proliferation in some cancers, while in others

it may contribute but not drive tumorigenesis, and in yet others, it may trigger compensatory responses leading to cell death. In any case, we have in general a relatively limited understanding of why particular genetic abnormalities are associated with tissue-specific tumorigenesis.

Driver and Passenger Genetic Abnormalities in Cancer Pathogenesis

Most human cancers, particularly adult cancers, harbor dozens to hundreds of genetic abnormalities. In one study, Vogelstein and colleagues performed large-scale DNA sequencing from a series of breast and colon carcinomas [5]. They found a median of approximately 80 mutations per tumor that give rise to premature truncation or a change in protein sequence. However, only a minority of these mutations (about 15 per tumor) were observed recurrently in multiple cancers and thought to be "significant." These mutations, many of which were found in well-established cancer genes such as p53 and K-Ras, have been termed "drivers" because they are thought to drive malignant transformation and progression. The majority of the mutations, however, were not observed repeatedly in multiple tumors. These mutations are assumed to be the chance result of genetic instability which occurs during the process of tumorigenesis. They have therefore been termed "passenger" mutations. Determining definitively which tumor-associated genetic abnormalities are drivers and which are passengers involves both large-scale analysis of tumor genomes and functional studies of cancer pathways. Identifying cancer driver abnormalities has important implications for the new generation of cancer therapies that selectively target particular cancer driver pathways.

Activation of Oncogenes and Proto-oncogenes

The first cancer genes were identified within the genomes of retroviruses known to cause tumors in rodents and birds. The viral genes responsible for tumor formation were found to be activated homologues of mammalian genes (proto-oncogenes), which had been co-opted during evolution as a means of promoting cellular proliferation and thus viral replication [2]. Subsequently, it was found that some human cancers harbored analogously activated alleles of these endogenous proto-oncogenes, even though no virus was involved (Table 1.1). Among the first proto-oncogenes to be identified were receptors for cellular growth factors (e.g., platelet-derived growth factor (PDGF) receptor or epidermal growth factor receptor (EGFR)), in which oncogenic activation

Table 1.1 Selected oncogene mutations in human cancer

Gene	Activation mechanism	Protein properties	Cancer types	Germline mutations
K-*Ras*	PM	p21 GTPase	Pancreatic, colorectal, lung, endometrial, other carcinomas	ND
N-*Ras*	PM	p21 GTPase	Myeloid leukemia	ND
H-*Ras*	PM	p21 GTPase	Bladder	ND
EGFR (erb B)	PM, GA	Growth factor (EGF) receptor	Lung and other carcinomas, gliomas	ND
NEU (erb B2)	GA	Growth factor receptor	Breast, ovarian, gastric, other carcinomas	ND
c-*Myc*	CT, GA	Transcription factor	Burkitt lymphoma, SCLC, other carcinomas	ND
N-*Myc*	GA	Transcription factor	Neuroblastoma, SCLC	ND
L-*Myc*	GA	Transcription factor	SCLC	ND
Bcl-2	CT	Antiapoptosis protein	B cell lymphoma (follicular type)	ND
CYCD1	GA, CT	Cyclin D, cell cycle control	Breast and other carcinomas, B cell lymphoma, parathyroid adenomas	ND
bcr-abl	CT	Chimeric nonreceptor tyrosine kinase	CML, ALL (T cell)	ND
RET	CT, PM	GNDF-receptor tyrosine kinase	Thyroid (papillary and medullary types)	Yes (MEN2)
CDK4	GA, PM	Cyclin-dependent kinase	Sarcoma	Yes (familial melanoma)
MET	PM, GA	HGF-receptor tyrosine kinase	Gastric, colorectal, lung carcinomas	Yes
PIK3CA	PM	Lipid kinase/growth factor signaling	Breast, colon, endometrial carcinomas	ND
SMO	PM	Transmembrane signaling molecule in sonic hedgehog pathway	Basal cell skin	ND
β-CAT	PM, in-frame deletion	Transcriptional coactivator, links E-cadherin to cytoskeleton	Melanoma, colorectal	ND
BRAF	PM	Signaling kinase downstream of Ras	Melanoma, colorectal	ND
HST	GA	Growth factor (FGF-like)	Gastric	ND
PML-RAR-α	CT	Chimeric transcription factor	APL	ND
W2A-PBX1	CT	Chimeric transcription factor	Pre-B ALL	ND
MDM-2	GA	p53-binding protein	Sarcoma	ND
GLI	GA	Transcription factor	Sarcoma, glioma	ND
KIT	PM	Growth factor receptor	GIST, acral melanoma	ND
Notch	CT, PM	Cell surface receptor/transcription factor	T cell ALL	ND
ERG/ETV	CT	Transcription factor	Prostate carcinoma	ND

PM point mutation, *GA* gene amplification, *CT* chromosomal translocation, *ALL* acute lymphocytic leukemia, *APL* acute promyelocytic leukemia, *CML* chronic myelogenous leukemia, *GIST* gastrointestinal stromal tumor, *EGF* epidermal growth factor, *FGF* fibroblast growth factor, *GDNF* glial cell line-derived neurotrophic factor, *GTPase* guanosine triphosphatase, *HGF* hepatocyte growth factor, *ND* not determined, *SCLC* small cell lung carcinoma

resulted in ligand-independent activation. Another early described class of oncogenes were G-protein-coupled receptors (e.g., H-Ras, K-Ras, N-Ras), for which activation resulted in constitutive "on" signaling rather than transient on/off shuttling [6]. Molecules involved in various steps of growth factor signaling are now known to be among the most common targets for cancer-associated activation. Multiple potential mechanisms are involved in the activation of normal cellular proto-oncogenes in human cancer. These include point mutations, genetic deletion or amplification, and structural rearrangements such as chromosomal translocations (Fig. 1.1). All of these can result in an altered or additional functional property of the encoded protein which is dominant over the wild-type protein. For this reason, these mutations are commonly referred to as "gain-of-function" mutations.

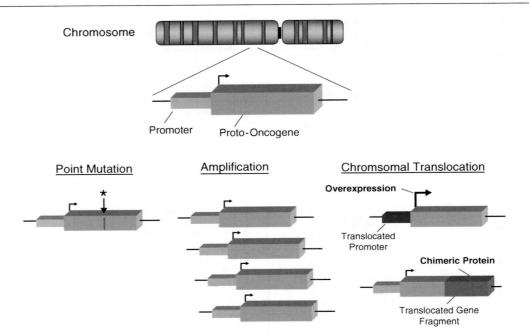

Fig. 1.1 Mechanisms of oncogene activation. Cellular oncogenes (also known as proto-oncogenes) may be activated in cancer as a result of (**a**) point mutations (including small deletions and insertions) that alter the amino acid sequence and thereby result in a protein that may be constitutively activated; (**b**) amplification of the cellular gene, resulting in higher levels of protein expression; or (**c**) chromosomal translocations that lead to the juxtaposition of a strong promoter and cause increased protein expression, or that produce a novel chimeric fusion protein encoded from fragments of two different genes normally present on different chromosomes

Point Mutations

Point mutations that result in oncogene activation occur at highly selective residues and induce specific amino acid changes. In most cases, this is because only a restricted set of changes can give rise to an activated rather than defective protein. For example, the vast majority of tumor-associated changes in the K-Ras oncogene are found within two amino acid residues that are critical for GTPase activity [6]. Similarly, mutations which are found in growth factor receptors and which give rise to ligand-independent activation of these receptors are highly selective and produce proteins with increased tyrosine kinase catalytic activity. Presumably, these mutations are selected because they confer an advantage during tumorigenesis, while other silent or deleterious mutations are lost within the population of cells. Because these mutant proteins are dominant in their action and have profound effects on cellular function, most of them are acquired somatically and are not passed through the germline. They are therefore not involved in hereditary cancer. The single best-described example of an activated oncogene that is in fact involved in hereditary cancer is the RET receptor tyrosine kinase gene. Germline mutations in different domains of this gene give rise to somewhat different clinical phenotypes (MEN 2A and 2B), although both involve early-onset medullary thyroid carcinoma [7]. Remarkably, loss-of-function mutations in this same gene are associated with

Hirschspring's disease, a profound deficiency of colonic innervation. These different clinical phenotypes associated with mutations within the same gene likely reflect both the effects of distinct mutations and the diverse functional and tissue-specific properties of the Ret tyrosine kinase itself.

Gene Amplifications and Chromosomal Translocations

Structural alterations of chromosomes can also lead to gain of function of proto-oncogenes. Activation of oncogenes by this mechanism usually involves either gene amplification, a gain in gene copy number, or translocation, a structural rearrangement of the genes. Gene amplification results from aberrant replication of specific chromosomal loci and gives rise to dramatically elevated expression of the amplified gene [8]. These amplified genetic loci, which in some cases are present in hundreds of extra copies, may be maintained as extra-chromosomal elements (double minute chromosomes) or may be apparent as homogenously staining loci within the normal chromosome. Normal cells are protected against these chromosomal aberrations by genes such as p53 which serve to monitor and repair such events. Loss of p53 function in cancer cells enhances subsequent abnormal genetic events, such as gene amplification of growth factor receptors, which are then potent drivers of cellular proliferation. One of the best-studied cancer gene amplification events involves the N-Myc gene, which is amplified in childhood neuroblastoma and confers a particularly poor prognosis [9]. The Myc family of oncogenes control the transcription of several hundreds of downstream genes, through which they regulate protein translation, cellular proliferation, and cell survival.

In contrast to gene amplification, which increases gene expression through additional gene copies, chromosomal translocations can increase oncogene expression levels by juxtaposing the relevant gene to a highly active promoter usually directing expression of a different gene [10]. In Burkitt's Lymphoma, another Myc family member, c-Myc, is translocated and thereby juxtaposed to the promoter and enhancer elements of either the heavy or light immunoglobulin chains [11, 12]. Levels of c-Myc then become dramatically elevated, as these promoters are highly active within the B lymphocytes that give rise to this tumor. Similarly, in some T lymphocytic leukemias, a fragment of a gene known as Notch becomes overexpressed as a result of a translocation which juxtaposes it to regulatory elements for the β T-cell receptor, which is highly active in these lymphocytes [13]. More commonly, the Notch gene, which is important for cell proliferation and cell fate decisions in many tissues, is activated by point mutations in these tumors [14]. Therefore, Notch presents an example of an oncogene that may be activated in the same tumor type through distinct genetic mechanisms.

Many cancer-associated chromosomal translocations, rather than leading to overexpression of an oncogene, result in the creation of a fusion or hybrid protein product with cancer-promoting properties. The first-identified chromosomal translocation in human cancer occurs in chronic myelogenous leukemia (CML) and juxtaposes the c-abl protein kinase on chromosome 9 to a gene called BCR (for "breakpoint cluster region") on chromosome 22 [15]. This abnormal translocated chromosome was evident karyotypically in tumor cells and was initially called the Philadelphia chromosome. The fusion protein product results in dysregulation and activation of c-abl, promoting leukemogenesis. In late-stage "blast-crisis" of CML, the translocated chromosome is often duplicated, underscoring its contribution as a cancer driver. Furthermore, this fusion oncoprotein exhibits remarkable tissue specificity, as a subtle alteration in the breakpoint for this translocation gives rise to an aggressive form of pediatric lymphoid leukemia [16]. The relevance of this fusion has also been demonstrated in a mouse model, in which expression of a fusion gene that mimics the translocation product in mouse bone marrow cells is sufficient to induce a leukemia resembling CML when these cells are reintroduced in vivo [17]. This activated oncoprotein was also among the first to be successfully targeted by a therapeutic inhibitor, imatinib mesylate (Gleevec), which blocks the function of the activated kinase and induces dramatic responses [18]. Use of Imatinib is now a clinical standard in treatment of CML.

Several other chromosomal translocations that result in creation of fusion proteins have been identified in human leukemia. Acute promyelocytic leukemia (APML) is defined by the presence of a translocation that fuses the retinoic acid receptor (RAR) to the PML oncoprotein [19]. While the specific mechanism of this protein product remains under investigation, its presence leads to a block in cellular differentiation which can be relieved by treatment with all-trans retinoic acid (ATRA). Induction of tumor cell differentiation with ATRA is now an important component of therapy in APML [20]. In addition to providing treatment opportunities, certain chromosomal translocations are also used to define prognosis in particular leukemias. For example, the TEL–AML1 fusion observed in pediatric leukemia results from a chromosomal translocation whose presence confers a more favorable prognosis than does the absence of any recognizable translocation [21].

The identification of chromosomal translocations in cancer was initially facilitated by the ease with which cytogenetic analysis could be performed on hematologic malignancies. More recently, it has been recognized that solid tumors also harbor such translocations. Among the first to be identified were a group of translocations in a group of pediatric tumors including Ewing's sarcoma and the family of peripheral neuroepithelial tumors. These involve a fusion of the EWS gene (or its related family members) to one of the ETS-family transcription factors, the most common being an EWS–FLI1 fusion [3]. The chimeric transcription factor product is thought to directly regulate the expression of a set of genes involved in cellular proliferation and differentiation. Clinically, these translocations are useful in the diagnosis of these tumors. Moreover, they are useful in directing therapy, as these translocations define a group of tumors with similar clinical behavior and therapeutic response.

Until recently, it was not clear whether chromosomal translocations were important contributors to the common adult carcinomas. A recent series of studies, however, has demonstrated that the majority of prostate carcinomas harbor translocations between one of two ETS-related transcription factors ERG or ETV1, and the promoter of the androgen-regulated gene TMPRSS2 [22]. The translocation therefore results in dysregulation and overexpression of ERG/ETV1 expression in an androgen-dependent manner, thus providing a tissue specific mechanism of cellular transformation. Underscoring the relevance of these ETS transcription factors to prostate tumorigenesis is the finding that ETV1 is also found to be overexpressed in an androgen-independent manner in a subset of cases [23]. Ongoing studies seek to determine whether androgen-dependent versus independent expression of this oncoprotein in prostate cancer is a determinant of the response to anti-androgen therapy.

Tumor Suppressor Genes

The concept of tumor suppressor genes is that these cellular genes function at least in part to suppress malignant transformation in normal cells, and that these genes are targeted for inactivation (loss-of-function) through various genetic abnormalities in human cancer (Table 1.2). The identification of these genes was the product of three convergent fields of investigation: cell fusion studies of normal and tumor cells demonstrating "reversion of tumorigenesis"; epidemiologic analysis of familial pediatric cancer incidence; and molecular studies of cancer-associated chromosomal abnormalities. One early finding supporting this concept was the observation that the fusion of a normal cell to a cancer cell suppressed the malignant properties of the tumor cell [24]. This experiment therefore suggested that the malignant state was

Table 1.2 Selected tumor suppressor genes associated with cancer predisposition syndromes and mutated in human cancers

Gene	Function of protein product	Cancers with somatic mutations	Germline mutations
RB1	Transcriptional regulator, E2F1 binding	Retinoblastoma, osteosarcoma, SCLC, breast, prostate, and bladder	Familial retinoblastoma
TP53	Transcription factor	~50% of all cancers (rare in some cancer types – e.g., prostate carcinoma, neuroblastoma)	Li-Fraumeni syndrome
CDKN2A	p16-INK4a, Cyclin-dependent kinase inhibitor	~20–25% of many different cancer types (e.g., breast, lung, pancreatic, bladder)	Familial melanoma, familial pancreatic carcinoma
APC	Regulates β-catenin function, ?microtubule binding	Colorectal, rare or absent in most other cancers	Familial adenomatous polyposis, Gardner syndrome, Turcot syndrome, familial desmoid disease
MSH2, MLH1, MSH6, PMS1, PMS2	DNA-mismatch repair	Colorectal, endometrial, gastric	Hereditary nonpolyposis colorectal cancer
WT-1	Transcription factor	Wilms tumor	WAGR and Denys-Drash
NF-1	Regulator of Ras-GTPase	Melanoma, neuroblastoma	Neurofibromatosis type 1
NF-2	Juxtamembrane link to cytoskeleton	Schwannomas, meningiomas, ependymomas	Neurofibromatosis type 2
VHL	Regulator of protein stability	Renal (clear-cell type), hemangioblastoma	von Hippel-Lindau disease
BRCA1	DNA repair, complexes with Rad51, transcriptional regulation	Ovarian (<10%), rare in breast	Inherited breast and ovarian carcinoma
BRCA2	DNA repair, binds to Rad51	Not known	Inherited breast (female and male), pancreatic, and ovarian carcinoma
MEN1	Histone Methylation	Parathyroid adenomas, pituitary adenomas, endocrine tumors of pancreas	Multiple endocrine neoplasia type I
PTCH	Transmembrane receptor for sonic hedgehog;	Basal cell skin, medulloblastoma	Gorlin syndrome, hereditary basal cell syndrome
PTEN	Lipid-phosphatase	Glioma, breast, prostate, head and neck, squamous cell, follicular thyroid cancer	Cowden disease
STK11	LKB1 kinase regulating cell growth and polarity	Lung carcinoma, squamous cell carcinoma	Peutz-Jeghers syndrome
TSC1, TSC2	GTPase activating protein complex	Transitional cell carcinoma	Tuberous sclerosis
SMAD4	Downstream signaling in TGF-β pathway	Pancreatic, mutations rare in others (e.g., colon, gastric)	Juvenile Polyposis
CDH1	Transmembrane cell–cell adhesion molecule	Gastric cancer/lobular breast cancer; rare in endometrial and ovarian	Hereditary diffuse gastric cancer syndrome
α-CAT	Links E-cadherin to the cytoskeleton	Some prostate and lung	Not known
TGF-βII R	Transmembrane receptor TGF-β	Colorectal and gastric	Not known
MYH	Base excision repair protein	Not known	MYH-associated polyposis

AML acute myeloid leukemia, *SCLC* small cell lung carcinoma, *TGF-β* transforming growth factor-β, *WAGR* Wilms tumor, aniridia, genitourinary abnormalities, mental retardation syndrome genetically recessive. Subsequent work demonstrated that transfer of a single chromosome from a normal cell to a tumor cell was in some cases capable of suppressing malignant behavior [25]. Once the technology was developed to isolate and express individual genes, it was established that transfer of a single gene, in theory a gene whose function was lost in the tumor cells, was capable of suppressing malignancy.

Studies of DNA tumor viruses also lent support to the existence of key endogenous tumor suppressor genes within normal cells. Unlike transforming retroviruses, which commonly harbor activated versions of normal cellular genes (oncogenes), DNA tumor viruses encode their own unique proteins which are capable of transforming mammalian cells. These proteins, which include the T antigen encoded by SV40 virus, the E1A and E1B proteins of adenovirus, and the E6 and E7 proteins of human papilloma virus, promote proliferation and transformation in many human cell types. The fields of tumor virology and human cancer genetics essentially converged when it was discovered that these viral proteins function by specifically inactivating two key cellular tumor suppressor proteins: p53 and pRb [26]. Thus, transforming retroviruses express modified versions of mammalian proto-oncogenes, while DNA tumor viruses express viral genes that inactivate cellular tumor suppressor genes. These studies of viral genetic mechanisms provide a clear demonstration that tumorigenesis can result from both activation of oncogenes and loss of tumor suppressors.

The Knudson Model for Loss of Tumor Suppressor Gene Function

Most common cancers occur in adulthood, and their frequency increases with age. These facts are assumed to reflect the time required for the accumulation of a sufficient number of genetic events within a target cell to induce tumorigenesis. A subset of cancers, however, occurs exclusively in children and is thought to result from a limited number of genetic abnormalities acquired in particular stem cells or maturing progenitor cells. Two examples are retinoblastoma, thought to arise through the transformation of retinal stem cells, and Wilms tumor, which arises from primitive renal stem cells. Although these tumors most commonly occur in a sporadic pattern, in some cases they are clustered within families, and in these cases the tumors that arise are often multicentric or bilateral. By developing a statistical model that accounted for the earlier age of onset of tumors in familial versus sporadic cases, Alfred Knudson proposed a hypothesis of "hit kinetics," now understood to represent biallelic tumor suppressor gene inactivation, which today forms the foundation of human cancer genetics (Fig. 1.2) [27].

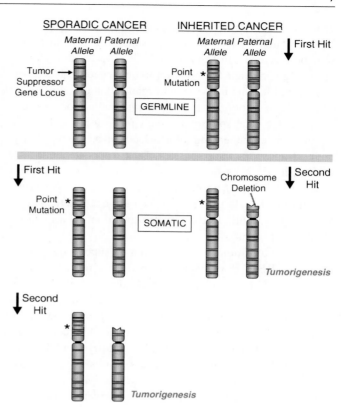

Fig. 1.2 The Knudson two-hit model of tumor initiation. This model predicts that inactivation of both alleles of a tumor suppressor gene are required and rate-limiting for the initiation of cancer. In sporadic cancer, the inactivation of these two alleles depends on two independent rare genetic events that must occur within the same somatic cell. In contrast, persons who have one mutated tumor suppressor gene allele in their germline, either inherited from one parent or as a result of a de novo germline mutation, require only one genetic event in a somatic cell (i.e., loss of the second allele) for tumor initiation. This single mutation may occur in any cell within the target organ, which explains the earlier onset and high frequency of cancer, and its frequent multicentric presentation in individuals with genetic predisposition to cancer

The model proposed by Knudson states that tumor formation requires two genetic "hits" within a cancer-associated gene. In sporadic cases, both hits are acquired somatically, resulting in a relatively low frequency for tumorigenesis. In familial cases, however, the first hit is harbored within the germline, and a single somatic hit is therefore sufficient to induce tumorigenesis. The two hits postulated by Knudson are now understood to constitute mutations or chromosomal deletions targeting each allele of a tumor suppressor gene. The probability of this single mutational event is so much higher than the probability of two independent hits striking both alleles within the same cell that it accounts for the increased frequency, earlier onset and multicentricity observed for familial versus sporadic cancers. This model also predicts that tumor suppressor genes mutations, while resulting in gene inactivation or "loss of function," are genetically transmitted as autosomal dominant traits with high penetrance. This paradox results from the fact that somatic inactivation of the second allele occurs at high frequency (given single hit mutation frequency and the number of susceptible cells in the target organ), thus initiating tumorigenesis in carriers of a germline mutated tumor suppressor gene. Of note, some individuals may harbor a de novo germline mutation leading to increased cancer susceptibility in the absence of a family history. These cases are evident in some pediatric syndromes, such as WAGR Syndrome associated with Wilms Tumor, in which a de novo germline chromosomal deletion leads to constitutional genetic abnormalities, in addition to cancer predisposition in children of unaffected parents.

The identification of the first tumor suppressor genes, including RB1, responsible for pediatric retinoblastoma [28], and WT1, associated with childhood Wilms tumor [29], validated Knudson's model. In most cases, the germline hit corresponded to a point mutation with the tumor suppressor, while the second, somatic hit commonly involved a deletion of the remaining wild-type allele. The somatic deletion could in some cases be observed on cytogenetic analysis. More commonly, the deletion was identifiable as loss of a polymorphic genetic marker (a variant in which one form is inherited from each parent) that was within the region of the tumor suppressor gene [30]. The mapping of the specific chromosomal loci exhibiting this so-called "loss of heterozygosity" (LOH) in tumors allowed the localization and eventual identification of the first tumor suppressor genes (Fig. 1.3). Advances in microchip technology and the sequencing of the entire human genome have now made possible rapid, genome-wide approaches to identifying tumor suppressor loci. In one technique, genome-wide analysis of single-nucleotide polymorphisms can be carried out to identify regions of LOH in tumor DNA versus matched normal tissue. Another approach is to use quantitative DNA hybridization analysis in order to find regions of genomic deletion in tumors that may correspond to tumor suppressor loci.

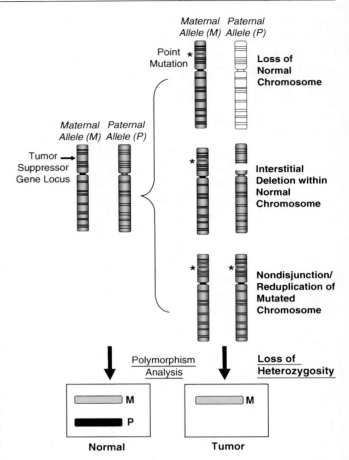

Fig. 1.3 Allelic losses in tumors and loss of heterozygosity (LOH). Loss of genetic material accompanies tumor development, and mapping regions of chromosomal loss has been used to identify the location of tumor suppressor genes. The initial genetic hit typically results from a point mutation within a tumor suppressor gene, while the second gene inactivation event commonly involves a gross chromosomal loss. This may include loss of the entire normal chromosome, a deletion that removes a chromosomal segment containing the gene, or a duplication of the chromosome carrying the mutant allele, with loss of the normal chromosome. These chromosomal events can be mapped using restriction fragment length polymorphisms (RFLPs) or other molecular methods that distinguish maternally inherited alleles from paternally inherited alleles. In traditional cancer gene mapping studies, the identification of chromosomal loci that are subject to LOH has formed the starting point for the identification of cancer predisposition genes

Tumor Suppressors and Cell Cycle Dysregulation: The RB1 Pathway

The first tumor suppressor to be identified was the RB1 gene, which is associated with pediatric retinoblastoma [28]. RB1 validated Knudson's postulates, as the majority of sporadic cases exhibit bi-allelic inactivation of RB1 within tumor cells but not normal cells. In familial cases, a single mutant RB1 allele is found in the germline, while tumor cells show inactivation of the remaining wild-type allele. The RB1 gene functions as a key regulator of cell cycle progression, a

finding which highlights the link between dysregulated proliferation and tumorigenesis. Further supporting this link is the finding that RB1 functions within a cell cycle regulatory pathway that involves a number of other important oncogenes and tumor suppressors.

The protein encoded by RB1, pRb, is a nuclear phosphoprotein, whose key function is to serve as a gatekeeper, blocking progression from the G1 phase of the cell cycle (Fig. 1.4). The pRb protein physically associates with a family of transcription factors known as E2F, which are in turn associated with a protein known as DP [31]. The E2F–DP

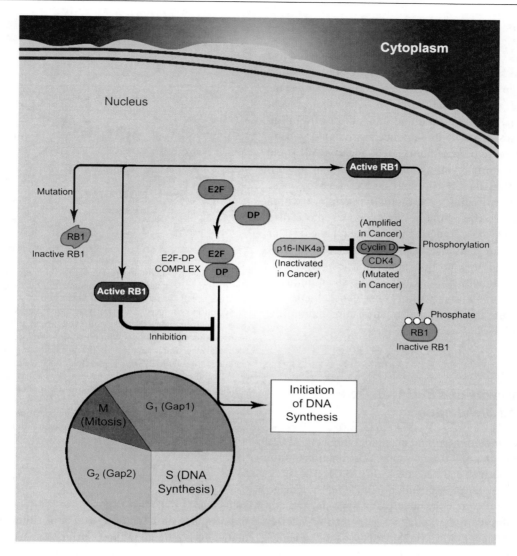

Fig. 1.4 The retinoblastoma gene (RB1) cell cycle pathway. The events leading to cellular division in mammalian cells are triggered by a critical checkpoint between the G1 phase and DNA synthesis (S phase). The RB1 tumor suppressor protein blocks progression to S phase by inhibiting the E2F-DP protein complex, which activates genes required for DNA synthesis. Normal cell cycle progression requires the reversible inactivation of RB1 protein by phosphorylation induced by protein complexes including cyclin D and Cyclin-Dependent Kinase 4 (CDK4). Mutations in RB1 prevent its normal inhibition of cell cycle progression, contributing to deregulated cellular division. The RB1 pathway is disrupted in human cancers not only through inactivation of RB1 itself, but also through amplification of cyclin D, activating mutations in CDK4, and inactivation of the CDK4 inhibitor p16-INK4a

complex regulates a set of genes that are essential for DNA synthesis and cell cycle progression. In noncycling cells, pRb is dephosphorylated, bound to E2F–DP, and represses E2F–DP-dependent transcription and cell cycle entry. In normal cycling cells, pRb is phosphorylated by a series of cyclin-dependent kinases (CDKs), including CDK4, to allow cell cycle entry. The phosphorylation of pRb is reversible and therefore allows for appropriate cell cycle regulation. In contrast, genetic mutation or deletion of RB1 results in permanent cell cycle dysregulation that contributes to tumorigenesis. As noted above, transforming proteins from several DNA tumor viruses (SV40 T antigen, adenovirus E1A protein, and HPV E7 protein) all function by binding and inactivating pRb, which underscores its role as a key cell cycle regulator.

Studies of the biochemical pathway for RB1 function have uncovered additional cancer genes whose identification points to the fundamental role of cell cycle regulation in tumorigenesis. CCND1, which encodes cyclin D1, a protein required for CDK function and thus for pRb inactivation, is subject to genomic amplification in a subset of breast cancers. The CDKN2A gene, which encodes an inhibitor of cyclin D1/CDK4 called p16-INK4a, is subject to genomic deletion or epigenetic gene silencing in many human cancers. Germline mutation of CDKN2A gives rise to FAMMM, a familial syndrome involving predisposition to multiple atypical moles, melanoma, and pancreatic cancer [32]. Finally, specific mutations in CDK4 that prevent inhibition by p16-INK4a are found in a subset of familial melanoma cases. Each of these cancer-associated genetic events promotes hyperphosphorylated, inactive pRb and therefore inappropriate cell cycling. The fact that they all converge on pRb function is likely to explain why these genetic events are found to be mutually exclusive within individual tumors (i.e., tumors never display more than one mutation in these functionally related genes). This striking finding suggests that no additional selective advantage is conferred by multiple abnormalities within the same genetic pathway [33]. Uncovering such mutually exclusive driver mutations within other cancer pathways has helped define the functional relationships among the genes involved.

The P53 Pathway and BRCA1 in Genome Stability and DNA Repair

While the pRb protein is a fundamental component of cell cycle regulation, the p53 tumor suppressor functions in the response to abnormal cellular stress (Fig. 1.5). The stress conditions that trigger p53 activation include DNA damage, oncogene activation ("oncogenic stress"), hypoxia, and others. The central role of p53 in maintaining genome stability had led to its designation as the "guardian of the genome" [34]. p53 functions as a transcription factor that orchestrates the cellular response to stress by inducing target genes involved in a wide variety of cellular processes, including cell cycle regulation, cell death (apoptosis), DNA repair, and cellular metabolism. For example, induction of p53 in response to DNA damage leads to upregulation of p21, a protein that induces G1 phase cell cycle arrest, which in turn is thought to be required to allow DNA repair to occur before proceeding to DNA replication in S phase. Depending on the cell type and the extent of DNA damage, p53 may also induce a variety of proteins involved in a cell death process known as apoptosis. Loss of p53 during tumorigenesis induces genomic instability, abnormal proliferation, and abnormal cellular survival, all of which may explain the finding that p53 is the most commonly inactivated gene in human cancer. Loss or mutation of p53 is observed in 50% or more of a broad spectrum of human cancers.

The mutations observed in p53 can in some cases be correlated with the mechanism of carcinogenesis. For example, specific mutations have been observed in liver cancers whose

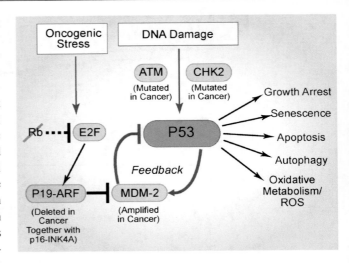

Fig. 1.5 The p53 cellular stress and DNA damage response pathway. The p53 protein is activated in response to DNA damage, oncogenic stress (e.g., RB1 inactivation) and other cellular stresses. P53 induces transcription of a large variety of genes that mediate its diverse functions, which include G1-phase cell cycle arrest and programmed cell death (apoptosis). In tumors with mutations of p53, DNA damage is not adequately repaired, leading to the accumulation of mutations and genetic rearrangements. Two key cellular genes regulate p53 activation: MDM2 and p19-ARF. MDM2 induces the normal degradation of p53 protein, and amplification of MDM2 in some tumors results in loss of p53 function. p19-ARF, which is induced by E2F, inhibits the effects of MDM2 and contributes to the activation of p53 following RB1 inactivation. The p19-ARF gene is commonly deleted in human cancers along with p16-INK4a, as these genes are expressed from overlapping chromosomal loci

incidence is linked to exposure to the potent carcinogenic fungus aflatoxin in certain regions of China. Other specific mutations are found in lung cancers associated the exposure to polycyclic carcinogens in tobacco smoke. In colorectal carcinomas, however, p53 mutations are observed in DNA residues susceptible to methylation, which may be an intrinsic cellular mutation-prone mechanism [35].

The p53 gene frequently undergoes missense mutations in human cancers, unlike most tumor suppressors which predominantly undergo nonsense (truncating) mutations. These p53 missense mutants are often expressed at high levels in tumors due in part to the fact that p53 normally exerts negative control on its own expression. Thus, somewhat paradoxically, overexpression of p53 in tumor cells is commonly used as a marker of p53 mutation and consequent functional inactivation. Why p53 frequently undergoes such missense mutations has been a subject of intensive analysis. It is possible that these p53 missense mutants are able to exert a dominant effect (so-called "dominant-negative" effect) on the remaining wild-type p53 within the cell, thus inactivating whatever normal protein is produced by a second allele. Alternatively, the highly expressed mutant p53 proteins may themselves have specific oncogenic properties.

Mutant p53 bind to and inhibit the function of two p53-related proteins, p63 and p73, which themselves exhibit p53-like properties. Thus, mutant p53 could suppress tumor suppressor activity by other members of the p53 gene family. The unique properties of mutant p53 were most clearly shown in a mouse model, in which the effect of nonsense versus missense mutants in endogenous p53 was compared. Mice expressing the missense mutants had a higher frequency of epithelial tumors and an increased frequency of metastasis compared to those expressing truncating (null) p53 mutants [36, 37].

Like RB1, p53 is targeted for inactivation by viral onco-proteins, including the SV40 T Antigen, Adenovirus E1B protein, and HPV E6 protein. By inactivating both RB1 pathways and p53 pathways, these viruses therefore promote abnormal proliferation through loss of pRb, while blocking p53-dependent cell death that might ensue as a result of cell cycle dysregulation (i.e., loss of the "checkpoint") [38]. Endogenous cellular proteins that regulate p53 are also targeted for genetic alteration in cancer. The MDM-2 gene, encoding a potent negative regulator of p53 protein stability, undergoes genomic amplification and consequent overexpression in a subset of sarcomas [39]. That p53 and MDM-2 function in a common pathway is strongly supported by the observation that MDM-2 amplification and p53 mutation are mutually exclusive in individual sarcomas – suggesting that either genetic event is sufficient to functionally inactivate p53. MDM-2 is also absolutely required to control p53 levels during normal embryonic development, as mice lacking this gene exhibit an early embryonic lethal phenotype which can be fully rescued by simultaneous deletion of p53 [40].

Another key protein in the p53/MDM-2 pathway is p19-ARF. The ARF (Alternative Reading Frame) protein is, strangely enough, encoded within the same CDKN2A genetic locus as p16-INK4a, although these two proteins are read in a different nucleotide codon frame and hence share no amino acid homology [41]. Many human cancers exhibit deletions of this locus and therefore inactivation of both p16-INK4a and ARF proteins, consistent with the idea that both proteins function as tumor suppressors. A major function of the ARF protein is to induce p53 protein stabilization by inhibiting MDM-2. ARF itself is induced by E2F transcription factors, which suggests that it serves as means of "cross-talk" between RB1 and p53 pathways [42]. Thus, RB1 loss or mutation leads to aberrant E2F activation and cell cycle dysregulation, but at the same time it also results in ARF upregulation, inducing p53-dependent growth arrest or apoptosis. Loss of ARF or p53 removes this obstacle to proliferation induced by loss of the RB/p16 pathway. Mouse models have further supported the central role of the ARF/MDM-2/p53 pathway in tumor suppression. An increase in gene copies encoding either ARF or p53 leads to a decreased incidence of spontaneous cancers

in mice, and a similar decrease in tumors is seen in mice with a mutation causing decreased MDM-2 expression [43].

Mutation of p53 in the germline is associated with Li-Fraumeni syndrome, which is manifested as a high frequency of many types of cancer, including sarcomas, breast cancer, brain tumors, and leukemia [44]. The contribution of p53 to maintaining genomic stability is thought to explain much of its tumor suppressor properties. Consistent with this view, several other inherited cancer predisposition syndromes result from germline mutational inactivation of DNA damage response and repair proteins. Chk2 is a kinase that phosphorylates p53 and induces its stabilization in response to DNA damage. Unlike p53 mutations, however, germline Chk2 mutations are associated with only a modest increase in predisposition to breast cancer [45]. Presumably, this observation reflects the presence of many proteins that may function upstream to regulate p53. Another example is the ATM kinase gene, which is mutated in ataxia telangiectasia (AT), a syndrome involving cerebellar degeneration, immunologic dysfunction, and cancer predisposition [46]. ATM is an early sensor of DNA damage, particularly in response to ionizing radiation, which signals to p53 upstream and in parallel to Chk2. ATM also phosphorylates the NBS1 protein, one of three sub-units of a key DNA repair complex. Germline mutations of NBS1 are responsible for Nijmegen Breakage Syndrome, which shares many phenotypic features with AT, supporting the finding that these proteins function in a common DNA damage response and repair pathway [47].

A major proportion of familial early-onset breast and ovarian cancer is caused by germline mutation in one of two key genes involved in DNA repair, BRCA1 and BRCA2 [48, 49]. These genes encode very large proteins whose role in maintaining genomic stability is still poorly understood. Nevertheless, tumors arising in BRCA1 and BRCA2 mutation carriers exhibit distinct clinical characteristics and responses to therapy compared with the far more common sporadic breast cancers. Biochemical studies have recently uncovered a functional link between BRCA1/2 and Fanconi Anemia. This cancer predisposition syndrome results from germline mutations in one of several FA genes, which encode repair proteins that function in overlapping pathways with BRCA1/2 [50].

DNA Mismatch Repair and Microsatellite Instability

A distinct pathway for DNA repair is subject to cancer-associated mutations in Lynch syndrome, or hereditary nonpolyposis colorectal cancer (HNPCC). This syndrome, which includes predisposition to cancers of the colon, ovary,

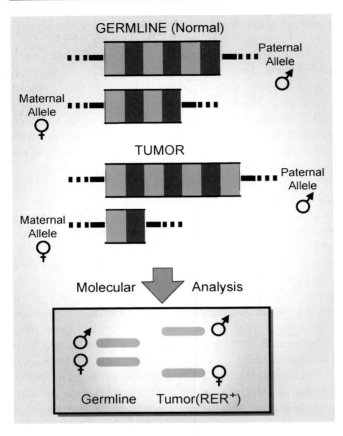

Fig. 1.6 DNA mismatch repair and microsatellite instability. Microsatellites are short repeated sequences of DNA that are distributed throughout the genome. These sequences are of highly variable length, facilitating the distinction between maternally inherited alleles and paternally inherited alleles. Unlike tumors showing LOH, which have loss of one allele compared with the germline, tumors that have microsatellite instability (so-called RER+ tumors) demonstrate altered lengths for microsatellite markers compared to normal (germline) DNA. This results from errors in DNA mismatch repair. When microsatellite sequences are present within the coding region of a gene, mismatch repair errors lead to mutations and loss of gene function that may promote tumor initiation and progression

and endometrium, results from mutations in genes including MSH2 and MLH1 that are required for DNA mismatch repair [51] (Fig. 1.6). A hallmark of tumors with a mismatch repair defect is so-called microsatellite instability (MSI). Microsatellites are stretches of repetitive nucleotides whose length varies from one individual to another. Tumors with MSI are found to have microsatellites that differ in size from those within the normal cells of the same patient [52]. Since these microsatellite variations result from errors introduced during DNA replication, these tumors are referred to as replication-error positive (RER+). In addition to HNPCC associated with germline mismatch repair mutations, approximately 10% of sporadic colorectal cancers demonstrate MSI, suggesting that disruption of mismatch repair also contributes to colorectal cancer in the absence of familial predisposition [53]. Although MSI is a marker of mismatch repair deficiency, microsatellite changes themselves are not oncogenic. Instead, mismatch repair deficiency is thought to lead to mutations in other genes associated with key cell signaling pathways. In colon cancer, for example, MSI can be associated with mutations within the TGF-β receptor gene, which harbors a microsatellite repeat within its coding sequence [54]. Mutation of this sequence, as a consequence of impaired mismatch repair, results in the disruption of TGF-β signaling that may be a key early event in colon carcinogenesis. An important feature that distinguishes mismatch repair defects from other tumor suppressor mechanisms is that the former promote tumors indirectly through mutation of other genes. Thus, reintroduction of p53 into a p53-deficient tumor is expected to induce growth arrest and/or apoptosis. In contrast, restoration of a mismatch repair gene would in theory not be of therapeutic value because it would presumably occur too late to reverse the malignant phenotype. Tumor suppressor genes of this class have been described as "caretakers" of the genome, rather than "gatekeepers" of specific pathways that drive cancer cell proliferation.

Tumor Suppressors Involved in Cellular Signaling and Differentiation

The identification of tumor suppressor genes that function in critical cellular signaling pathways has provided important insights into tumor cell metabolism. In particular, these studies have revealed that several such tumor suppressor genes function within common regulatory pathways. A prime example of this principle is the signaling pathway that controls the activity of a kinase called mTORC1 (mammalian target of rapamycin complex 1) (Fig. 1.7) [55]. The mTORC1 kinase is a master integrator of growth factor signals and regulator of cell growth and proliferation through its control of protein translation, autophagy (self-catabolism), and angiogenesis. The PTEN tumor suppressor encodes a protein that functions as an upstream inhibitor of mTORC1 and is among the most commonly mutated genes in a wide variety of sporadic human cancers. Additionally, germline mutations of PTEN are associated with several syndromes including Cowden disease, characterized by benign tumors known as hamartomas and breast cancer predisposition [56]. PTEN encodes a phosphatase that catalyzes the removal of phosphate residues from key lipids (phosphoinositides), thereby negatively regulating the phosphoinositide 3-kinase (PI3K) pathway. The PI3K pathway is activated in response to growth factor stimulation and in turn activates mTORC1 through two other tumor suppressor proteins, TSC1 (hamartin) and TSC2 (tuberin). The TSC1 and TSC2 genes

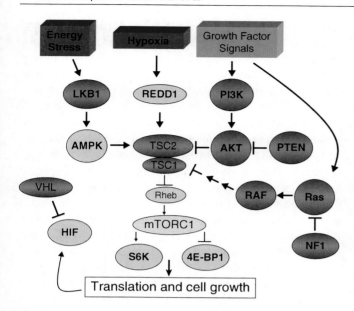

Fig. 1.7 Human cancer genes involved in linked cellular signaling pathways. Growth factors signals and certain cellular stress signals regulate cellular metabolism in part through the mTOR complex 1 (mTORC1) kinase. Genes involved in this signaling pathway and mutated in cancer (shown in blue) include the LKB1 kinase, which is mutated in Peutz–Jeghers syndrome (PJS) and functions via the AMPK kinase as an activator of the TSC1/2 complex. The PTEN tumor suppressor protein activates TSC1/2 indirectly by inhibiting the PI3 kinase pathway, while the genes encoding TSC1 and TSC2 are mutated in Tuberous Sclerosis Syndrome (TSC). This pathway converges on the regulation of mTORC1, which promotes protein translation and cell growth by phosphorylating its substrates including ribosomal S6 kinase (S6K). mTORC1 can also be regulated via the Ras pathway and the neurofibromatosis type I (NF1) tumor suppressor. Activation of mTOR induces up-regulation of the hypoxia-inducible factor (HIF), which is also upregulated through mutation of the von Hippel-Lindau tumor suppressor VHL. Tumor suppressor syndromes involving these genes share a predisposition for benign hamartomas and a variable incidence of malignant tumors. Analogues of rapamycin, a small-molecule inhibitor of mTOR, are currently being tested in clinical trials for a variety of benign and malignant tumors

Several other tumor suppressor syndromes associated with hamartoma development have less direct, but probable, links to mTORC1 signaling. One example is the von Hippel-Lindau (VHL) gene, which is frequently mutated in adult renal cell cancers and in the germline of persons with a syndrome that includes both benign and malignant vascular tumors. The VHL protein controls the degradation of certain proteins including the hypoxia-inducible factor (HIF), a key regulator of angiogenesis [59]. Because HIF is also positively regulated by mTORC1, the syndromes described above share some phenotypic similarities with VHL, including highly vascular tumors. The NF1 gene, which is responsible for neurofibromatosis (von Recklinghausen disease) and whose gene product normally downregulates the proto-oncogene Ras, may function at least in part through upstream suppression of mTORC1 [60]. Finally the NF2 gene, which is frequently mutated in mesotheliomas and schwannomas, encodes a structural protein that may be involved in cellular adhesion and control of growth factor receptors such as EGFR [61].

Important tumor suppressors are also involved in other key signaling pathways. The familial adenomatous polyposis syndrome (FAP), characterized by the development of numerous colonic polyps and very high risk of malignant transformation, results from germline mutations in the APC gene. In addition to germline mutations, sporadic APC mutation is perhaps the earliest recognized event in the development of colon carcinomas. The APC protein regulates the WNT signaling pathway by controlling β-catenin, a key protein cofactor for TCF/LEF transcription factors [62]. The TGF-β signaling pathway is dysregulated as a result of germline mutations in the SMAD 4 gene, which are associated with juvenile polyposis and gastrointestinal malignancy [63]. The PTCH gene is involved in yet another growth factor signaling cascade known as hedgehog. Mutations in PTCH, which encodes a receptor for hedgehog, convey an increased risk of skin cancer in the basal cell nevus syndrome [64].

While pathways including TGF-β and WNT play a role in normal cellular development and differentiation in many tissues, other tumor suppressor genes affect organ-specific differentiation. The best example is the WT1 gene, which has a relatively selective role in the developing kidney and testes. Germline mutations in WT1 are associated with both genitourinary developmental defects and Wilms tumor, an embryonic kidney cancer. WT1 is a transcription factor that is required for normal kidney differentiation, but whose inactivation leads to tumorigenesis [29]. A second gene associated with Wilms tumor has been identified, residing on the X chromosome [65]. This gene, WTX, also appears to regulate kidney differentiation, and its inactivation by a "single somatic hit" (which targets the single X chromosome in males and the active X chromosome in females) is unique among tumor suppressor genes.

encode inhibitors of mTORC1 and are mutated in tuberous sclerosis, a syndrome characterized by multifocal hamartomas of the CNS, kidney, and other tissues [57]. Thus, in the absence of PTEN or TSC1/2, mTORC1 activity is inappropriately increased, leading to aberrant cell growth. These observations have led to the use of the potent mTORC1 inhibitor, rapamycin, as a therapeutic strategy for patients with tuberous sclerosis, with at least some early success. Another important tumor suppressor functioning upstream of mTORC1 is the LKB1 kinase, which signals through TSC1/2 to inhibit mTORC1 activity in the setting of limited cellular ATP. LKB1 is encoded by the STK11 gene, which is mutated in Peutz–Jeghers syndrome, associated with intestinal hamartomas as well as malignant tumors of the intestine, pancreas and other sites [58].

Tumor Progression

The Accumulation of Genetic Lesions

Stepwise Accumulation of Genetic Abnormalities

Malignant transformation can be initiated by a single genetic hit in a rate-limiting gene. Nevertheless multiple genetic hits are almost always required for progression to invasive and metastatic cancer. These genetic changes are thought to occur in a stepwise fashion, with each hit occurring in one or a few cells, providing a selective advantage and eventually becoming dominant within the population. The identity and order of these genetic hits may be characteristic of a particular tumor type, and a particular genetic event that is rate-limiting in one tissue may not be in another. The best-studied example of stepwise genetic progression in tumorigenesis involves work by Kinzler and Vogelstein on the genetic evolution of colon carcinoma [66]. The earliest step is an inactivating mutation in the APC gene, which induces epithelial hyperplasia, followed by K-Ras mutation and changes in DNA methylation which induce progression to low-grade adenomatous polyps. Changes in one or more genes residing on chromosome 18q, including SMAD4, are associated with high-grade adenoma, and finally mutation of p53 accompanies progression to invasive carcinoma. This model was discernable in part because these preneoplastic lesions are histologically apparent on biopsies of colonic mucosa. While some cancers do not exhibit multiple readily identifiable preneoplastic lesions, many other cancers do; these include bladder, head and neck, and esophageal carcinomas. Genetic progression in these cases is currently under investigation.

Epigenetic Lesions and Gene Silencing

In addition to genetic events, it is now established that tumorigenesis also involves dramatic changes in the epigenetic profile of cancer cells. Epigenetic changes refer to nonheritable chromosomal modifications that affect gene expression. Two types of epigenetic changes have been most intensively studied and are thought to play a role in tumor progression: methylation of DNA itself, and methylation or acetylation of histone proteins that serve to package DNA within the cell nucleus [67]. DNA methylation occurs at cytosine (C) residues, most commonly within cytosine/guanine-rich regions of the genome known as CpG islands, as this dinucleotide is the target of DNA methyltransferases. CpG islands frequently comprise gene regulatory regions and are hypomethylated in many normal cells, leading to active gene transcription. In tumor cells, hypermethylation of the CpG island regulatory regions of particular tumor

suppressor loci, including CDKN2A, MLH1, and many others, is common and serves as an important mechanism for tumor suppressor silencing. Paradoxically, despite having increased methylation at specific CpG islands, tumor cells exhibit global hypomethylation which becomes more pronounced during progression, for example, from colonic polyps to carcinoma. A second mechanism for epigenetic gene silencing important in tumor cells involves methylation and acetylation of DNA-associated histone proteins. These modifications occur on specific amino acid residues of specific histones, and their pattern is tightly correlated with gene expression such that these patterns are sometimes referred to as the "histone code," analogous to the genetic (DNA) code itself. In both tumor and normal cells, DNA methylation and histone methylation/acetylation are interdependent regulatory mechanisms [68]. The fact that these epigenetic changes in tumor cells are potentially reversible opens the door to new therapeutic opportunities. For example, restoration of tumor suppressor gene expression in several mouse models has dramatic effects, either eliminating cancer cells or reversing the malignant phenotype. Therapies that promote reversal of epigenetic silencing of such genes in human tumors might in the future produce similar results.

MicroRNAs and Cancer Progression

Genetic studies in lower organisms recently uncovered the surprising finding that certain phenotypes are associated with genes that do not encode proteins. Among the most interesting of these genes are those encoding microRNAs (miRNAs), which are synthesized and processed into very small RNA molecules (16–29 nucleotides in length, in contrast to the average 1,500 nucleotide processed messenger RNA). These miRNAs function to inhibit RNA and protein expression by pairing to sequences within protein-coding RNA molecules themselves. It is believed that miRNAs evolved initially as a defense against foreign RNA species associated with viral infection; they are now known to regulate a wide variety of cellular processes including cellular proliferation, differentiation, and survival [69]. Hundreds of human miRNAs have now been identified, and global miRNA analysis has demonstrated that tumor cells exhibit dramatic changes in miRNA expression compared to normal cells. The view that these changes may be a cause rather than effect of the malignant phenotype is supported by specific examples, in which miRNAs appear to function as classical oncogenes and tumor suppressor genes. A significant subset of B cell chronic lymphocytic leukemia (B-CLL) cases, for example, exhibit loss of a region on chromosome 13q14. The only expressed genes in this locus are two miRNAs known as miR-15a and -16-1. These miRNAs are believed to inhibit the expression of the Bcl-2 oncogene, a key survival factor in malignant lymphocytes [70]. Loss or silencing of these miRNAs, which is observed in the majority of B-CLL as well as in other tumors, may therefore promote abnormal tumor cell survival. Similarly, the let-7 family of miRNAs may function as tumor suppressors given that they inhibit expression of the Ras oncogene. Indeed, expression of let-7 is inversely correlated with that of Ras in non-small cell lung carcinomas [71]. Other miRNAs appear to function as oncogenes, including miR-372 and miR-373. These miR-NAs are inhibitors of p53-mediated cell cycle arrest and are overexpressed in testicular carcinomas, which could potentially explain in part why p53 itself is infrequently mutated in these tumors [72]. In addition to their contribution to tumor progression, miRNAs are being investigated as potentially important predictors of prognosis and response to therapy.

Evasion of Cell Death and Acquisition of Immortality

Initial genetic events in tumorigenesis that drive cellular proliferation are often associated with cell death, which must be overcome to allow tumor progression. One example is loss of the RB1 tumor suppressor, which induces proliferation driven by E2F factors, but which may also trigger activation of p53-dependent death through upregulation of the p19-ARF protein. Nascent tumors must therefore inactivate p53 (or p19-ARF) in order to survive and expand. Another well-established example is the Bcl-2 protein, mentioned above as a target of tumor-suppressive miRNAs. Bcl-2 is a member of a family of proteins (the Bcl-2 family) that regulate cell death through the mitochondrial pathway for apoptosis [73]. In slow-growing follicular B-cell lymphomas, Bcl-2 is highly overexpressed through a chromosomal translocation that juxtaposes the gene to the strong promoter and enhancer elements of immunoglobulin genes [74]. In more aggressive lymphomas and in animal models, Bcl-2 cooperates with the c-Myc oncogene, as c-Myc activation induces proliferation but also cell death which can be attenuated by overexpression of Bcl-2.

In addition to bypassing controls on proliferation and evading cell death mechanisms, tumor cells must attain cellular immortality, the ability to undergo unlimited cell divisions. The normal limitation on cell division is most apparent in cultured normal cells, which undergo a finite number of cell divisions before entering a state of senescence, or irreversible growth arrest [75] (Fig. 1.8). Among the mediator pathways that may induce senescence in normal cells are p16-INK4A/p19-ARF and p53. Human cells which have bypassed these pathways are not immortal, however, due to the limitation on cellular lifespan imposed by chromosomal

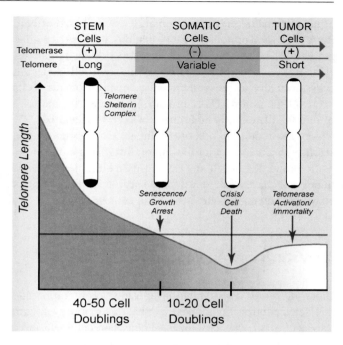

Fig. 1.8 Cellular senescence and the activation of telomerase. Normal cellular division requires the maintenance of telomeres at the ends of chromosomes. In germ cells and stem cells, this telomere maintenance results from the activity of the enzyme telomerase. Many somatic cells lack telomerase, and their growth in culture therefore results in progressive telomere shortening, until such time as cellular division ceases and senescence is reached. Cells driven to proliferate past that point by the expression of transforming genes continue to shrink their telomeres until they reach crisis, a point at which chromosomes become unstable and massive cell death results. In rare cells, telomerase may be activated at the time of crisis, producing immortal cells capable of indefinite growth in vitro. The majority of human cancers express high levels of telomerase, suggesting that a similar selection pressure in vivo contributes to their unlimited growth potential

telomeres. Telomeres constitute the ends of each chromosome, comprising multiple copies of a short, repeated DNA sequence and protected by a "cap" composed of a group of telomere-associated proteins known as the shelterin complex [76]. Telomeres function as a cellular counting mechanism because they shorten slightly with each cellular division, resulting from loss of nucleotides required for priming during initiation of DNA synthesis. Critically short telomeres trigger senescence, which if bypassed leads to further telomere shortening and a state known as crisis, characterized by substantial cell death. Crisis arises when telomeres become so short that the protein cap is disrupted, inducing a DNA damage response as cells try to repair or recombine telomeric DNA. Examination of human samples and mouse models suggests that the genetic instability which occurs during crisis may be an important mechanism for introducing chromosomal aberrations that drive tumor progression [77].

Arising from crisis are rare, immortal cells which have stabilized their telomeres, commonly through upregulation of the enzyme telomerase. Telomerase is composed of both RNA (hTR) and protein (hTERT) subunits and has the unique property of being able to add length to cellular telomeres, using RNA as a template [78, 79]. While stem cells and germ cells normally express telomerase, many somatic cells express little if any hTERT protein. In contrast, the majority of tumor cells express high levels of both hTR and hTERT, which they require in order to maintain telomere length and stability that are essential for immortality. The unique enzymatic properties of telomerase and its requirement in most tumor cells have made developing specific inhibitors of this enzyme a potentially attractive therapeutic approach.

Metastasis and Angiogenesis

Immortal tumor cells which have evaded proliferation and cell death controls do not pose a lethal threat, however, until they acquire the capacity for tissue invasion and metastasis. These latter processes involve the ability of cells to mobilize, invade basement membrane, travel to distant sites, and reestablish themselves as viable clones in a foreign environment. Tumor cells adapt at each of these steps in the metastatic process; both genetic and epigenetic changes in multiple genes are required, and only very rare cells eventually acquire full metastatic potential. Gene expression changes involved in initial invasion include upregulation of the Rho family of small GTPases, which regulate cytoskeletal architecture and cell mobility; increases in matrix metalloproteinases such as MMP-9 that are capable of digesting the basement membrane, facilitating tissue invasion and seeding of the bloodstream [80]; and suppression of cell–cell adhesion molecules such as E-cadherin. Paradoxically, TGF-β signaling, which in early tumorigenesis functions as a tumor suppressor mechanism, is found to be activated and to contribute to metastatic progression through both paracrine (through secretion by stromal cells) and autocrine effects. Current efforts are focused on inhibiting TGF-β signaling as a therapeutic strategy [81]. In addition to general metastasis promoters, recent studies have begun to uncover factors which mediate metastasis to specific organs such as lung and bone.

A key barrier to tumor progression for both the primary tumor and its metastatic derivatives is the establishment of an adequate supply of oxygen and nutrients. This concept led Folkman to propose that growing tumors must undergo an "angiogenic switch" in order to induce development of the tumor-specific vasculature, and that targeting tumor-specific angiogenesis might be an effective therapeutic strategy (Fig. 1.9) [82]. The pathways that mediate tumor-specific angiogenesis are now known to involve many of the same factors activated in response to physiologic hypoxia, including HIF and its downstream activated target vascular

endothelial growth factor (VEGF). Metabolic pathways regulating HIF stability and thus its activity are involved in at least three distinct tumor predisposition syndromes, which result from germline mutations in the VHL gene, the D-subunit of succinate dehydrogenase (SDHD) gene, and the fumarate hydratase (FH) gene [83]. These findings demonstrate the fundamental role of angiogenic factors in cancer, and they emphasize the potential of exploiting tumor angiogenesis therapeutically. An antibody directed against VEGF, bevacizumab (Avastin), has shown significant benefits in some cancer settings, as has a small molecule inhibitor of the VEGF receptor, sunitinib (Sutent) [84]. In addition to inducing angiogenesis, hypoxia itself is thought to drive tumor progression by promoting genetic instability (through altered reactive oxygen species) and inducing adaptations that promote tumor cell survival. Recent studies have shown that angiogenic tumors have a highly disordered vasculature, and that the effect of therapeutic inhibitors is not to eliminate the vasculature but to "normalize" its structure, thereby alleviating tumor hypoxia and improving tumor perfusion by chemotherapeutic agents [85].

Genetic Mechanisms of Treatment Resistance

Current cancer therapeutic approaches attempt to exploit particular vulnerabilities of tumor cells. Chemotherapy and radiation function by inducing various forms of DNA damage, inhibiting DNA replication or blocking mitosis. Tumor cells are more susceptible than normal cells to these insults due to more rapid cell division, defective repair pathways, and metabolic stress that can lower their apoptotic threshold. While these therapies exploit general properties of tumor cells, a new generation of so-called "targeted" therapeutics inhibits particular pathways that are activated in individual tumors through specific genetic mechanisms. Treatment resistance in human cancer results from a combination of host factors (variations in enzymes that metabolize therapeutic agents, for example), intrinsic properties of certain tumor types which reflect their tissue of origin (general drug resistance of the renal epithelium due to its ability to withstand naturally occurring toxins), and tumor-specific factors.

One mechanism of tumor-specific resistance to a broad variety of chemotherapeutic agents is the upregulation of the multidrug resistance (mdr) transporter genes (Fig. 1.10) [86]. These genes encode adenosine triphosphate (ATP)-dependent pumps that span the cell membrane and appear to be involved in the transport of large organic compounds. The most intensively studied gene implicated in this chemotherapy resistance mechanism is mdr-1, whose gene product is capable of exporting a wide range of compounds, including anthracyclines and vinca alkaloids. Expression of mdr-1 is expected

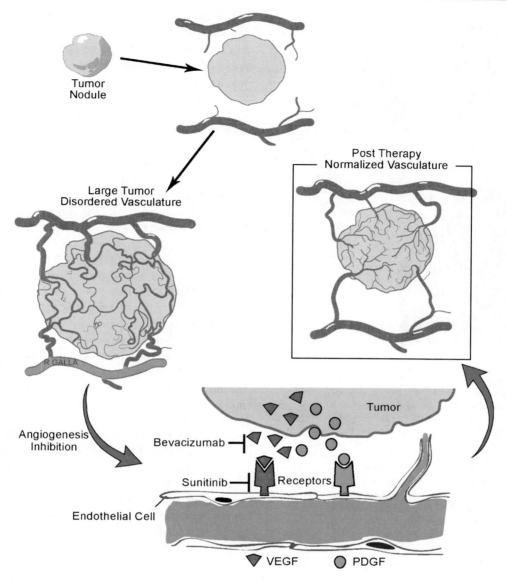

Fig. 1.9 Tumor angiogenesis and therapeutic angiogenesis inhibitors. Among the most important properties of tumors is their ability to recruit blood vessels, providing nutrients that allow their growth beyond a minimal size. Angiogenic recruitment depends on the secretion by tumors of endothelial growth factors such as VEGF and PDGF. Tumor vessels are leaky and disorganized, resulting in tumor-associated edema and hypoxia that contribute to therapeutic resistance. Current clinically available approaches to inhibit angiogenesis as cancer therapy include blocking VEGF itself (Bevacizumab) or inhibiting the receptors for VEGF and PDGF (Sunitinib). Anti-angiogenic therapies result in normalization of the tumor vasculature that may improve drug delivery and therapeutic response

to be associated with resistance to multiple agents in the absence of prior exposure. However, in some cancers, such as multiple myeloma, repeated exposure to anthracyclines and vinca alkaloids does appear to be correlated with further increases in mdr-1 expression and progressive chemoresistance. A well-described example of acquired chemoresistance occurs following exposure to the drug methotrexate, which specifically inhibits the enzyme dihydrofolate reductase (DHFR), required for DNA synthesis [87]. Tumors may become methotrexate resistant by acquiring defects in the intracellular transport of methotrexate; by mutations in the DHFR gene, resulting in an enzyme that fails to bind methotrexate; or by amplification of the DHFR gene itself, which increases the amount of protein made and thereby acts to overcome the intracellular concentration of the inhibitory drug.

The use of effective targeted therapeutics provides strong selection within tumors for genetic changes which confer specific resistance to particular drugs. Imatinib (Gleevec), a small-molecule selective inhibitor of the Bcr–Abl fusion

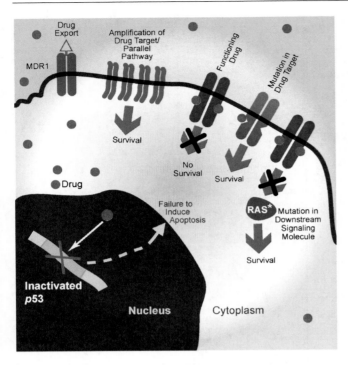

Fig. 1.10 Genetic mechanisms of resistance to anti-cancer therapy. Mechanisms of resistance to traditional chemotherapeutic drugs may include mutations in the p53 gene, which preclude the physiologic cellular apoptotic response to DNA injury mediated by these drugs; decreased drug uptake; or increased drug export by MDR1-related proteins. Specific resistance mechanisms have been identified for targeted therapeutics that function by blocking survival signals from activated growth factor receptors (e.g., EGFR). Mutations within the receptor active site can confer resistance to drugs that bind within that site. Alternatively, gene amplification of a receptor (e.g., c-MET) that signals in a parallel pathway, or mutational activation of a downstream signaling component (e.g., Ras) may promote tumor cell survival and resistance to targeted therapy

EGFR inhibitory antibody cetuximab (Erbitux) (Fig. 1.10). Mutations in the K-Ras oncogene are highly predictive of a lack of response to this agent, presumably because K-Ras mutation induces functional activation of the MAPK pathway irrespective of upstream EGFR signaling [90]. Molecular testing of colon cancers for this mutation is now becoming part of standard clinical practice for patients considering cetuximab therapy.

Specific therapeutic targets and associated resistance mechanisms are not as well established for tumor suppressor pathways as they are for the oncogene pathways described above. One exception, however, is breast and ovarian cancers associated with germline BRCA1 and BRCA2 mutations. BRCA1/2-deficient tumor cells have a specific defect in a DNA repair mechanism known as homologous recombination. These tumors are therefore dependent on the base-excision repair pathway to remedy spontaneous and induced DNA damage. This dependence can be exploited by treating these tumors with inhibitors of poly ADP ribose polymerase (PARP), an enzyme required for base-excision repair, either alone or in combination with chemotherapy. Remarkably, however, a subset of tumors becomes resistant to both PARP and chemotherapy by acquiring a small DNA deletion within the mutant BRCA2 allele [91]. This deletion excises the mutant stop codon, restores the BRCA2 reading frame for protein translation, and results in the production of a functional BRCA2 protein. These BRCA2-"restored" tumor cells are assumed to be DNA repair-competent and therefore no longer sensitive to therapy. A similar mechanism has been described in BRCA1-associated tumors. While this is an uncommon mechanism of resistance, it highlights the ability of tumor cells to adapt to specific selective pressures through genetic events that overcome treatment susceptibility.

protein kinase which drives CML, is initially highly effective in eliminating the bulk population of tumor cells [18]. In many cases, however, resistance develops through mutations within the kinase domain of Bcr–Abl that is targeted by imatinib. These observations have led to the successful introduction of so-called second generation inhibitors, dasatinib and nilotinib, which have higher affinity for the kinase domain and therefore increased potency, particularly against imatinib-resistant Bcr–Abl mutants [88]. Other important mechanisms of resistance occur through genetic alterations not in the therapeutic target itself, but in a parallel or downstream pathway. For example, an additional mechanism of imatinib resistance in CML is through overexpression of related Src-family kinases [89]. These proteins may function in common tumor-promoting pathways as Bcr–Abl, and at high levels they may also titrate away the inhibitory compound from Bcr–Abl. A clear example of a genetic event in a downstream pathway which confers resistance to a targeted inhibitor has recently been observed for colon cancers treated with the

Techniques for Cancer Genetic and Genomic Analysis

Two key advances have made is possible to analyze genetic abnormalities in tumor cells on a genome-wide scale: the sequencing of the entire human genome, and the development of high-density microarray technology. The most common of these types of analyses fall into two general categories: gene expression profiling and genome-wide DNA analysis. Gene expression profiling can be used to examine the levels of RNA for all human genes (approximately 30,000 genes) simultaneously in a tumor or other sample. The technique involves hybridization of RNA from the test sample to complementary probes attached to the microarray. The amount of hybridized RNA, which is proportional to the level of each RNA species, can then be determined by optical scanning. The entire set of probes corresponding to known human genes can be included on two microarrays which are each approximately the size of a nickel. Gene expression profiles have proven useful for both diagnostic and prognostic applications in human cancer, and are now being tested for their utility as predictors of response to particular therapies. For example, expression profiling has provided new insights into the classification of lymphomas and leukemias that have clinical implications and that would not have been possible through single-gene analysis [92]. Similarly, expression profiling has demonstrated the biologic basis for breast cancer classification and treatment. Specific gene "signatures" have been identified that are associated with prognosis but are independent of recognized clinical parameters. Clinical trials are now underway in breast and other cancers in order to test whether the application of these signatures to guide clinical decision-making can lead to improved outcomes [93]. It is also expected that analysis of these signatures may lead to the identification of potentially new and therapeutically relevant cancer driver pathways.

The second general class of genome-wide analysis uses microarrays to examine cellular DNA rather than RNA. The most widely used applications seek to uncover genome-wide patterns of chromosomal gains and losses within tumor cells at very high resolution. One approach used for this purpose, known as competitive genomic hybridization (CGH), is conceptually similar to gene expression analysis but assesses copy number of DNA rather than RNA [94]. The other commonly used method analyzes LOH by using high-density microarrays to detect single nucleotide polymorphisms (SNPs) across the genome [95]. LOH for a polymorphic marker in a tumor sample compared with normal tissue from the same individual is taken to indicate loss of the corresponding chromosomal locus. Most common human epithelial cancers are found to have numerous gains and losses, some of which are recurrent and correspond to oncogene and tumor suppressor loci, respectively. Both CGH and SNP arrays have been used to identify global patterns of DNA gains and losses which appear to correlate with clinical outcome in individual tumors. Combining these DNA-based approaches with gene expression profiling holds significant promise as a means to sort through and uncover the most relevant genetic changes in tumor cells [96]. In addition to these techniques, rapid advances in DNA sequencing technology will soon make it possible to sequence entire tumor genomes on a relatively cost-effective scale. Such studies may lead to a new appreciation of similarities and differences between tumor types that is based on shared genetic pathways and mutations, rather than tissue type or histologic appearance – so-called molecular taxonomy [97]. Furthermore, the emerging link between tumor-specific driver mutations and the clinical response to targeted therapeutics provides a clear rationale for integrating wide-scale

tumor sequence analysis into oncology clinical research and clinical practice.

As technologies for somatic genetic analyses of tumors have evolved, so has the capacity to conduct genome-wide studies to predict cancer susceptibility. The genome-wide scoring of SNPs present in populations from different ethnic groups has provided fundamental information about inheritance patterns of chromosomal loci and genetic recombinational events over generations [98]. Thus, groups of SNPs that tend to be co-inherited constitute "haplotype blocks," large regions of chromosomes ranging from 100 to 1,000 kilobases that are consistently linked across generations (Fig. 1.11). Chromosomal recombination events that occur outside of these haplotype blocks can lead to scrambling of haplotype inheritance patterns. The size of haplotype blocks may vary within different chromosomes, as well as with the evolutionary ancestry and divergence of human ethnic groups. The ability to group SNPs into haplotype blocks has allowed the patterns of human genomic variation to be interrogated in a manageable high throughput format, thus allowing genome-wide screens for genetic associations with unprecedented power.

These screens, known as Genome-Wide Association Studies (GWAS), have now been initiated across many human diseases including cancer. Their power lies in the ability to test large numbers of affected but unrelated individuals for coinheritance of specific loci. The polymorphic markers that

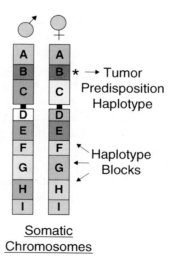

Fig. 1.11 Haplotype analysis and cancer predisposition. Blocks of DNA sequence are inherited in a linked fashion over generations, with chromosomal recombination events occurring between these blocks, giving rise to variable haplotype patterns between maternal and paternal alleles. Here, each haplotype block is shown as a letter, with different haplotype variants shown in different colors. Genome-wide association studies seek to identify the association of particular haplotype variants (in this case "B red" variant) with cancer predisposition. Detailed genetic studies are then required to identify the causative gene or sequence within a risk-associated haplotype variant

define such a locus are unlikely to be directly relevant to cancer susceptibility itself, but they define a haplotype which harbors a cancer causing "founder mutation" that arose at some time in the distant past. Thus, the power of GWAS studies is to identify relatively "common variants" in the population that are enriched among certain cancer patients, by virtue of their association with yet-unidentified disease causing mutations. Results of GWAS studies in common cancers have indeed revealed a number of previously unsuspected genetic loci which are potentially implicated in cancer susceptibility within the general population [99]. Two considerations are important to stress with respect to such studies: first, the specific deleterious mutation is not always readily identified by GWAS analyses. In fact, many loci identified by GWAS studies involve intergenic regions of the genome that are not well annotated, or promoter/regulatory sequences, whose effects on gene expression may be subtle. As such, considerable experimental analyses will be required before the functional consequences of many new cancer predisposing candidate loci are understood. Second, GWAS studies are specifically designed to identify common variants associated with a relatively low cancer risk, rather than the traditional rare "dominant acting" tumor suppressor gene mutations that are central to clinical genetic counseling. Most cancer susceptibility loci identified in GWAS studies to date are associated with relative risks of 1.1 to 1.5 over the general population (compared with 5- to 20-fold for traditional cancer predisposing alleles like p53 or BRCA1 mutations). This low relative risk renders them of epidemiological interest, but not appropriate for counseling individuals carrying a specific genetic variant. This consideration will become more relevant as "personal genomic profiles" become available in the future, undoubtedly including many such low risk factor variants that will need to be interpreted in the clinical setting. On the other hand, the relative cancer risk determined from GWAS studies may increase significantly as detailed studies identify the specific deleterious lesion that is associated with the flagged SNP. Taken together, the insights into cancer susceptibility provided by these whole genome analyses will continue to enhance our understanding of the entire breadth of genetic variation that together contributes to cancer risk within the population.

References

1. Lichtenstein P, Holm NV, Verkasalo PK et al (2000) Environmental and heritable factors in the causation of cancer – analyses of cohorts of twins from Sweden, Denmark, and Finland. N Engl J Med 343(2):78–85
2. Stehelin D, Varmus HE, Bishop JM, Vogt PK (1976) DNA related to the transforming gene(s) of avian sarcoma viruses is present in normal avian DNA. Nature 260(5547):170–173
3. Delattre O, Zucman J, Melot T et al (1994) The Ewing family of tumors – a subgroup of small-round-cell tumors defined by specific chimeric transcripts. N Engl J Med 331(5):294–299
4. Wistuba II, Gazdar AF, Minna JD (2001) Molecular genetics of small cell lung carcinoma. Semin Oncol 28(2 Suppl 4):3–13
5. Wood LD, Parsons DW, Jones S et al (2007) The genomic landscapes of human breast and colorectal cancers. Science 318(5853):1108–1113
6. Lowy DR, Willumsen BM (1993) Function and regulation of Ras. Annu Rev Biochem 62:851–891
7. Eng C, Clayton D, Schuffenecker I et al (1996) The relationship between specific RET proto-oncogene mutations and disease phenotype in multiple endocrine neoplasia type 2. International RET mutation consortium analysis. JAMA 276(19):1575–1579
8. Schimke RT (1984) Gene amplification, drug resistance, and cancer. Cancer Res 44(5):1735–1742
9. Brodeur GM, Seeger RC, Schwab M, Varmus HE, Bishop JM (1984) Amplification of N-Myc in untreated human neuroblastomas correlates with advanced disease stage. Science 224(4653):1121–1124
10. Rabbitts TH (1994) Chromosomal translocations in human cancer. Nature 372(6502):143–149
11. Dalla-Favera R, Bregni M, Erikson J, Patterson D, Gallo RC, Croce CM (1982) Human c-Myc onc gene is located on the region of chromosome 8 that is translocated in Burkitt lymphoma cells. Proc Natl Acad Sci U S A 79(24):7824–7827
12. Taub R, Kirsch I, Morton C et al (1982) Translocation of the c-Myc gene into the immunoglobulin heavy chain locus in human Burkitt lymphoma and murine plasmacytoma cells. Proc Natl Acad Sci U S A 79(24):7837–7841
13. Ellisen LW, Bird J, West DC et al (1991) TAN-1, the human homolog of the Drosophila notch gene, is broken by chromosomal translocations in T lymphoblastic neoplasms. Cell 66(4):649–661
14. Weng AP, Ferrando AA, Lee W et al (2004) Activating mutations of NOTCH1 in human T cell acute lymphoblastic leukemia. Science 306(5694):269–271
15. Shtivelman E, Lifshitz B, Gale RP, Canaani E (1985) Fused transcript of abl and bcr genes in chronic myelogenous leukaemia. Nature 315(6020):550–554
16. Rowley JD (1984) Biological implications of consistent chromosome rearrangements in leukemia and lymphoma. Cancer Res 44(8):3159–3168
17. Daley GQ, Van Etten RA, Baltimore D (1990) Induction of chronic myelogenous leukemia in mice by the P210bcr/abl gene of the Philadelphia chromosome. Science 247(4944):824–830
18. Druker BJ, Sawyers CL, Kantarjian H et al (2001) Activity of a specific inhibitor of the BCR-ABL tyrosine kinase in the blast crisis of chronic myeloid leukemia and acute lymphoblastic leukemia with the Philadelphia chromosome. N Engl J Med 344(14):1038–1042
19. Look AT (1997) Oncogenic transcription factors in the human acute leukemias. Science 278(5340):1059–1064
20. Warrell RP Jr, Frankel SR, Miller WH Jr et al (1991) Differentiation therapy of acute promyelocytic leukemia with tretinoin (all-trans-retinoic acid). N Engl J Med 324(20):1385–1393
21. Golub TR, Barker GF, Bohlander SK et al (1995) Fusion of the TEL gene on 12p13 to the AML1 gene on 21q22 in acute lymphoblastic leukemia. Proc Natl Acad Sci U S A 92(11):4917–4921
22. Tomlins SA, Rhodes DR, Perner S et al (2005) Recurrent fusion of TMPRSS2 and ETS transcription factor genes in prostate cancer. Science 310(5748):644–648
23. Tomlins SA, Laxman B, Dhanasekaran SM et al (2007) Distinct classes of chromosomal rearrangements create oncogenic ETS gene fusions in prostate cancer. Nature 448(7153):595–599
24. Ephrussi B, Davidson RL, Weiss MC, Harris H, Klein G (1969) Malignancy of somatic cell hybrids. Nature 224(5226):1314–1316

25. Saxon PJ, Srivatsan ES, Stanbridge EJ (1986) Introduction of human chromosome 11 via microcell transfer controls tumorigenic expression of HeLa cells. EMBO J 5(13):3461–3466

26. Whyte P, Buchkovich KJ, Horowitz JM et al (1988) Association between an oncogene and an anti-oncogene: the adenovirus E1A proteins bind to the retinoblastoma gene product. Nature 334(6178):124–129

27. Knudson AG Jr (1971) Mutation and cancer: statistical study of retinoblastoma. Proc Natl Acad Sci U S A 68(4):820–823

28. Friend SH, Bernards R, Rogelj S et al (1986) A human DNA segment with properties of the gene that predisposes to retinoblastoma and osteosarcoma. Nature 323(6089):643–646

29. Call KM, Glaser T, Ito CY et al (1990) Isolation and characterization of a zinc finger polypeptide gene at the human chromosome 11 Wilms' tumor locus. Cell 60(3):509–520

30. Cavenee WK, Dryja TP, Phillips RA et al (1983) Expression of recessive alleles by chromosomal mechanisms in retinoblastoma. Nature 305(5937):779–784

31. Weinberg RA (1995) The retinoblastoma protein and cell cycle control. Cell 81(3):323–330

32. Foulkes WD, Flanders TY, Pollock PM, Hayward NK (1997) The CDKN2A (p16) gene and human cancer. Mol Med 3(1):5–20

33. Sherr CJ (1996) Cancer cell cycles. Science 274(5293):1672–1677

34. Lane DP (1992) Cancer. p53, guardian of the genome. Nature 358(6381):15–16

35. Harris CC, Hollstein M (1993) Clinical implications of the p53 tumor-suppressor gene. N Engl J Med 329(18):1318–1327

36. Lang GA, Iwakuma T, Suh YA et al (2004) Gain of function of a p53 hot spot mutation in a mouse model of Li-Fraumeni syndrome. Cell 119(6):861–872

37. Olive KP, Tuveson DA, Ruhe ZC et al (2004) Mutant p53 gain of function in two mouse models of Li-Fraumeni syndrome. Cell 119(6):847–860

38. Debbas M, White E (1993) Wild-type p53 mediates apoptosis by E1A, which is inhibited by E1B. Genes Dev 7(4):546–554

39. Oliner JD, Kinzler KW, Meltzer PS, George DL, Vogelstein B (1992) Amplification of a gene encoding a p53-associated protein in human sarcomas. Nature 358(6381):80–83

40. Montes de Oca Luna R, Wagner DS, Lozano G (1995) Rescue of early embryonic lethality in mdm2-deficient mice by deletion of p53. Nature 378(6553):203–206

41. Quelle DE, Zindy F, Ashmun RA, Sherr CJ (1995) Alternative reading frames of the INK4a tumor suppressor gene encode two unrelated proteins capable of inducing cell cycle arrest. Cell 83(6):993–1000

42. Sherr CJ (1998) Tumor surveillance via the ARF-p53 pathway. Genes Dev 12(19):2984–2991

43. Matheu A, Maraver A, Klatt P et al (2007) Delayed ageing through damage protection by the Arf/p53 pathway. Nature 448(7151):375–379

44. Malkin D, Li FP, Strong LC et al (1990) Germ line p53 mutations in a familial syndrome of breast cancer, sarcomas, and other neoplasms. Science 250(4985):1233–8

45. Meijers-Heijboer H, van den Ouweland A, Klijn J et al (2002) Low-penetrance susceptibility to breast cancer due to CHEK2(*)1100delC in noncarriers of BRCA1 or BRCA2 mutations. Nat Genet 31(1):55–59

46. Savitsky K, Bar-Shira A, Gilad S et al (1995) A single ataxia telangiectasia gene with a product similar to PI-3 kinase. Science 268(5218):1749–1753

47. Featherstone C, Jackson SP (1998) DNA repair: the Nijmegen breakage syndrome protein. Curr Biol 8(17):R622–R625

48. Miki Y, Swensen J, Shattuck-Eidens D et al (1994) A strong candidate for the breast and ovarian cancer susceptibility gene BRCA1. Science 266(5182):66–71

49. Wooster R, Bignell G, Lancaster J et al (1995) Identification of the breast cancer susceptibility gene BRCA2. Nature 378(6559):789–792

50. Joenje H, Patel KJ (2001) The emerging genetic and molecular basis of Fanconi anaemia. Nat Rev 2(6):446–457

51. Lynch HT, Smyrk T, Lynch JF (1998) Molecular genetics and clinical-pathology features of hereditary nonpolyposis colorectal carcinoma (Lynch syndrome): historical journey from pedigree anecdote to molecular genetic confirmation. Oncology 55(2):103–108

52. Kolodner RD (1995) Mismatch repair: mechanisms and relationship to cancer susceptibility. Trends Biochem Sci 20(10):397–401

53. Aaltonen LA, Salovaara R, Kristo P et al (1998) Incidence of hereditary nonpolyposis colorectal cancer and the feasibility of molecular screening for the disease. N Engl J Med 338(21):1481–1487

54. Markowitz S, Wang J, Myeroff L et al (1995) Inactivation of the type II TGF-beta receptor in colon cancer cells with microsatellite instability. Science 268(5215):1336–1338

55. Inoki K, Corradetti MN, Guan KL (2005) Dysregulation of the TSC-mTOR pathway in human disease. Nat Genet 37(1):19–24

56. Sansal I, Sellers WR (2004) The biology and clinical relevance of the PTEN tumor suppressor pathway. J Clin Oncol 22(14):2954–2963

57. Crino PB, Nathanson KL, Henske EP (2006) The tuberous sclerosis complex. N Engl J Med 355(13):1345–1356

58. Hemminki A, Markie D, Tomlinson I et al (1998) A serine/threonine kinase gene defective in Peutz-Jeghers syndrome. Nature 391(6663):184–187

59. Iliopoulos O, Kaelin WG Jr (1997) The molecular basis of von Hippel-Lindau disease. Mol Med 3(5):289–293

60. McCormick F (1995) Ras signaling and NF1. Curr Opin Genet Dev 5(1):51–55

61. Gusella JF, Ramesh V, MacCollin M, Jacoby LB (1996) Neurofibromatosis 2: loss of merlin's protective spell. Curr Opin Genet Dev 6(1):87–92

62. Fearnhead NS, Britton MP, Bodmer WF (2001) The ABC of APC. Hum Mol Genet 10(7):721–733

63. Hahn SA, Schutte M, Hoque AT et al (1996) DPC4, a candidate tumor suppressor gene at human chromosome 18q21.1. Science 271(5247):350–353

64. Hahn H, Wicking C, Zaphiropoulous PG et al (1996) Mutations of the human homolog of Drosophila patched in the nevoid basal cell carcinoma syndrome. Cell 85(6):841–851

65. Rivera MN, Kim WJ, Wells J et al (2007) An X chromosome gene, WTX, is commonly inactivated in Wilms tumor. Science 315(5812):642–645

66. Kinzler KW, Vogelstein B (1996) Lessons from hereditary colorectal cancer. Cell 87(2):159–170

67. Ting AH, McGarvey KM, Baylin SB (2006) The cancer epigenome – components and functional correlates. Genes Dev 20(23):3215–3231

68. Esteller M (2007) Cancer epigenomics: DNA methylomes and histone-modification maps. Nat Rev 8(4):286–298

69. Wiemer EA (2007) The role of microRNAs in cancer: no small matter. Eur J Cancer 43(10):1529–1544

70. Calin GA, Dumitru CD, Shimizu M et al (2002) Frequent deletions and down-regulation of micro-RNA genes miR15 and miR16 at 13q14 in chronic lymphocytic leukemia. Proc Natl Acad Sci U S A 99(24):15524–15529

71. Johnson SM, Grosshans H, Shingara J et al (2005) Ras is regulated by the let-7 microRNA family. Cell 120(5):635–647

72. Voorhoeve PM, le Sage C, Schrier M et al (2006) A genetic screen implicates miRNA-372 and miRNA-373 as oncogenes in testicular germ cell tumors. Cell 124(6):1169–1181

73. Korsmeyer SJ (1995) Regulators of cell death. Trends Genet 11(3):101–105

74. Cleary ML, Smith SD, Sklar J (1986) Cloning and structural analysis of cDNAs for bcl-2 and a hybrid bcl-2/immunoglobulin transcript resulting from the t(14;18) translocation. Cell 47(1):19–28

75. Hayflick L, Moorhead PS (1961) The serial cultivation of human diploid cell strains. Exp Cell Res 25:585–621

76. Greider CW (1998) Telomeres and senescence: the history, the experiment, the future. Curr Biol 8(5):R178–R181

77. Artandi SE, DePinho RA (2000) Mice without telomerase: what can they teach us about human cancer? Nat Med 6(8):852–855

78. Meyerson M, Counter CM, Eaton EN et al (1997) hEST2, the putative human telomerase catalytic subunit gene, is up-regulated in tumor cells and during immortalization. Cell 90(4):785–795

79. Nakamura TM, Morin GB, Chapman KB et al (1997) Telomerase catalytic subunit homologs from fission yeast and human. Science 277(5328):955–9

80. Liotta LA, Tryggvason K, Garbisa S, Hart I, Foltz CM, Shafie S (1980) Metastatic potential correlates with enzymatic degradation of basement membrane collagen. Nature 284(5751):67–68

81. Bierie B, Moses HL (2006) Tumour microenvironment: TGFbeta: the molecular Jekyll and Hyde of cancer. Nat Rev 6(7):506–520

82. Folkman J (1996) Fighting cancer by attacking its blood supply. Sci Am 275(3):150–154

83. Gottlieb E, Tomlinson IP (2005) Mitochondrial tumour suppressors: a genetic and biochemical update. Nat Rev 5(11):857–866

84. Chow LQ, Eckhardt SG (2007) Sunitinib: from rational design to clinical efficacy. J Clin Oncol 25(7):884–896

85. Jain RK (2005) Normalization of tumor vasculature: an emerging concept in antiangiogenic therapy. Science 307(5706):58–62

86. Ling V (1997) Multidrug resistance: molecular mechanisms and clinical relevance. Cancer Chemother Pharmacol 40(Suppl):S3–S8

87. Kinsella AR, Smith D (1998) Tumor resistance to antimetabolites. Gen Pharmacol 30(5):623–626

88. Quintas-Cardama A, Cortes J (2008) Therapeutic options against BCR-ABL1 T315I-positive chronic myelogenous leukemia. Clin Cancer Res 14(14):4392–4399

89. Jabbour E, Cortes J, O'Brien S, Giles F, Kantarjian H (2007) New targeted therapies for chronic myelogenous leukemia: opportunities to overcome imatinib resistance. Semin Hematol 44(1 Suppl 1): S25–S31

90. Karapetis CS, Khambata-Ford S, Jonker DJ et al (2008) K-Ras mutations and benefit from cetuximab in advanced colorectal cancer. N Engl J Med 359(17):1757–1765

91. Edwards SL, Brough R, Lord CJ et al (2008) Resistance to therapy caused by intragenic deletion in BRCA2. Nature 451(7182): 1111–1115

92. Rosenwald A, Wright G, Chan WC et al (2002) The use of molecular profiling to predict survival after chemotherapy for diffuse large-B-cell lymphoma. N Engl J Med 346(25):1937–1947

93. Sotiriou C, Pusztai L (2009) Gene-expression signatures in breast cancer. N Engl J Med 360(8):790–800

94. Brown PO, Botstein D (1999) Exploring the new world of the genome with DNA microarrays. Nat Genet 21(1 Suppl):33–37

95. Fan JB, Chee MS, Gunderson KL (2006) Highly parallel genomic assays. Nat Rev 7(8):632–644

96. Kim SY, Hahn WC (2007) Cancer genomics: integrating form and function. Carcinogenesis 28(7):1387–1392

97. Lakhani SR, Ashworth A (2001) Microarray and histopathological analysis of tumours: the future and the past? Nat Rev 1(2):151–157

98. Gibbs JR, Singleton A (2006) Application of genome-wide single nucleotide polymorphism typing: simple association and beyond. PLoS Genet 2(10):e150

99. Gold B, Kirchhoff T, Stefanov S et al (2008) Genome-wide association study provides evidence for a breast cancer risk locus at 6q22.33. Proc Natl Acad Sci U S A 105(11): 4340–4345

Chapter 2
Principles of Cancer Genetic Counseling and Genetic Testing

Kristen M. Shannon and Devanshi Patel

Keywords Genetic testing • Informed consent • Autosomal dominant • Autosomal recessive • DNA banking • Germline mutations • Risk assessment • Confidentiality

Introduction

Although only 5–10% of all cases of cancer are attributable to a highly penetrant cancer predisposition gene, the identification of individuals at inherited risk for cancer has become an integral part of the practice of predictive and preventative medicine. Identifying those individuals with a significantly higher risk of developing specific cancers allows health-care providers to intervene with appropriate counseling and education, increased cancer surveillance, and sometimes even cancer prevention. This chapter focuses on the identification of patients at high risk for cancer and the importance of referral to genetic counselors and other genetics professionals. The chapter also discusses the intricacies surrounding genetic testing, including the ethical, legal, and social implications of identifying those at increased risk for cancer.

Identification of At-Risk Individuals

The accurate identification of individuals at increased risk for developing cancer is essential. There are various models to aid providers in this process of identification, and they all rely on an individual's personal and/or family history of cancer. The National Comprehensive Cancer Network (NCCN) has established criteria for those individuals that need further genetics risk assessment for breast cancer and gastrointestinal cancer (Table 2.1) and recommends that individuals meeting

these criteria be referred to a cancer genetics professional for further workup and potential genetic testing [1, 2].

The process of identifying those requiring genetics assessment varies among institutions. Some programs rely on physicians to recognize these individuals. Caution should be exercised with this approach, because the success will rely on other nonphysician factors – the strongest of which is patient inquiry about their need for genetic testing for cancer [3, 4]. In one study of family practitioners [5], the information present in the individual's medical record was insufficient to permit risk assessment in over two thirds of cases with a significant family history of colon cancer. In this same study, the appropriate level of cancer screening was not achieved in half of the patients with a family history of colon cancer, individuals at moderate or high cancer risk were not identified as such, and those at high risk were not offered cancer genetics referral.

Other institutions will implement a more rudimentary screening program and use a "pen and paper" family history questionnaire that is reviewed by a trained staff member to identify and refer patients for genetic counseling. Still others utilize a more complex approach, where a patient inputs his or her personal and family history into a computerized program and the software identifies those needing genetic counseling [6, 7]. Use of the Internet to provide family history information is a potentially powerful tool, and interest in this modality is high [8]. Data are lacking, however, on which approach is most efficient at identifying individuals at risk [9].

Once an individual is recognized as being at increased risk, it is important that they are referred to a cancer genetics professional [1], as the importance of pretest and posttest genetic counseling for cancer susceptibility testing is widely recognized [10]. The provider must understand the complexities of genetic testing and the appropriate interpretation of the test results. One study reported that patients undergoing genetic testing for *APC* mutations frequently received inadequate counseling from their health-care provider and 32% had their test results incorrectly interpreted [11]. The authors concluded that physicians should be prepared to offer appropriate genetic counseling if they order genetic tests. Some states, such as Massachusetts, mandate that part of the

K.M. Shannon(✉)
Center for Cancer Risk Assessment,
Massachusetts General Hospital, Boston, MA, USA
e-mail: keshannon@partners.org

D.C. Chung and D.A. Haber (eds.), *Principles of Clinical Cancer Genetics: A Handbook from the Massachusetts General Hospital*,
DOI 10.1007/978-0-387-93846-2_2, © Springer Science+Business Media, LLC 2010

Table 2.1 Criteria for Referral to a Genetics Professional [1, 2]

For breast cancer risk assessment	For colon cancer risk assessment
Early onset breast cancer* (<50 years)	Early-age-onset (<50 years) colorectal or endometrial cancer OR
Two breast primaries or breast and ovarian cancer** in a single individual OR two or more breast primaries or breast and ovarian cancers in close relative(s) from the same side of a family (maternal or paternal)	Individuals with multiple primary HNPCC-related cancers (see below) OR
Clustering of breast cancer with one or more of the following: thyroid cancer, sarcoma, adrenocortical carcinoma, endometrial cancer, pancreatic cancer, brain tumors, dermatologic manifestations or leukemia/lymphoma on same side of the family	Individuals with an HNPCC-related cancer who have one or more first-degree relatives with an HNPCC-related cancer prior to age 50 or two or more first- or second-degree relatives with an HNPCC-related cancer diagnosed at any age
Member of a family with a known mutation in a cancer susceptibility gene	HNPCC-related cancers include: • Colorectal
Populations at risk***	• Endometrial
Any male breast cancer	• Ovarian
Ovarian cancer**: one or more on same side of family	• Duodenal/small bowel
	• Gastric
	• Sebaceous adenomas or sebaceous carcinomas
	• Ureteral/renal pelvis
	• Hepatobiliary/pancreas
	Brain tumors (particularly glioblastomas) OR
	Multiple colorectal carcinomas or >10 adenomas in same individuals OR
	Family with known hereditary syndrome associated with cancer with or without mutation (e.g., polyposis)

*DCIS included

**Fallopian tube cancer and primary peritoneal cancer included

***For populations at risk, the guidelines may be lessened (e.g., women of Ashkenazi Jewish ancestry with breast or ovarian cancer at any age)

informed consent procedure for genetic testing includes the identification and referral to a genetic counselor or geneticist (Mass. Gen. Laws Ch. 111, § 70G).

The Genetic Counseling Process

Genetic counseling is the process of interpreting and communicating information with respect to medical, psychological, and familial implications of genetic disease [12]. This practice is specifically aimed at assessing a patient's personal and family history to determine whether there is an underlying cancer predisposition. Ascertaining and communicating this information helps patients and their health-care providers better understand an individual's cancer risk. This information is then used to help establish the best medical management for a patient with respect to cancer surveillance and/or risk reduction [13].

The process of cancer genetic counseling can be divided into distinct components that include contracting, obtaining medical information, risk assessment, genetic testing, informed consent, education, and psychosocial support. These seven components are outlined in the following pages.

Contracting

Contracting is the term used to describe the beginning of the encounter when the counselor and counselee share their intentions for the session. Contracting provides the opportunity to communicate expectations of what will occur during the appointment. Patients are sometimes unaware of what a genetic counseling session entails [14] and may have conflicting expectations for the visit. Contracting also provides the genetic counselor with the opportunity to describe their role in the process. This is particularly important for patients who want to pursue testing but do not expect comprehensive education and counseling to accompany the practice [14].

Contracting also provides the genetic counselor the opportunity to assess the patient's knowledge and comfort level. Assessing the comfort level is particularly important as some patients are ambivalent toward pursuing genetic counseling due to underlying anxiety of cancer [15–17]. Determining all of this information from the outset allows for the organization of a session that best meets the patient's needs.

It is believed that contracting may actually shorten the length of a genetic counseling session, as it can potentially prevent the "doorknob syndrome". The phenomenon of "doorknob syndrome" is common and results when patients are not given the opportunity to share their thoughts and concerns with providers and choose to do so only near the end of the session [18]. Allowing these issues to fall to the end of the session can lengthen the time of the consultation.

Obtaining Medical Information

Obtaining the Family History

After the brief contracting, the genetics professional will most often begin the assessment with a detailed family history. Typically, a detailed three-generation family history is constructed in the form of a pedigree [19, 20]. It is important to gather information on both maternal and paternal lineages, with particular focus on individuals with malignancies (affected) and noncancer phenotypes associated with inherited cancer predisposition syndromes.

Information on All Individuals

When taking the family history, it is important to document each individual's age or age at death as well as his/her personal history of cancer or benign tumors. It is imperative to include those family members without a personal history of cancer (unaffected) because the ratio and pattern of affected and unaffected influences risk assessment. It is equally important to include the presence of nonmalignant findings in the proband and family members, as some inherited cancer syndromes have other physical characteristics associated with them (e.g., trichilimommas with Cowden Syndrome). When a syndrome with such nonmalignant findings is suspected, direct follow-up questions with respect to other features associated with the disease in question are warranted. For example, if Cowden syndrome is suspected, the provider should ask for a history of thyroid disease, large head size, and abnormal skin findings in each family member individually.

General medical information can also be pertinent to the patient's future medical management. For example, in women worked up for hereditary breast and ovarian cancer syndrome (HBOCS), it would be important to determine if their ovaries are intact as this affects risk assessment as well as potential screening/surgical recommendations (prophylactic bilateral salpingo oophorectomy has been shown to reduce the risk of developing breast cancer in HBOCS patients [21, 22]).

It is also important to determine whether there are lifestyle factors that can influence their hereditary cancer risk, such as smoking for pancreatic cancer or increased sun exposure for melanoma.

Information on Affected Individuals

When gathering information on an individual who has been diagnosed with cancer, information on the specifics of the cancer diagnosis is important and should include the primary site of the tumor, the age at diagnosis with cancer, and the number of primary tumors. It is important to recognize that some patients will not distinguish among a primary tumor, a recurrence, or a metastasis, so it is important for the provider to probe with appropriate questioning. It is also important to ask about environmental exposures that may have contributed to the development of the individual's diagnosis with cancer.

Details about the pathology of the tumor can be very helpful and can guide the differential diagnosis. For example,

breast cancers are associated with many hereditary cancer syndromes. Invasive ductal breast cancers that are ER, PR, and HER2 negative on pathology ("triple negative" or "basaloid type") are typically can be associated with *BRCA1* mutations [23, 24], while lobular breast cancer can be associated with *CDH1* mutations [25, 26]. Intestinal-type cancers of the stomach can be associated with Lynch syndrome, whereas diffuse gastric cancer can be associated with *CDH1* mutations [27]. The pathology of "colon polyps" is often critical to risk assessment. Most patients will report a history of "colon polyps" and it is important to determine the number (e.g., 1 vs. 5–10 vs. >100) and type (e.g., adenomatous vs. hamartomatous vs. hyperplastic) as the differential diagnosis will hinge upon these characteristics.

Most patients will not be aware of the specific pathology or histology of their tumor, and in some cases, confirming the diagnosis with pathology reports is essential [13]. This process can be very time-consuming on the part of both provider and patient – especially when trying to obtain medical records from relatives.

Accuracy of Information

When taking the family history, the accuracy of the information obtained should be considered. Many factors can influence an individual's knowledge of the family history [28]. Information on relatives may not be available because of estrangement, adoption, or simply because the patient has lost contact with his or her family members. In many families, cancer is simply not discussed, so the information available may be incomplete. The information provided can be incorrect because he or she is mistaken about the diagnosis or confused between a malignant and benign tumor, for example. A recent study indicates that individuals are often confident that a family member has had cancer, but are typically unsure of the details surrounding that diagnosis [9, 29]. Reports of breast cancer tend to be accurate, while reports of ovarian cancer are less trustworthy [30, 31]. It is also important to note that family histories can change over time, with new diagnoses arising in family members as time passes. All of these factors must be considered during the consultation, as the risk assessment and differential diagnosis are based primarily on this information.

Risk Assessment

There are some published guidelines on when to recommend genetic testing. American Society of Clinical Oncology (ASCO) recommends that genetic testing be offered when (1) the individual has personal or family history features suggestive of a genetic cancer susceptibility condition,

(2) the test can be adequately interpreted, and (3) the results will aid in diagnosis or influence the medical or surgical management of the patient or family members at hereditary risk of cancer [10]. The NCCN provides guidelines for individuals who should be offered genetic testing for Hereditary Breast/Ovarian Cancer Syndrome, Li-Fraumeni Syndrome, Cowden Syndrome, Lynch syndrome, Familial Adenomatous Polyposis, Attenuated Familial Adenomatous Polyposis, MYH-Associated Polyposis and Puetz–Jeghers syndrome [1]. Ultimately, it is up to the individual provider to determine whether genetic testing is indicated.

Patient Reaction to High Risk Status

The patient's reaction to the designation of "high risk" status can vary greatly depending on their personal and family history and their underlying emotional well-being [28]. Some individuals may feel validated that their fears regarding cancer are real. Others who have lived in denial may react with disbelief, anger, and fear. The individual's experience with cancer also will be a factor in their reaction. Those who have lost many family members to cancer are more likely to be anxious, while those whose family members have survived cancer may be less worried about cancer mortality.

Patient Reaction to Low Risk Assessment

When the provider feels that genetic testing is not indicated because the patient has a low risk of being a mutation carrier, the patient can react in a variety of ways. Patients who learn that their personal and/or family history of cancer is similar to the general public can react with relief, surprise, and sometimes anger [28]. The mere presence of cancer in the family can often lead patients to believe that they are at increased risk of developing cancer. Once it is explained that since one out of two American males and one out of three American females are diagnosed with cancer in their lifetime [32], having a family history of some cancer is not unusual. This along with an explanation that features associated with hereditary cancers are absent in their family often leave patients with a sense of relief that their cancer risk is most likely that of the general population.

On the other hand, those motivated to pursue a genetic test to help better determine their personal cancer risk, even in the absence of a significant family history of cancer, can sometimes feel frustrated and angry when a genetic test is not recommended. Educating these individuals to the fact that genetic testing in the context of a negative family history will most likely yield an uninformative negative test result

and not add any information in personal cancer risk assessment is essential.

Principles of Genetic Testing

Ideal Testing Candidate

Once it has been determined that the family history is suggestive of a hereditary cancer predisposition, the next step is to determine whether genetic testing is appropriate and who in the family is the best person to test first.

In the past, genetic testing was generally offered to patients who exceeded the threshold of a 10% likelihood of being a carrier of a cancer predisposition mutation [33]. However, in 2003, ASCO deleted this threshold in their statement on genetic testing for cancer susceptibility [13, 34]. Within a family, the individual with the highest a priori risk is the ideal person to test first. This is typically an individual who diagnosed with a component tumor at a young age or an individual who has two primary component tumors. This is preferred because it allows for the best interpretation of test results. Unaffected individuals are usually offered genetic testing only when the ideal testing candidate cannot or does not want to be tested. When a family mutation is identified, unaffected individuals should then be offered testing, as interpretation of test results are clear in this scenario.

For most inherited cancer syndromes, there are diagnostic criteria and/or guidance as to whom should be tested for genetic susceptibility. The details of these criteria will be discussed further in this book.

Timing of Genetic Testing

For most of the inherited cancer syndromes, genetic testing takes 4–12 weeks and results are typically not available quickly enough to impact the treatment of a newly diagnosed cancer. There are some exceptions to this that warrant attention.

BRCA1/2 genetic test results are typically available within 14 days of blood draw. The information gleaned has the potential to affect surgical decision making if the results are available prior to definitive surgery. If a woman tests positive for a deleterious mutation, for example, she may choose mastectomy to treat her cancer and also undergo contralateral prophylactic mastectomy to reduce the ≤60% risk of developing a second breast malignancy. Studies have revealed that women are interested in obtaining this information at the time of diagnosis, as it may help them plan their surgery [35]. However, some women who would not consider bilateral mastectomies even with a *BRCA* mutation are likely to proceed with breast conserving surgery regardless of the *BRCA* result [36]. For several reasons, it is important to identify women who are interested in using this testing information in their surgical decision. When women undergo genetic counseling after definitive surgery, they are less likely to consider genetic testing [37]. In addition, one study showed that women who had *BRCA1/2* testing and initially had undergone breast-conserving surgery chose to undergo subsequent bilateral prophylactic mastectomy prior to receiving radiation therapy [38]. This subjects these women to an additional surgical procedure and associated risks. Finally, many women with a family history of breast cancer are advised to consider prophylactic mastectomy for treatment of their newly diagnosed breast cancer. Silva reported that in a group of such women, learning that they are not mutation carriers *after* the prophylactic procedure leads many to question their earlier decision to undergo prophylactic surgery. This, in turn, is often associated with complications and quality of life issues [39].

Genetic testing for *p53* mutations can take as little as 3 weeks if ordered as an urgent test. It is well known that *p53* mutant cells are extremely sensitive to DNA damage [40, 41]. In vivo studies suggest that DNA damaging agents (e.g., chemotherapy and radiotherapy) used for treatment of a cancer in an individual with LFS can cause a second malignancy [42]. One study showed the risk of developing second cancer after radiotherapy was as high as 57% [43]. Although avoidance of chemotherapy in many situations is not realistic, radiotherapy can sometimes be avoided depending on the surgical techniques employed (e.g., mastectomy rather than lumpectomy for surgical treatment of breast cancer). It is important that oncologists recognize that radiation should be avoided if possible (e.g., choosing mastectomy over lumpectomy) in LFS. In cases where radiation therapy is necessary, though, it is imperative that the physicians and patient be aware of the risk of a second primary in the radiation field [42, 44].

Implication for At-Risk Family Members

First-degree relatives of individuals with an autosomal dominant hereditary cancer predisposition have a 50% chance of inheriting the cancer predisposition gene/condition. It is important to determine which parent carries the mutation, so that the relatives from the respective lineage can be informed of the family mutation and can consider the option of testing. Sometimes the family history is limited and such a judgment cannot be readily made. In this case, testing both parents may be necessary. If neither parent is available, offering testing to family members on both sides of the family is indicated until a mutation is found in either lineage.

It is unusual but possible that both parents may test negative for their child's mutation. The possible explanations for this scenario include non-paternity, a "de novo" genetic event, or one of the parents is a germline mosaic. The "de novo" mutation rates for certain genes are fairly high. For example, the de novo mutation rate for *APC* can be up to ~25% [45], and the de novo mutation rate for *p53* is estimated at ~20% [46]. In a true "de novo" case, only the offspring of the affected individual are at risk for inheriting the cancer predisposition. However, if germline mosaicism is suspected, testing the affected individual's siblings may be warranted. Germline mosaicism refers to two or more genetic cell lines confined to the precursor cells (eggs or sperm) in the affected individual's parents. One way to rule out germline mosaicism is to test the parents' gametes, but this option is not generally recommended.

Individuals with an autosomal recessive cancer predisposition are informed that their siblings are at a 25% risk having the condition and a 50% risk of carrying one copy of the mutation. Children of individuals with autosomal recessive cancer predisposition condition are at 100% risk of carrying one copy of a mutation. Although the carrier frequency for autosomal recessive cancer predisposition genes such as *MYH* is not firmly established, the likelihood that the partner of an individual with *MYH*-Associated Polyposis (MAP) carries a mutation in the *MYH* gene is expected to be very low. Nonetheless, genetic testing of the partner or the children of an individual with MAP should be considered.

The conventional view in clinical genetics is that carriers of mutations of autosomal recessive genetic conditions are not affected with the condition. However, it is not clear that this is true in recessive cancer predisposition syndromes such as MYH-Associated Polyposis (MAP) syndrome, where it may be prudent not to abandon screening of single-mutation carriers [47].

Choosing the Right Test

Once the most appropriate index testing candidate is identified, it is important to determine which test to order. For some populations, founder mutations have been identified and are sometimes useful in the initial screening process for cancer predisposition. For instance, if an individual of Ashkenazi Jewish descent has a family history suggestive of hereditary breast and ovarian cancer, testing for the founder mutations 185delAG and 53282insC in *BRCA1* and 6174delT in *BRCA2* is indicated as an initial step. If this testing is negative, full gene sequencing of *BRCA1/2* may then be considered. It is important to note that individuals who are not of Ashkenazi Jewish descent should not be screened for the Ashkenazi founder mutations.

It is equally important to recognize that germline (blood) genetic testing is not always the most appropriate first step in the genetic testing process. In the genetic workup for Lynch syndrome, tumor testing can help determine which mismatch repair gene is responsible. This screening tool is called immunohistochemistry (IHC) testing. In Lynch syndrome, one of four genes can be altered: *MLH1*, *MSH2*, *MSH6*, or *PMS2* [48–51]. IHC testing detects whether proteins from these genes are present in the tumor [49]. If IHC of *MLH1*, *MSH2*, *MSH6*, and *PMS2* indicates that one of these proteins is missing, it suggests that particular gene is not functional and germline testing of just that specific gene would be recommended. Using this screening tool as an initial step predetermines which gene should be analyzed by germline genetic testing, thereby providing a cost benefit [52].

Choosing the Right Laboratory

Things to consider when choosing the laboratory are:

- The sensitivity of the test at various laboratories. Many laboratories may offer genetic testing for a particular gene, but the technology for screening may vary from laboratory to laboratory. In genetic testing for *p53*, for example, some laboratories sequence only specific exons within the gene and may miss mutations that exist outside of these exons. With genetic testing for DNA mismatch repair genes, some laboratories will include Southern blot analysis to detect genomic rearrangements, where other laboratories will perform Multiplex Ligation-dependent Probe Amplification (MLPA) for the same purpose. Different technologies have different specificities and sensitivities, and therefore it is important review the technologies offered at each laboratory in order to offer the most appropriate test to the patient.
- Turnaround time will also vary from laboratory to laboratory. This is important to consider especially if the results are going to be used for immediate medical management as in the case of breast cancer.
- Costs and payment options are important to review with patients.

Research Testing

In certain cases, genetic testing can be pursued via a research laboratory. Usually, research laboratories are not CLIA-approved; therefore, any genetic testing results from a non-CLIA approved research laboratory should be confirmed through a CLIA-approved laboratory. Limitations of research labs include a lengthier turnaround time for test results and additional participation (additional consent forms, questionnaires, interviews, etc.) on the part of the patient. The benefit is usually that the patient will receive the testing at low or no cost [13].

DNA Banking

In certain cases, assessment of a family history reveals an increased number of cancer cases, but the cluster of cancers does not suggest a recognized cancer syndrome. When this is the case, genetic testing is likely to be unrevealing. However, DNA banking may be appropriate so that testing may be pursued at a later date. It is important to note that DNA banking has costs associated with it. Typically, there is an initial set up fee, an annual fee and a fee when a sample is released from the lab for testing. These costs are not generally covered by health insurance, so it is imperative that the patient's family understands these inherent costs.

When Testing Is Declined

When patients decline genetic testing, it is important to refer back to the family history to make medical management recommendations for the patient. For example, a young woman who decides that she does not want to learn her carrier status for the *BRCA* mutation that her mother carries should be screened as if she is positive.

Disclosure of Test Results

Historically, it has been standard to disclose test results in person, but the practice has evolved to include phone disclosure of genetic test results. A randomized study of disclosure of genetic test results showed no difference in anxiety or satisfaction between those randomized to the phone arm versus the in-person arm and also found a slight preference for phone results [53]. Current practice is generally to offer the patient in-person or phone disclosure and have them decide, as this procedure leads to greater patient satisfaction with the testing process [53, 54]. Regardless, it should be clarified that the results will be disclosed verbally (in person or over the telephone) and then mailed to them along with a letter interpreting their test results.

The Process of Informed Consent

Genetic counselors are integral in obtaining informed consent for genetic testing. Informed consent is "the process of obtaining a patient's permission for a procedure after the

Table 2.2 Elements of Informed Consent

Purpose of the test and who to test
General information about the gene(s)
Possible test results
Positive result
Negative result: no mutation in the family (i.e., uninformative negative)
Negative results: known mutation in the family (i.e., true negative)
Variant of uncertain significance
Likelihood of positive result
Technical aspects and accuracy of the test
Economic considerations
Risks of genetic discrimination
Psychosocial aspects
Anticipated reaction to results
Timing and readiness for testing
Family issues
Preparing for results
Confidentiality issues
Utilization of test results
Alternatives to genetic testing
Storage and potential reuse of genetic material

Adapted from ref. [13]

patient and doctor have discussed the risks, benefits, and alternatives of the procedure and the patient understands them" [55]. This is distinct from an Informed Consent Document, which is "a form listing the most common and worst possible risks of a procedure, the alternatives to the procedure, and the possible benefits of the procedure, which the patient signs to document their agreement to have the procedure at the end of the Informed Consent process" [56]. The Informed Consent Document will be discussed in more detail later in this chapter.

Most health-care providers agree that informed consent should be obtained prior to genetic testing [10, 57–60], but debate exists over the essential elements of this process [57, 61, 62]. Table 2.2 lists the components of informed consent endorsed by the National Society of Genetic Counselors (NSGC) [13].

Education About Genetics and Cancer

The education portion of the cancer genetic counseling session includes information about the role of genes in tumorigenesis, genetic conditions and their inheritance patterns, possible test results, risk reduction options, and the benefits, risks, and limitations of genetic testing. The role of the genetic counselor in this component of the session is to effectively communicate scientific information to meet the patient's level of understanding [63]. As patients have diverse learning styles, it is important to be able to communicate the same information in different ways to accommodate a patient's specific learning method. The education portion is typically the longest portion of a genetic counseling section.

Education About Genes, Tumorigenesis, and Inheritance Patterns

All cancer is the result of accumulated mutations in a cell's DNA. The predisposition to cancer can be attributable to several categories of genes. Most cancer predisposition syndromes are due to mutations in tumor suppressor genes, where affected individuals are already born with one mutated copy of a gene and the likelihood of acquiring the second somatic "hit" is very high [64, 65]. Although not essential to the understanding of genetic testing, most genetic counselors will describe tumor suppressor genes and utilize this "two hit" hypothesis to describe the difference between hereditary and sporadic cancer (see Fig. 2.1). Some cancer predisposition syndromes (like MEN2A) are due to mutations in oncogenes, where inheritance of one mutated copy of a gene that "turns on" the mutagenic process is sufficient for tumorogenesis. Still other syndromes (like *MYH*-Associated polyposis) require inheritance of biallelic mutations, which hinders the DNA repair mechanism in the cell, leading to increased susceptibility to mutations and cancer. A patient's understanding the differences in the types of genes that give rise to predisposition to cancer is not imperative to the informed consent process. However, the manner in which these genes are inherited in families is essential to understanding the familial implications of genetic testing, which is imperative in the informed consent process. It is important to note that some mutations in cancer predisposition gene occur as a de novo mutation in an individual. To date, there is no known cancer predisposition inherited in a sex-linked pattern [28].

Education About the Disease and Risk Reduction Options

The education portion of the genetic counseling encounter extends into a thorough discussion of the disease that is suspected in the family. This will include a discussion of the cancer risks associated with the disease as well as cancer screening and prevention options. Risk reduction options for individuals at risk for hereditary cancers include increased screening or prophylactic removal of at risk organs. Medications to reduce cancer risk, such as tamoxifen for breast cancer risk reduction, are not routinely prescribed. The genetic counselor's role is to introduce these concepts during the pretest session. Although a detailed discussion is generally provided by the respective specialists (surgeons, oncologists, gastroenterologists, etc.), the genetic counselor has the unique opportunity to introduce these concepts to the patients.

Two Hit Hypothesis

In sporadic cancer, each gene is damaged individually.

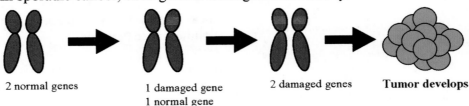

2 normal genes   1 damaged gene   2 damaged genes   **Tumor develops**
                        1 normal gene

In hereditary cancer, one damaged gene is inherited.

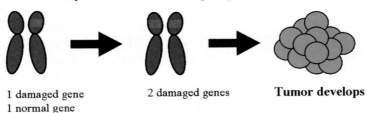

1 damaged gene   2 damaged genes   **Tumor develops**
1 normal gene

Fig. 2.1 Sample counseling aid

Education About Possible Test Results

Genetic testing is often not straightforward. When performing germline genetic testing, there are four possible test results.

Mutation detected (i.e., "Positive"): The individual has an increased chance of developing specific types of cancer in his/her lifetime. The individual can pass this gene mutation on to his/her children.

No mutation detected, and a gene mutation has previously been found in another family member (i.e., "True Negative"): The individual's family history does *not* increase his/her chance of getting certain cancers. The individual has the same cancer risk as anyone else with a similar personal medical history. In addition, the individual cannot pass the mutation on to his/her children.

No mutation detected, but a mutation has not been found in another family member (i.e., "Inconclusive Negative"). The test has provided little new information about the individual's cancer risk. He/she may still have an inherited risk for cancer because:

- The individual may still have a mutation in the gene being tested, but it was not detectable with testing technology that was used,
- The individual may have a gene mutation in another gene that was not analyzed in this test.
- The individual may not have an inherited risk for cancer at all.

A mutation is found, but its meaning is unknown (i.e., variant of uncertain significance (VUS)): This is considered an inconclusive result and is typically a missense mutation.

There is insufficient data to classify whether the variant is deleterious to gene function or is a benign polymorphism that has no bearing on gene function. Testing affected family members to determine if the VUS is tracking with the cancers may help in predicting the significance of the VUS. However, until enough data are collected to confidently determine this, a VUS result should not be used to guide medical management and clinicians should defer to the family history to determine the best management protocol for the patient and their family.

Education About the Benefits, Risks, and Limitations of Testing

There are benefits, risks, and limitations to genetic testing that should be reviewed with patients. They are outlined as follows:

Benefits

- Test results may help explain the pattern of cancer in a family. If an individual has been diagnosed with cancer, testing may explain his/her own cancer history.
- An individual's test results may provide additional information in assessing his/her personal cancer risk. This information may help the individual and health-care providers determine the best plan for medical management with respect to cancer surveillance or risk reduction.

- Results may give other family members information about their chance of having inherited a mutation and chance of developing certain cancers.
- If an individual learns that he/she is a true negative, it means there is no increased risk of cancer due to their family history. Their cancer risk is that of the general population.
- For some patients, test results may relieve anxiety and the worry of not knowing their gene status. It may reduce feelings of uncertainty. For some people, knowing is better than not knowing.

Risks

- If an individual is found to have a gene mutation, they may have feelings of depression, anxiety, and vulnerability, and they are about to embark on a journey that will have them make difficult decisions about their medical care.
- Sharing information about a positive test result may affect relationships with family members. This information may be upsetting to family members and strain relationships.
- It is possible that testing will reveal a variant of uncertain significance which can be disconcerting to patients as we do not know if this variant increases an individual's risk of cancer or not. Patients may have increased feelings of distress and uncertainty.
- If an individual is found to be a true negative, it may cause feelings of survivor guilt over not having inherited the gene mutation that other family members have.
- There is a possibility of learning sensitive information about the family. For instance, if more than one family member is tested, there is a chance of learning about non-paternity or unknown adoption.
- Genetic discrimination occurs when a genetic test result is used as a preexisting condition by insurance providers and employers. The current view is that those patients who already have a cancer diagnosis may not be affected by genetic discrimination as they already have a pre-existing condition. However, those who are unaffected should know that most are protected by law with respect to discrimination by their health insurance company or employer. However, limited legislation exists to protect individuals from life insurance or disability insurance companies to use this information. Unaffected patients may want to consider this before having their blood drawn for genetic testing. The section on confidentiality later in this chapter provides a more detailed discussion of legislation.

Limitations

- Test results provide cancer risk, but cannot predict if an individual will actually develop cancer.
- Results cannot determine how effective treatment might be.

- If an individual is a true negative, it does not mean that they will never develop cancer.
- If an individual is not found to have a mutation and no one in the family has a gene mutation, this "negative" test is uninformative.

Psychosocial Assessment and Support

Although genetic testing can be regarded as a 'simple' blood draw and analysis of genes, the psychosocial implications for patients and their families are substantial. Psychosocial assessment should be provided throughout the entire genetic testing process.

Pre-test Support

During the pretest counseling, the genetics professional should help the patient understand the information and support his/her decision to proceed or not proceed with the genetic testing. Although there have been no studies that formally address whether genetic counseling leads to genetic testing decisions that are consistent with patient preferences [66], the role of the health-care professional is to provide emotional support and empathy. Patient-perceived provider empathy has been shown to increase patient satisfaction and compliance by way of the mediating factors of information exchange, perceived expertise, inter-personal trust, and partnership [67]. In order for the full benefit of genetic testing to be realized, patients must ultimately be compliant with the recommendations for cancer screening and prevention.

It is also important that the patient's support system and readiness for testing be identified prior to the test initiation. The pretest counseling session is also the time to gather more information about family dynamics. Whether an individual wants it to be or not, genetic testing is a family affair, and there are family issues that will be brought forth. Various factors can influence patient decisions about which family members to share the genetic testing information with [68, 69]. It is important to determine if a patient will be comfortable doing this and if not, provide guidance and support. Identifying individuals with insufficient sources of support and addressing family communication concerning hereditary cancer in genetic counseling may help the counselee to adjust better to genetic testing [70].

An additional psychological issue that should be addressed in the pretest counseling session is the anticipation of test results. Waiting for test results can be stressful for some patients. It is important to offer a reliable estimate of when the results will be available as anxiety tends to heighten around the end of this timeline.

Patient Reaction to Test Results

Positive Test Result

It is very difficult for people to predict how they will react to learning about the presence of a mutation in their families and in themselves. Unaffected individuals in cancer-predisposition testing programs are generally accurate in anticipating emotional reactions to test results while cancer patients may underestimate their distress after disclosure of positive results [71]. A variety of feelings may occur after learning that one carries a mutation that increases the chance of developing certain cancers. Some patients may experience short term distress but most develop long term coping skills [72, 73].

For individuals who have had cancer, memories of being diagnosed with cancer or going through cancer treatment may increase in intensity. Testing may also bring up feelings about family members who have had cancer. Anxiety, sleeplessness, or depression may increase as a result of worries about one's current medical care and future health. Individuals who have children may worry about whether they might have inherited the gene and, thus, be at increased risk for certain cancers. Questions may arise, too, about how best to talk to other family members about the availability of testing or about the test results.

Consultation with a psychologist, social worker, or psychiatrist may be helpful in dealing with feelings that may arise from genetic testing. Some individuals express a desire and willingness to talk with others who have been tested.

Negative Test Result

For individuals who have a low pretest probability, a negative test result may be reassuring as they are pursuing the option of testing to rule out the small chance that a mutation is present. However, for patients who come with a strong family history of cancer, an inconclusive negative test result may leave them frustrated. Studies have shown that individuals from such families often hope for a positive test results because they provide an explanation for why cancers are occurring in their family [74].

A negative test result in the context of a positive family mutation is a true negative. Patients often express a great sense of relief with this test result. However, there are reports of a phenomenon that is similar to survivor's guilt whereby the person who tests negative for the family mutation feels guilty that they have not inherited the family mutation.

True negatives also may have to deal with the notion of a new identity. Most of these individuals have worried their entire lives that they are at increased risk of developing cancer. Their true negative result reassures them that they will most likely not suffer the fate of their carrier relatives. They then need to consolidate this new identity with the one they have held for years. On-going follow-up and support may be recommended for true negatives as well [75].

Claes et al. reported that with time, non-carriers report relief and personal growth with respect to their negative test result [76, 77].

Variant of Uncertain Significance

It is particularly important to educate patients about this result, as they often are unaware of the possibility of a variant. If not informed, a patient may find this type of result unsettling, particularly if they were seeking a clear cut answer. Educating them about this prior to administering the test allows the necessary time to become comfortable with this possibility [78].

Post-test Support

Although most individuals cope well with the results of genetic testing, some will require additional support after the test results are given. Studies have indicated that there are factors, such as high anxiety at time of blood draw for genetic testing, that predict who will be distressed 6 months after receiving a test result [71, 79]. Health-care providers should be aware of these factors and identify these individuals who will need additional support, so as to maximize opportunities for prevention, early detection, and healthy coping [80]. Support groups for people found to have cancer predisposition gene mutations can be helpful, and some have suggested that such support groups should be a priority [81].

The Informed Consent Document

Some states have legislation that dictates many of the elements necessary in the informed consent document itself. For example, the Commonwealth of Massachusetts [82] requires that a genetics professional be identified as a resource for the individual undergoing genetic testing. Figure 2.2 is the informed consent document used in the MGH Cancer Center's Center for Cancer Risk Assessment (CCRA) to fulfill the necessary Massachusetts statute requirements along with "information sheets," written in lay material for the patient. Figure 2.3 is one example of the information sheet used, which serves as supplemental for *BRCA1/2* genetic testing.

It is imperative that providers who order a genetic test be familiar with the laws that govern the informed consent

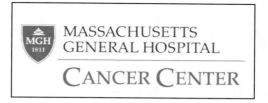

**CONSENT FOR GENETIC TESTING AND PLACEMENT OF RESULTS INTO THE
PATIENT'S MEDICAL RECORD**

Genetic Counselor:

I have explained the purpose, possible risks, benefits and limitations of genetic testing for
_____and have answered any questions regarding the test(s) to the best of my
ability. Specifically, I have described to the patient and/or their designee the meaning of a positive or
negative test result, as well as the accuracy of a positive or negative test result in predicting the
development of the disease or condition associated with this genetic test. I have also provided to, and
reviewed with, this patient and/or their designee written information about this genetic test and its
associated disease or disorder, and I have communicated to the patient and/or their designee the
importance and availability of genetic counseling following genetic testing.

_____   _____
        Genetic Counselor/Clinician   Date

Patient and/or Designee:

I confirm that the purpose, possible risks, benefits and limitations of genetic testing for_____
_____have been explained to me. I understand the meaning of a positive or negative test
result and the certainty associated with the test result that I may receive. All of my current questions have
been answered. I have reviewed the written information about the test(s) and relevant diseases that are
being tested for and have been given a copy of this information. I have been given the name and contact
information of a genetics counselor who will discuss the meaning of my test results with me, as well as any
follow up questions that I may have.

Brochure: _____ Version date:_____

Brochure: _____ Version date:_____

Brochure: _____ Version date:_____

I recognize that a copy of the test result will be put into my electronic medical record. Because my test results
will be placed into the electronic medical record, they may be viewed by any healthcare provider involved in
my care.

My signature below indicates my willingness to have this type of genetic testing.

_____   _____
     Signature of Patient/Designee   Date

Version Date: 03/09

Fig. 2.2 MGH/CCRA informed consent document for genetic testing

practices in their state. A useful resource for this information can be found at http://www.ncsl.org/programs/health/Genetics/ndishlth.htm. It is also important that each provider work with his or her general counsel, so that the required elements of the informed consent document are present in the institution's consent form.

Confidentiality

The confidentiality issues surrounding genetic testing are of utmost importance. Most patients and providers in the US are concerned about confidentiality and its relationship to genetic discrimination [83]. In some cases, providers may

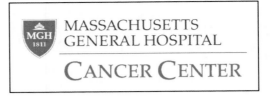

BRCA1 and *BRCA2* genes: What You Need to Know

What does it mean to carry a *BRCA1* or *BRCA2* gene mutation?
Mutations in the *BRCA1* and BRCA2 genes cause a cancer predisposition condition called Hereditary Breast and Ovarian Cancer (HBOC) syndrome.

What is my risk for cancer if I have a *BRCA1* or *BRCA2* mutation?
If you have a BRCA1 or BRCA2 mutation, you have an increased risk of getting certain types of cancer. However, not everyone who has a gene mutation will develop cancer.

BRCA1 gene mutations:
- A woman with a *BRCA1* gene mutation has a 50-85% chance of developing breast cancer. In comparison, women in the general population have a 10-12% risk for breast cancer.
- A woman with a *BRCA1* gene mutation and a history of breast cancer has a 40-60% chance of developing a second primary breast cancer.
- A woman with a *BRCA1* gene mutation has a 20-54% chance of developing ovarian cancer. In comparison, women in the general population have a 1-2% risk for ovarian cancer.
- Men who have a *BRCA1* gene mutation may have a slightly increased risk for breast and prostate cancer, although these risks are not well defined.

BRCA2 gene mutations:
- A woman with a *BRCA2* gene mutation has a 50-85% chance of developing breast cancer. In comparison, women in the general population have a 10-12% risk for breast cancer.
- A woman with a *BRCA2* gene mutation and a history of breast cancer has a 40-60% chance of developing a second primary breast cancer. A woman with a *BRCA2* gene mutation has a 10-27% chance of developing ovarian cancer. In comparison, women in the general population have a 1-2% risk for ovarian cancer.
- A man with a *BRCA2* gene mutation has about a 6-10% risk of developing breast cancer. In comparison, men in the general population have a less than 1% chance of developing breast cancer.
- A man with a *BRCA2* gene mutation also has a slightly increased chance of developing prostate cancer.
- There may also be a slightly increased chance of developing other cancers, such as pancreatic cancer.

What is the chance that I will pass a BRCA1 or BRCA 2 mutation to my child?
Both men and women who have a *BRCA1* or *BRCA2* gene mutation have a 50% chance of passing it on to their child.

Handout: BRCA
Version Date: 04/09

Fig. 2.3 Sample information sheet for BRCA1/2 genetic testing

not even refer for genetic counseling and testing because of this fear [84, 85]. Other studies have shown that uptake of genetic testing is diminished because of concerns about genetic discrimination [86, 87]. In countries with socialized medicine, however, issues of confidentiality are of less importance [88].

The federal Genetic Information Nondiscrimination Act (GINA) was signed on May 21, 2008. This law prohibits genetic discrimination in health insurance and employment, but "is unlikely to resolve the uncertainty surrounding the lawful uses of genetic information" [89]. Concerns about this federal law include its lack of applicability with regard to life insurance, disability insurance, or long-term care insurance and the fact that it is only applicable to individuals who are not symptomatic. Concerns over the effect of genetic discrimination on life insurability are genuine. At this time, there are few states that provide protection against life insurance companies from using genetic information to determine premiums. There is debate about whether or not this practice should change and how important it will be in the future [34, 90, 91]. In addition to the federal legislation, many states have their own laws that protect against discrimination. A useful resource for this information can be found at http://www.ncsl.org/programs/health/Genetics/ndishlth.htm.

While no documented cases of insurance discrimination exist in the U.S. [92], several incidents of genetic discrimination in life insurance access, underwriting and coercion, as well as applications for worker's compensation and early release from prison have been reported in Australia [93].

It is imperative that both patients and providers are educated about the reality of these confidentiality concerns. Often, misconceptions about the risks associated with genetic testing are barriers to genetic testing [94]. It would be unfortunate if a person declined genetic testing based on this misconception, particularly when the benefit of knowing one's genetic status is crucial in clinical management.

Costs and Billing Practices

In today's health-care system, the issue of cost is of paramount importance. To that end, it is imperative that both the provider and the patient understand the cost and billing practices surrounding genetic counseling and testing. The cost of any given genetic test varies widely depending on the size of the gene, the type of laboratory technique used to detect mutations, the cost of labor associated with performing the technique, and royalty/patent costs associated with the test [95]. The cost of genetic testing is often higher than the simple price tag on the gene test because of the cost of the clinical visit associated with the testing (so that informed consent can be obtained). In some instances, cost of testing for a gene will vary widely between two laboratories. Likewise, the cost of the genetic counseling visit will vary widely between two institutions. It is important that the provider be upfront about the consultation fees and the patient be well informed about the cost issues associated with the genetic test.

Paying for genetic testing is also an important concept to consider. At the present time, no state requires health insurance coverage of genetic testing for adult onset disorders (which most inherited cancer predisposition genes are classified as) [96]. Many third party payers (i.e., private health insurance companies) will cover the cost of a genetic test, when the test is ordered by a contracted provider and is deemed "medically necessary". However, caution should be used for patients who have deductibles or copayments.

Since many genetic tests for cancer predisposition cost upward of $1,200/gene, a copayment of 20%, for example, can be quite significant. In addition, it is important to note that not all private health insurance companies will pay for the associated cost of genetic counseling. This genetic counseling cost can vary widely depending on the type of provider offering the service and may include blood draw fees and shipping costs.

For various reasons, some individuals will consider paying for genetic counseling and testing out of pocket. Much of the time, this is founded on fears of genetic discrimination and other confidentiality issues [83]. An upfront and frank discussion of the pros and cons is warranted. It is important to review the fact that genetic testing information needs to be readily available to health-care providers in order to realize its maximum clinical utility.

Ethical Issues

Testing Minors

Traditionally, testing individuals under the age of 18 for genetic conditions is not an ethical matter when treatment and/or beneficial surveillance for the condition exists [97]. For example, testing for PKU in the newborn period identifies children who can be targeted for a specific diet that will reduce the likelihood that they will manifest the mental deficiencies associated with PKU when left untreated. However, ethical concerns are raised in testing children for diseases that do not have any definitive therapeutic or effective screening methods [98]. When considering whether or not to offer childhood testing for inherited cancer susceptibility, certain ethical issues for the minor, their family, and their health-care providers must be considered. These include: (1) obtaining informed consent from a minor, (2) eliminating the child's right "not to know" their individual genetic status, and (3) concerns about social stigmatization and discrimination. There has been little scholarship on genetic testing of children. This discrepancy is significant because ethical decision-making principles are different for children than for adults. More specifically, beneficence supersedes autonomy for pediatric patients, while autonomy is usually the most important consideration for adult patients. The ethics of genetic testing for cancer predisposition in children is challenged by this difference in prioritization of such principles [99].

In 1995, the American Society of Human Genetics in conjunction with the American College of Medical Genetics published a position statement maintaining that genetic testing which confers no immediate benefits to a child should be deferred until adulthood. The statement also affirmed that timely medical benefits to the child should be the primary justification for genetic testing in children and adolescents and that if the medical benefits are or will not accrue until a later time, genetic testing should generally be deferred [100]. Essentially, if the child's medical management will not be altered based on the results of the genetic testing, then this testing is not indicated in childhood. ASCO recommends that "the decision to offer testing to potentially affected children should take into account the availability of evidence-based risk-reduction strategies and the probability of developing a malignancy during childhood. Where risk-reduction strategies are available or cancer predominantly develops in childhood, ASCO believes that the scope of parental authority encompasses the right to decide for or against testing. In the absence of increased risk of a childhood malignancy, ASCO recommends delaying genetic testing until an individual is of sufficient age to make an informed decision regarding such tests. As in other areas of pediatric care, the clinical cancer genetics professional should be an advocate for the best interests of the child" [34].

Testing a child for a familial RET mutation, for example, can effectively distinguish those children who require prophylactic thyroidectomy to prevent medullary thyroid cancer associated with MEN2 from those children who do not need this life altering surgery. In contrast, children who are at risk for inheriting a *BRCA1* or *BRCA2* mutation should arguably not be tested for the mutation because their medical management would not be altered until they are in their twenties. The difficulty lies in testing children for conditions such as Li-Fraumeni syndrome, where the medical community has not reached a consensus on how medical management may change based upon test results. Children with LFS are at risk of developing a number of malignancies, but effective screening methods have not been validated. It is difficult to initiate costly and potentially insensitive screening such as MRIs and CT scans because they are of questionable benefit to decreasing morbidity and mortality in LFS children [97]. Conversely, one would be hard pressed to argue that one should not do anything beyond routine pediatric care for LFS children who have such a high risk of developing a malignancy.

It is important for the genetics provider to consider all of these issues when faced with parents that push the issue of testing minors for inherited cancer susceptibility. Typically, a thoughtful discussion about the pros and cons of testing minors with parents will lead to a mutually agreeable decision. Providers are encouraged to seek counsel from their institutions' Ethics Board and Office of General Counsel when necessary.

Preimplantation Genetic Diagnosis

Preimplantation genetic diagnosis is (PGD) is an assisted reproductive technology (ART) where an embryo is tested for a genetic disorder prior to transfer to a womb for implantation. This entails in vitro fertilization (IVF), including intracytoplasmic sperm injection. The DNA for genetic testing is acquired through embryo biopsy or polar body biopsy [101]. The Society of American Reproductive Technology and American Society for Reproductive Medicine states that PGD is indicated for couples who are at risk of transmitting a specific genetic disease to offspring [102]. The American Society of Obstetricians and Gynecologists recommends that PGD decisions should be based on the idea of creating the "best life" for the child [103]. Controversy surrounds the definition of "best life" for a child. How does one determine what will be best for the child? And perhaps the more important question is *who* decides what is best for the child?

Many of the ethical issues surrounding PGD for inherited cancer susceptibility are similar to those discussed previously with regard to the genetic testing of minors. PGD has been used in a number of cancer predisposition conditions (see Table 2.3) [101]. Studies of patient opinions about PGD for cancer susceptibility yield fairly consistent results. A study of *BRCA* carriers in Spain showed that the majority (61%) approve of PGD but interestingly, fewer (48%) would personally consider it [104]. A similar study from the United Kingdom also found that the majority (75%) felt PGD was acceptable for *BRCA* carriers. In this study, some PGD supporters expressed concerns with respect to quality of life, value to society, effective management and treatment, and cost and only 1 (14%) would consider PGD for future pregnancy [105]. In a study from Israel that studied 10 *BRCA* carriers who opted for further PGD counseling, 6/10 women opted for PGD, but it is important to note that 5/6 required IVF to conceive [106].

It is important to recognize that patient opinion about PGD for cancer predisposition may differ between diseases. A study from Boston showed that 100% of individuals with Familial Adenomatous Polyposis (FAP), for example, consider PGD and PND ethical as it provides early reassurance of an unaffected pregnancy and avoids the issue of pregnancy termination. Ninety percent personally would consider PGD because they have an affected child or experienced the death of a relative due to FAP [107].

In summary, most patients support the idea of PGD but fewer would actually pursue the option. If a patient decides to pursue this option, counseling should be extensive. The discussion should include the impact of the disorder on quality of life, the inheritance of the disorder, the risks associated with IVF, risks associated with embryo biopsy and extended culture, technical limitations of PGD, cost of PGD, low

Table 2.3 Reports of prenatal diagnosis (PND) or pre-implantation genetic diagnosis (PGD) for dominantly inherited cancer susceptibility syndromes

Syndrome	Genes	PND	PGD
Hereditary non-polyposis colorectal cancer	MLH1, MSH2, MSH6, PMS2		✓
Li-Fraumeni syndrome	TP53	✓	✓
Familial adenomatous polyposis	APC	✓	✓
Gorlin syndrome	PTCH	✓	✓
Neurofibromatosis 1	NF1	✓	✓
Neurofibromatosis 2	NF2/merlin	✓	✓
Tuberous sclerosis complex	TSC1, TSC2	✓	✓
Von Hippel-Lindau disease	pVHL		✓
Retinoblastoma	RB1	✓	✓
Multiple edocrine neoplasia type 2A	RET	✓	✓
Rhabdoid tumors	hSNF5		✓
Breast ovarian Caner syndrome	BRCA1, BRCA2		✓

success rate for pregnancy, false negatives, prenatal diagnosis options, and alternative methods of avoiding affected children [102].

The current recommendation from various consensus groups, including the NCCN, is that this option should be discussed with cancer predisposition mutation carriers that are considering future pregnancy [1]. It is important to understand a patient's motivation for pursuing or declining PGD. For patients who pursue PGD, a multidisciplinary approach to care is recommended.

Duty to Warn

When a patient tests positive for a gene mutation, there are inherent implications for family members. Historically, mutation carriers were informed of the benefit of disseminating this information to family members, but it was reinforced that this choice was ultimately theirs to make. Today, although the patient's right to share this information is still highly regarded, individuals are strongly encouraged to share test results with family members.

In 1998 the American Society of Human Genetics (ASHG) stated that in exceptional cases "disclosure should be permissible where attempts to encourage disclosure on the part of the patient have failed; where harm is highly likely to occur and is serious and foreseeable; where the at risk relative(s) is identifiable; and where either the disease is preventable/treatable or medically acceptable standards indicate that early monitoring will reduce genetic risk. Furthermore, the harm from failing to disclose should outweigh the harm from disclosure" [108]. However, providers are not able to disseminate this information without patient permission, because the Health Insurance Portability and Accountability Act (HIPAA) restricts the dissemination of genetics information without proper consent [109].

Although the majority of patients do share positive test results with close family members [68, 69, 110], health-care providers can be faced with difficulties when patients choose not to share. This is especially complex when one health-care provider is the caretaker for multiple family members [111].

It may be important to seek counsel (risk management or the ethics boards of a hospital) to help determine the best way to proceed if a clinician is faced with this situation. In our experience, the best outcome is achieved when the implications of the patient's genetic test result for at risk family members, including dissemination of the results, is discussed at the pretest counseling session.

The genetic counselor can be vital in this regard as they can explore ways in which family members can be informed of genetic test results. A successful approach is for patients to share with the family that they have started the process of genetic testing before test results have returned [111]. This way the patient may be able to gain some insight as to whether or not family members would want to learn the results prior to actually knowing their own personal genetic status. It provides for an honest exchange between family members without the burden of the knowledge of a genetic test result that may not be welcome. Another strategy that is helpful is to provide patients with written information detailing the implications of the test results so that the patient can easily share this information with family members.

Summary

Cancer genetic counseling and genetic testing have become integral to the practice of preventative medicine and oncology. Genetic counselors are uniquely trained and have expertise in obtaining and assessing the family history. The importance of genetic counseling in the genetic testing informed consent process is clear. The identification of individuals at risk for inherited cancer susceptibility allows health-care professionals to intervene with appropriate counseling and education, increase cancer surveillance and thereby reduce the risk of developing an advanced malignancy.

References

1. NCCN. 2008. NCCN Clinical practice guidelines in oncology: high-risk assessment: breast and ovarian. V.1.2008.
2. NCCN. 2009. NCCN Clinical Practice in Oncology: Colorectal Screening. V.1.2009.
3. Sifri R et al (2003) Use of cancer susceptibility testing among primary care physicians. Clin Genet 64(4):355–360
4. Wideroff L et al (2003) Physician use of genetic testing for cancer susceptibility: results of a national survey. Cancer Epidemiol Biomarkers Prev 12(4):295–303
5. Tyler CV Jr, Snyder CW (2006) Cancer risk assessment: examining the family physician's role. J Am Board Fam Med 19(5):468–477
6. Acheson LS et al (2006) Validation of a self-administered, computerized tool for collecting and displaying the family history of cancer. J Clin Oncol 24(34):5395–5402
7. Sweet KM, Bradley TL, Westman JA (2002) Identification and referral of families at high risk for cancer susceptibility. J Clin Oncol 20(2):528–537
8. Simon C et al (2008) Patient interest in recording family histories of cancer via the Internet. Genet Med 10(12):895–902
9. Reid GT et al (2009) Family history questionnaires designed for clinical use: a systematic review. Public Health Genomics 12(2):73–83
10. ASCO (2003) American Society of Clinical Oncology policy statement update: genetic testing for cancer susceptibility. J Clin Oncol 21(12):2397–2406
11. Giardiello FM et al (1997) The use and interpretation of commercial APC gene testing for familial adenomatous polyposis. N Engl J Med 336(12):823–827
12. Resta R et al (2006) A new definition of Genetic Counseling: National Society of Genetic Counselors' Task Force report. J Genet Couns 15(2):77–83
13. Trepanier A et al (2004) Genetic cancer risk assessment and counseling: recommendations of the national society of genetic counselors. J Genet Couns 13(2):83–114
14. Bernhardt BA, Biesecker BB, Mastromarino CL (2000) Goals, benefits, and outcomes of genetic counseling: client and genetic counselor assessment. Am J Med Genet 94(3):189–197
15. Dorval M et al (2008) Health behaviors and psychological distress in women initiating BRCA1/2 genetic testing: comparison with control population. J Genet Couns 17(4):314–326
16. Tessaro I et al (1997) Genetic testing for susceptibility to breast cancer: findings from women's focus groups. J Womens Health 6(3):317–327
17. McDaniel SH (2005) The psychotherapy of genetics. Fam Process 44(1):25–44
18. Jackson G (2005) "Oh ... by the way ... ": doorknob syndrome. Int J Clin Pract 59(8):869
19. Bennett RL et al (2008) Standardized human pedigree nomenclature: update and assessment of the recommendations of the National Society of Genetic Counselors. J Genet Couns 17(5):424–433
20. Bennett RL et al (1995) Recommendations for standardized human pedigree nomenclature. Pedigree Standardization Task Force of the National Society of Genetic Counselors. Am J Hum Genet 56(3):745–752
21. Rebbeck TR et al (1999) Breast cancer risk after bilateral prophylactic oophorectomy in BRCA1 mutation carriers. J Natl Cancer Inst 91(17):1475–1479
22. Olopade OI, Artioli G (2004) Efficacy of risk-reducing salpingo-oophorectomy in women with BRCA-1 and BRCA-2 mutations. Breast J 10(Suppl 1):S5–S9
23. Turner NC, Reis-Filho JS (2006) Basal-like breast cancer and the BRCA1 phenotype. Oncogene 25(43):5846–5853
24. Foulkes WD et al (2004) The prognostic implication of the basal-like (cyclin E high/p27 low/p53+/glomeruloid-microvascular-proliferation+) phenotype of BRCA1-related breast cancer. Cancer Res 64(3):830–835
25. Kaurah P et al (2007) Founder and recurrent CDH1 mutations in families with hereditary diffuse gastric cancer. JAMA 297(21):2360–2372
26. Masciari S et al (2007) Germline E-cadherin mutations in familial lobular breast cancer. J Med Genet 44(11):726–731
27. Richards FM et al (1999) Germline E-cadherin gene (CDH1) mutations predispose to familial gastric cancer and colorectal cancer. Hum Mol Genet 8(4):607–610
28. Schneider KA (2002) Counseling about cancer: strategies for genetic counseling, 2nd edn. Wiley-Liss, New York, p Xviii, p. 333
29. Jefferies S, Goldgar D, Eeles R (2008) The accuracy of cancer diagnoses as reported in families with head and neck cancer: a case-control study. Clin Oncol (R Coll Radiol) 20(4):309–314
30. Murff HJ, Spigel DR, Syngal S (2004) Does this patient have a family history of cancer? An evidence-based analysis of the accuracy of family cancer history. JAMA 292(12):1480–1489
31. Chang ET et al (2006) Reliability of self-reported family history of cancer in a large case-control study of lymphoma. J Natl Cancer Inst 98(1):61–68
32. (2009) American Cancer Society: Cancer Facts and Figures 2008. http://www.cancer.org. Accessed April 2009
33. (1996) Statement of the American Society of Clinical Oncology: genetic testing for cancer susceptibility, Adopted on February 20, 1996. J Clin Oncol 14(5):1730-1736, discussion 1737-1740.
34. Armstrong K et al (2003) Life insurance and breast cancer risk assessment: adverse selection, genetic testing decisions, and discrimination. Am J Med Genet A 120A(3):359–364
35. Schwartz MD et al (2004) Impact of BRCA1/BRCA2 counseling and testing on newly diagnosed breast cancer patients. J Clin Oncol 22(10):1823–1829
36. Ray JA, Loescher LJ, Brewer M (2005) Risk-reduction surgery decisions in high-risk women seen for genetic counseling. J Genet Couns 14(6):473–484
37. Vadaparampil ST et al (2008) Experiences of genetic counseling for BRCA1/2 among recently diagnosed breast cancer patients: a qualitative inquiry. J Psychosoc Oncol 26(4):33–52
38. Stolier AJ, Corsetti RL (2005) Newly diagnosed breast cancer patients choose bilateral mastectomy over breast-conserving surgery when testing positive for a BRCA1/2 mutation. Am Surg 71(12):1031–1033
39. Silva E (2008) Genetic counseling and clinical management of newly diagnosed breast cancer patients at genetic risk for BRCA germline mutations: perspective of a surgical oncologist. Fam Cancer 7(1):91–95
40. Liang L et al (2002) Radiation-induced genetic instability in vivo depends on p53 status. Mutat Res 502(1–2):69–80
41. Shay JW et al (1995) Spontaneous in vitro immortalization of breast epithelial cells from a patient with Li-Fraumeni syndrome. Mol Cell Biol 15(1):425–432
42. Heyn R et al (1993) Second malignant neoplasms in children treated for rhabdomyosarcoma. Intergroup Rhabdomyosarcoma Study Committee. J Clin Oncol 11(2):262–270

43. Hisada M et al (1998) Multiple primary cancers in families with Li-Fraumeni syndrome. J Natl Cancer Inst 90(8):606–611

44. Salmon A et al (2007) Rapid development of post-radiotherapy sarcoma and breast cancer in a patient with a novel germline 'denovo' TP53 mutation. Clin Oncol (R Coll Radiol) 19(7):490–493

45. Hes FJ et al (2008) Somatic APC mosaicism: an underestimated cause of polyposis coli. Gut 57(1):71–76

46. Chompret A et al (2000) P53 germline mutations in childhood cancers and cancer risk for carrier individuals. Br J Cancer 82(12):1932–1937

47. Lipton L, Tomlinson I (2004) The multiple colorectal adenoma phenotype and MYH, a base excision repair gene. Clin Gastroenterol Hepatol 2(8):633–638

48. Peltomaki P (2003) Role of DNA mismatch repair defects in the pathogenesis of human cancer. J Clin Oncol 21(6):1174–1179

49. Hendriks YM et al (2004) Cancer risk in hereditary nonpolyposis colorectal cancer due to MSH6 mutations: impact on counseling and surveillance. Gastroenterology 127(1):17–25

50. Lynch HT, de la Chapelle A (2003) Hereditary colorectal cancer. N Engl J Med 348(10):919–932

51. Schweizer P et al (2001) Lack of MSH2 and MSH6 characterizes endometrial but not colon carcinomas in hereditary nonpolyposis colorectal cancer. Cancer Res 61(7):2813–2815

52. Engel C et al (2006) Novel strategy for optimal sequential application of clinical criteria, immunohistochemistry and microsatellite analysis in the diagnosis of hereditary nonpolyposis colorectal cancer. Int J Cancer 118(1):115–122

53. Jenkins J et al (2007) Randomized comparison of phone versus in-person BRCA1/2 predisposition genetic test result disclosure counseling. Genet Med 9(8):487–495

54. Baumanis L et al (2009) Telephoned BRCA1/2 genetic test results: prevalence, practice, and patient satisfaction. J Genet Couns 18(5):447–463

55. FDA U (2005) "Informed Consent".

56. FDA U (2005) "Informed Consent Document".

57. Harris M, Winship I, Spriggs M (2005) Controversies and ethical issues in cancer-genetics clinics. Lancet Oncol 6(5):301–310

58. NSGC (1991) Disclosure and Informed Consent.

59. Bove CM, Fry ST, MacDonald DJ (1997) Presymptomatic and predisposition genetic testing: ethical and social considerations. Semin Oncol Nurs 13(2):135–140

60. Rieger PT, Pentz RD (1999) Genetic testing and informed consent. Semin Oncol Nurs 15(2):104–115

61. Marsick R, Limwongse C, Kodish E (1998) Genetic testing for renal diseases: medical and ethical considerations. Am J Kidney Dis 32(6):934–945

62. Dickens BM, Pei N, Taylor KM (1996) Legal and ethical issues in genetic testing and counseling for susceptibility to breast, ovarian and colon cancer. CMAJ 154(6):813–818

63. Bennett RL et al (2003) Genetic counselors: translating genomic science into clinical practice. J Clin Invest 112(9):1274–1279

64. Knudson AG Jr (1971) Mutation and cancer: statistical study of retinoblastoma. Proc Natl Acad Sci U S A 68(4):820–823

65. Vogelstein B, Kinzler K (1998) The genetic basis of human cancer. McGraw-Hill, New York

66. Braithwaite D et al (2004) Psychological impact of genetic counseling for familial cancer: a systematic review and meta-analysis. J Natl Cancer Inst 96(2):122–133

67. Kim SS, Kaplowitz S, Johnston MV (2004) The effects of physician empathy on patient satisfaction and compliance. Eval Health Prof 27(3):237–251

68. Stoffel EM et al (2008) Sharing genetic test results in Lynch syndrome: communication with close and distant relatives. Clin Gastroenterol Hepatol 6(3):333–338

69. Patenaude AF et al (2006) Sharing BRCA1/2 test results with first-degree relatives: factors predicting who women tell. J Clin Oncol 24(4):700–706

70. van Oostrom I et al (2007) Family system characteristics and psychological adjustment to cancer susceptibility genetic testing: a prospective study. Clin Genet 71(1):35–42

71. Dorval M et al (2000) Anticipated versus actual emotional reactions to disclosure of results of genetic tests for cancer susceptibility: findings from p53 and BRCA1 testing programs. J Clin Oncol 18(10):2135–2142

72. Shiloh S et al (2008) Monitoring coping style moderates emotional reactions to genetic testing for hereditary nonpolyposis colorectal cancer: a longitudinal study. Psychooncology 17(8):746–755

73. Broadstock M, Michie S, Marteau T (2000) Psychological consequences of predictive genetic testing: a systematic review. Eur J Hum Genet 8(10):731–738

74. van Dijk S et al (2006) Clinical characteristics affect the impact of an uninformative DNA test result: the course of worry and distress experienced by women who apply for genetic testing for breast cancer. J Clin Oncol 24(22):3672–3677

75. Bakos AD et al (2008) BRCA mutation-negative women from hereditary breast and ovarian cancer families: a qualitative study of the BRCA-negative experience. Health Expect 11(3):220–231

76. Claes E et al (2005) Predictive genetic testing for hereditary breast and ovarian cancer: psychological distress and illness representations 1 year following disclosure. J Genet Couns 14(5):349–363

77. Valverde KD (2006) Why me? Why not me? J Genet Couns 15(6):461–463

78. Frost CJ et al (2004) Decision making with uncertain information: learning from women in a high risk breast cancer clinic. J Genet Couns 13(3):221–236

79. van Oostrom I et al (2007) Prognostic factors for hereditary cancer distress six months after BRCA1/2 or HNPCC genetic susceptibility testing. Eur J Cancer 43(1):71–77

80. Vadaparampil ST et al (2006) Psychosocial and behavioral impact of genetic counseling and testing. Breast Dis 27:97–108

81. Di Prospero LS et al (2001) Psychosocial issues following a positive result of genetic testing for BRCA1 and BRCA2 mutations: findings from a focus group and a needs-assessment survey. CMAJ 164(7):1005–1009

82. MGL (2005) Mass. Gen. Laws Ch. 111 70G

83. Hall MA et al (2005) Concerns in a primary care population about genetic discrimination by insurers. Genet Med 7(5):311–316

84. Lowstuter KJ et al (2008) Influence of genetic discrimination perceptions and knowledge on cancer genetics referral practice among clinicians. Genet Med 10(9):691–698

85. Nedelcu R et al (2004) Genetic discrimination: the clinician perspective. Clin Genet 66(4):311–317

86. Apse KA et al (2004) Perceptions of genetic discrimination among at-risk relatives of colorectal cancer patients. Genet Med 6(6):510–516

87. Peterson EA et al (2002) Health insurance and discrimination concerns and BRCA1/2 testing in a clinic population. Cancer Epidemiol Biomarkers Prev 11(1):79–87

88. Godard B et al (2007) Factors associated with an individual's decision to withdraw from genetic testing for breast and ovarian cancer susceptibility: implications for counseling. Genet Test 11(1):45–54

89. Rothstein MA (2008) Putting the Genetic Information Nondiscrimination Act in context. Genet Med 10(9):655–656

90. Lemaire J, Subramanian K, Asch DA (2000) Genetic testing for breast and ovarian cancer: implications for life insurance. LDI Issue Brief 5(6):1–4

91. Lynch EL et al (2003) "Cancer in the family" and genetic testing: implications for life insurance. Med J Aust 179(9):480–483

92. McKinnon W, Banks K, Skelly J, Kohlmann W, Bennett R, Shannon KM, Larson-Haidle J, Ashakaga T, Weitzel JN, Wood M (2009) Survey of unaffected BRCA and mismatch repair (MMR) mutation positive individuals: insurance outcomes. Fam Cancer 8(6):363–369

93. Barlow-Stewart K et al (2009) Verification of consumers' experiences and perceptions of genetic discrimination and its impact on utilization of genetic testing. Genet Med 11(3):193–201

94. Rose AL et al (2005) Attitudes and misconceptions about predictive genetic testing for cancer risk. Community Genet 8(3):145–151

95. Toland AE (2000) Costs of genetic testing. http://www.genetichealth. com/gt_genetic_testing_costs_of_genetic_testing.shtml

96. Johnson A (2002) Genetics and health insurance. Genetics Brief 2002(VII)

97. Hoffmann DE, Wulfsberg EA (1995) Testing children for genetic predispositions: is it in their best interest? J Law Med Ethics 23(4):331–344

98. Lustbader ED et al (1992) Segregation analysis of cancer in families of childhood soft-tissue-sarcoma patients. Am J Hum Genet 51(2):344–356

99. Kodish ED (1999) Testing children for cancer genes: the rule of earliest onset. J Pediatr 135(3):390–395

100. (1995) Points to consider: ethical, legal, and psychosocial implications of genetic testing in children and adolescents. American Society of Human Genetics Board of Directors, American College of Medical Genetics Board of Directors. Am J Hum Genet 57(5):1233–1241.

101. Offit K et al (2006) Cancer genetic testing and assisted reproduction. J Clin Oncol 24(29):4775–4782

102. (2007) Preimplantation genetic testing: a Practice Committee opinion. Fertil Steril 88(6):1497–1504.

103. (2008) ACOG Committee Opinion No. 410: Ethical issues in genetic testing. Obstet Gynecol 111(6):1495–1502.

104. Fortuny D et al (2009) Opinion about reproductive decision making among individuals undergoing BRCA1/2 genetic testing in a multicentre Spanish cohort. Hum Reprod 24(4):1000–1006

105. Menon U et al (2007) Views of BRCA gene mutation carriers on preimplantation genetic diagnosis as a reproductive option for hereditary breast and ovarian cancer. Hum Reprod 22(6): 1573–1577

106. Sagi M et al (2009) Preimplantation genetic diagnosis for BRCA1/2-a novel clinical experience. Prenat Diagn 29(5): 508–513

107. Kastrinos F et al (2007) Attitudes toward prenatal genetic testing in patients with familial adenomatous polyposis. Am J Gastroenterol 102(6):1284–1290

108. (1998) ASHG statement. Professional disclosure of familial genetic information. The American Society of Human Genetics Social Issues Subcommittee on Familial Disclosure. Am J Hum Genet 62(2):474-483

109. (2009) United States Department of Health and Human Services: Summary of the HIPAA Privacy Rule. http://www.hhs.gov/ocr/ privacy. Accessed April 2009

110. Claes E et al (2003) Communication with close and distant relatives in the context of genetic testing for hereditary breast and ovarian cancer in cancer patients. Am J Med Genet A 116A(1):11–19

111. Chan-Smutko G et al (2008) Professional challenges in cancer genetic testing: who is the patient? Oncologist 13(3): 232–238

Chapter 3
Genetics of Hereditary Breast Cancer

Paula D. Ryan

Keywords Breast cancer • Hereditary Breast Ovarian Cancer (HBOC) • BRCA1 • BRCA2 • p53 • Li–Fraumeni syndrome • Cowden's disease • PTEN gene • PARP inhibitor • Mammography

Introduction

The identification and clinical management of patients at inherited risk for breast cancer has become an integral part of the practice of preventative medicine and oncology. Although only about 5–10% of all cases of breast cancer are attributable to a highly penetrant cancer predisposition gene, individuals who carry a cancer susceptibility gene mutation have a significantly higher risk of developing breast cancer, as well as other cancers, over their lifetime compared to the general population. The ability to distinguish those individuals at high risk allows physicians and other health-care providers to intervene with appropriate counseling and education, surveillance, and prevention – with the overall goal of improved survival for these individuals. Recently, a number of germline alleles have been identified that have a modest impact on the risk of breast cancer [1] but there remain only a handful of genes in which a mutation substantially elevates the risk of breast cancer. These include *BRCA1, BRCA2, TP53, PTEN,* and *CDH1.* This chapter will provide an overview of the clinical features, cancer risks, causative genes, and medical management for the most clearly described hereditary breast cancer syndromes with particular attention to the most frequently encountered hereditary breast and ovarian cancer syndrome (HBOC) due to an underlying mutation in *BRCA1* or *BRCA2.* The surgical management of HBOC will be discussed in Chap. 4.

Hereditary Breast Cancer Syndromes

Four of the most clearly described hereditary breast cancer syndromes for which genetic testing is available are hereditary breast and ovarian cancer syndrome (HBOC), Li–Fraumeni syndrome (LFS), Cowden syndrome (CS), and hereditary diffuse gastric cancer syndrome (HDGC) (Table 3.1). All of these syndromes are inherited in an autosomal dominant pattern and are associated with other cancers and clinical features. Genetic testing for each of the genes associated with these syndromes is available through commercial and research laboratories (Table 3.2) that allows for appropriate genetic counseling and testing, and appropriate clinical care for at-risk individuals.

Hereditary Breast and Ovarian Cancer Syndrome

Clinical Features and Genetics

HBOC syndrome is associated with a significantly increased risk for breast cancer and ovarian cancer compared to the general population risk. Mutations in *BRCA1* and *BRCA2* account for 80–90% of cases of HBOCs [2]. Features of the HBOC syndrome include premenopausal breast cancer, ovarian cancer (at any age), bilateral breast cancer, both breast and ovarian cancer in the person, and male breast cancer. The cancer history is usually reported in several generations of the family related through the same bloodline, either maternal or paternal. Table 3.3 lists the testing criteria established by the National Comprehensive Cancer Network (NCCN) for HBOC.

Both *BRCA1* and *BRCA2* function as tumor suppressor genes and both are inherited in an autosomal dominant fashion with incomplete penetrance. Tumorigenesis in individuals with germline mutations in BRCA genes requires somatic inactivation of the remaining wild-type allele. The *BRCA1* and *BRCA2* genes encode large proteins that function in multiple cellular pathways, including transcription, cell cycle

P.D. Ryan (✉)
Breast and Ovarian Cancer Genetics and Risk Assessment Clinic, Massachusetts General Hospital, Boston, MA, USA
e-mail: pdryan@partners.org

Table 3.1 Genes associated with a hereditary predisposition to breast cancer

High penetrance gene	Syndrome	Breast cancer risk by age of 70 years (%)	Major associated cancers
BRCA1	Hereditary breast and ovarian cancer	39–87	Breast, ovary
BRCA2	Hereditary breast and ovarian cancer	26–91	Breast, ovary, prostate, pancreatic
p53	Li–Fraumeni syndrome	>90	Soft-tissue sarcoma, osteosarcoma, brain tumors, adrenocortical carcinoma, leukemia, colon cancer
PTEN	Cowden's; Bannayan-Riley-Ruvalcaba syndrome; Proteus syndrome; Proteus-like syndrome	25–50	Thyroid, endometrial, and genitourinary
CDH1	Hereditary diffuse gastric carcinoma	39	Lobular breast and diffuse gastric cancer; other tumors

Table 3.2 Clinical testing laboratories in the US

BRCA1/2	Myriad Genetics Laboratories (www.myriad.com)
	New Jersey Medical School (http://njms.umdnj.edu/genesweb2/diagnostic.html)
	UCLA Medical Center (http://www.pathnet.medsch.ucla.edu/referral/ODT%20Center/odtc_main.htm)
	UCSF (http://labmed.ucsf.edu/mdx2/)
	University of Chicago (http://genes.uchicago.edu/)
	University of North Carolina Hospitals (http://labs.unchealthcare.org/directory/molecular_pathology/index_html)
	University of Pittsburgh Medical Center (http://path.upmc.edu/divisions/mdx/diagnostics.html)
PTEN	Baylor College of Medicine (http://www.bcm.edu/geneticlabs/)
	Boston University School of Medicine (http://www.bumc.bu.edu/hg/)
	Emory University School of Medicine (http://www.genetics.emory.edu/egl/)
	GeneDx (http://www.genedx.com/)
	Greenwood Genetics Center (http://www.ggc.org/diagnostic.htm)
	Johns Hopkins Hospital (http://www.hopkinsmedicine.org/dnadiagnostic/)
	Signature Genomic Laboratories (http://www.signaturegenomics.com/)
	Ohio State University (http://www.pathology.med.ohio-state.edu/ext/Divisions/Clinical/molpath/)
	University of Michigan (http://sitemaker.umich.edu/michigan.medical.genetics.laboratories/home)
	University of Oklahoma Health Sciences Ctr (http://www.genetics.ouhsc.edu/)
	Yale University School of Medicine (http://www.genetics.ouhsc.edu/)
P53	Baylor College of Medicine (http://www.bcm.edu/geneticlabs/)
	Center for Genetic Testing at St. Francis (http://www.sfh-lab.com/)
	City of Hope National Medical Center (http://mdl.cityofhope.org/)
	Duke University Health System (http://manual.clinlabs.duke.edu/DukeMolecular/default.aspx)
	Emory University School of Medicine (http://www.genetics.emory.edu/egl/)
	Harvard Medical School (http://www.hpcgg.org/LMM/)
	Huntington Medical Research Institute (http://home.pacbell.net/genedoc/Eggspage.html)
CDH1	City of Hope National Medical Center (http://mdl.cityofhope.org/)
	Henry Ford Hospital
	Stanford Clinical Labs

Source: ref [116]

regulation, and the maintenance of genome integrity. The main role of BRCA2 appears to involve the regulation of RAD51 function in DNA repair by homologous recombination [3]. BRCA1 has a broader role, participating in cellular processes such as chromatin modeling, transcriptional regulation, and the DNA damage response [3] (Fig. 3.1).

Early studies of *BRCA2*-associated breast cancers found that they were similar in phenotype and clinical behavior in comparison to grade-matched sporadic cancers; [4, 5] however, more recent data have suggested that *BRCA2*-associated tumors are of higher grade with pushing margins, are more frequently estrogen receptor (ER) positive and are less likely

to express HER2 compared to control sporadic tumors matched for age and ethnicity [6]. *BRCA1*-associated breast cancers differ from other breast cancers in that they are usually high-grade, aneuploid carcinomas that do not express ER, progesterone receptor (PR), or HER2 (also referred to as "triple negative" phenotype). They often express cytokeratins 5 and 14, vimentin, epidermal growth factor receptor (EGFR), and P-cadherin (CDH3): features that predict clustering with the basal-like phenotype by gene expression profiling [7]. Atypical medullary carcinomas have also been observed more frequently in *BRCA1* carriers, a phenotype with abundant lymphocytic infiltrate and a smooth margin, which may

Table 3.3 Hereditary breast ovarian cancer syndrome testing criteria

- Individual from a family with a known BRCA1/2 mutation
- Personal history of breast cancer plus one or more of the following:
  - Diagnosed age ≤45 years
  - Diagnosed age ≤50 years with ≥1 close blood relative with breast cancer ≤50 years and/or ≥1 close blood relative with epithelial ovarian/fallopian tube/primary peritoneal cancer
  - Two breast primaries when first breast cancer diagnosis occurred prior to age 50
  - Diagnosed at any age, with ≥2 close blood relatives with breast and/or epithelial ovarian/fallopian tube/primary peritoneal cancer at any age
  - Close male blood relative with breast cancer
  - Personal history of epithelial ovarian/fallopian tube/primary peritoneal cancer
  - For an individual of ethnicity associated with higher mutation frequency (e.g., founder mutation populations of Ashkenazi Jewish, Icelandic, Swedish, Hungarian or other) no additional family history may be required
- Personal history of epithelial ovarian/fallopian tube/primary peritoneal cancer
- Personal history of male breast cancer
- Family history only – close family member meeting any of the above criteria

Source: National Comprehensive Cancer Network 2009 [79]

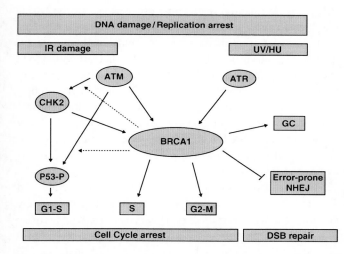

Fig. 3.1 BRCA1 in DNA damage signaling. DNA damage activates the kinases ATM, ATR, and CHK2, which in turn activate BRCA1 by phosphorylation. In response to IR induced damage, BRCA1 is phosphorylated by ATM and CHK2. ATR phosphorylates BRCA1 in response to UV damage or HU-induced replication arrest. BRCA1 participates in the G_1-S checkpoint response indirectly through several ways, including by affecting CHK2 and p53 phosphorylation. (Adapted by permission from Macmillan Publishers Ltd: Oncogene 25:5864–5874, copyright 2006.)

contribute to the poorer sensitivity of mammograms in mutation carriers [8]. A potential mechanism whereby loss of BRCA1 function might define the lack of ER and ER-regulated gene expression in BRCA1-associated tumors has been proposed: functional BRCA1 is necessary for the expression

of ER alpha by directly binding and transactivating the ESR1 gene promoter; when BRCA1 is lost in tumors, the ER alpha gene can no longer be expressed and as a result resistance to ER-targeted therapy is acquired [9].

The strong correlation between BRCA1 status and the triple-negative and basal-like phenotype should dictate the careful ascertainment of family history in women with tumors of this type. The Breast Cancer Linkage Consortium study suggests that patients with ER-negative and basal keratin-positive breast cancers have an odds ratio of approximately 148 of having a BRCA1 mutation when compared to age-matched controls [10].

The BRCA1 and BRCA2 genes were cloned in 1994 and 1995, respectively [11, 12]. Over 1,200 deleterious mutations have been identified throughout the length of these large genes: BRCA1, located on 17q11, encodes an 1863-amino acid polypeptide [11], and BRCA2, located on 13q12-q13, encodes 3,418 amino acids [12, 13]. Most pathogenic BRCA1 or BRCA2 mutations block protein production from the mutated allele and have been identified as frameshift or nonsense mutations or large genomic deletions or duplications [14, 15]. Missense mutations that interfere with critical regions of the gene, such as the RING finger motif or BRCT region of BRCA1 [16] or the PALB2 gene binding region of BRCA2 [17], behave like truncating mutations, whereas most missense mutations remain uncharacterized and are considered variants of uncertain significance [16]. BRCA1 and BRCA2 mutations are rare in most populations, occurring in approximately 1 of 400 persons, but much more common in the Ashkenazi Jewish population, in which 1 of 40 persons carries one of three main disease-causing mutations: two in BRCA1 (185delAG and 5382insC) and the 6174delT mutation in BRCA2 [18]. The prevalence of nonfounder mutations identified in Jewish women undergoing genetic testing is approximately 2% [19]. Other founder mutations have been identified, including the BRCA2 999del5 mutation in Iceland that is associated with an increased risk for prostate cancer in some kindreds and specific large BRCA1 deletions in the Dutch population [20, 21].

The penetrance or lifetime risk of developing breast or ovarian cancer remains an active area of research even 15 years after the discovery of BRCA1 and BRCA2. Women with mutations in BRCA1 have an estimated lifetime risk of breast cancer in the range of 50–80% and for women with BRCA2 mutations the range is 40–70% [2, 22, 23]. The range of breast cancer risk associated with mutations in BRCA1 and BRCA2 is influenced by the population under study: higher risk estimates have come from studies with affected families and somewhat lower risk estimates from studies in populations. The lifetime risk of ovarian cancer is 40% for BRCA1 mutation carriers and 20% for BRCA2 carriers [24]. The risk of ovarian cancer is not the same for all BRCA2 mutations, with mutations in the central ovarian cancer cluster region, conferring a higher lifetime risk [25]. Other factors, such as birth cohort, oral contraceptive use, age at first pregnancy, and exercise have all been shown to influence penetrance risk in populations [23]. The most robust risk modifier in *BRCA1* and *BRCA2* carriers has been prophylactic oophorectomy, which reduces the subsequent lifetime risk of breast cancer by about 50% [26, 27]. These clinical observations highlight the fact that risk associated with highly penetrant mutations can be modified or reduced by lifestyle factors, exogenous and endogenous hormone exposures, and other possible strategies.

Several studies have shown an association with *BRCA* mutations and increased risks for other cancers. The cancer risks for *BRCA1* carriers are confined largely to the breast and ovary, while pancreas, prostate, melanoma, and other cancer risks are associated with *BRCA2* carriers [28–31]. Serous papillary ovarian carcinoma is a key feature of hereditary cancers in *BRCA1* mutation carriers; it is less common in *BRCA2* carriers. Endometrioid and clear-cell subtypes of ovarian cancer have been observed [32], but borderline ovarian tumors do not seem to be a part of the HBOC phenotype [33]. Both primary tumors of the fallopian tubes and peritoneum occur with increased frequency in mutation carriers [34]. The prognosis of ovarian cancer in *BRCA1* and *BRCA2* carriers is better than age-matched controls [32, 35].

Based on genome-wide linkage studies for breast cancer susceptibility genes, it is thought that other genes with a population frequency and risk profile similar to *BRCA1* or *BRCA2* are unlikely to exist; [36] however, genome-wide association studies have identified a class of susceptibility genes in 15–40% of women with breast cancer that confer a minimal relative risk of breast cancer [16, 37–40]. The clinical utility of these findings is unclear, but these common, low-risk alleles may account for a measurable fraction of population risk through gene–gene interactions. Moderate risk alleles that are rare in most populations are associated with an approximate relative risk of breast cancer of 2.0, and have been identified and include *BRIP1*, *PALB2*, *ATM,* and *CHECK2*. These alleles may be more clinically significant in selected populations. For example, in *CHECK2*, the carrier frequency is approximately 1% for 1100delC in Dutch and Finnish populations, S428F mutant in the Ashkenazi Jewish population, and the founder mutation IVS2+1G→A in Slavic populations [41]. Founder mutations in *PALB2* occur in Finland and Quebec, Canada [42, 43].

The question of whether a mutation in *BRCA1* or *BRCA2* influences breast cancer prognosis has been studied extensively [44]. With the exception of the well-documented risk of a contralateral breast cancer among *BRCA1* and *BRCA2* carriers – which is substantial (approximately 3% per year) [45, 46], most studies have not found that *BRCA1* and *BRCA2* confer an adverse prognosis; however, there has been significant methodological heterogeneity in these studies.

In one analysis of 442 patients who developed breast cancer while enrolled in a prospective breast cancer surveillance study [47], *BRCA1* mutation status was associated with a worse prognosis even among node-negative patients. In a large population study in Israel (case records and pathological samples available on 1,545 women), there was no difference in overall or breast cancer specific survival among *BRCA1* or *BRCA2* carriers when compared to noncarriers [48], yet subgroup analysis showed that there was a statistically significant interaction between *BRCA1* mutation status and a more favorable prognosis in women receiving adjuvant chemotherapy when compared to noncarriers. Also, women who had tumors less than 2 cm had a worse prognosis if they were *BCRA1* carriers. It is also worth noting that *BRCA1*-associated breast cancers appear to lose the usual relationship between tumor size and the presence of lymph node metastases [49]. Another study of 505 Jewish women in New York and Montreal showed that the presence of an Ashkenazi Jewish founder mutation in *BRCA1* predicted adverse breast cancer survival when compared to noncarriers (62% at 10 years vs. 86%; $P<0.0001$) only among women who did not receive chemotherapy (HR 4.8, 95% CI 2.0–11.7; $P=0.001$) [50]. It is not clear if this phenomenon relates directly to *BRCA1* gene function or to some other aspect of the basal-like breast cancer phenotype. An adverse prognosis normalized by an apparent increase in sensitivity to chemotherapy in sporadic "basal-like" breast cancer has been reported [51] and sporadic "basal-like" breast cancers have been noted to have a high response rate to anthracycline-based chemotherapy [17]. Thus, these data suggest that *BRCA1* mutation carriers who present with small, node-negative breast cancers may be at increased risk for metastatic dissemination than noncarriers and explain a worse prognosis if chemotherapy is avoided in this situation.

A mature analysis of 160 *BRCA1* and *BRCA2* carriers and 445 matched controls treated with breast-conserving therapy and followed for a median of 6–8 years has shown no increase in ipsilateral breast tumor recurrence in carriers who had prophylactic oophorectomy when compared to matched controls; however, there was an increase in women who did not have prophylactic oophorectomy (HR 1.9, $P=0.03$) [12].

Clinical Management

Preclinical studies have begun to elucidate the question of whether there are conventional chemotherapeutic agents that are more effective in *BRCA1* or *BRCA2*-associated breast cancer. The DNA cross-linking agents, carboplatin, cisplatin, and mitomycin C appear to have the greatest genotype-specific effect in preclinical models [52–54]. A consistent theme in these studies is an increased sensitivity of these drugs to lesions that damage DNA in ways that arrest DNA replications forks and which subsequently require DNA repair by homologous recombination for fork repair and restart. This function is consistent with the integral role of *BRCA1* and *BRCA2* in the Fanconi anemia pathway, the hallmark of which is exquisite cellular sensitivity to DNA cross-linking agents [55].

Preclinical data have also suggested that *BRCA1* may be required to mediate paclitaxel-induced apoptosis with the loss of function of *BRCA1* leading to microtubule stabilizing and resistance to the drug [56]. However, data are mixed as a retrospective study from patients treated with taxane-based neoadjuvant therapy [57] suggested resistance to taxanes, whereas increased sensitivity to taxanes has been shown in preclinical *BRCA1* deficient models [58]. An international randomized phase II trial is now testing the efficacy of carboplatin versus docetaxel in *BRCA1* and *BRCA2* carriers with advanced breast cancer.

Is it possible to target *BRCA1* or *BRCA2* dysfunction with novel therapies? *BRCA1* and *BRCA2* are proteins with multiple functions, including repair of double-strand breaks in DNA by homologous recombination [59]. New therapeutic strategies have exploited this cellular function with the use of agents that cause DNA strand breaks that require repair through homologous recombination. Compounds such as PARP1 protein inhibitors, which block base excision repair, are emerging as potential therapeutic agents in cancers developing in *BRCA1* and *BRCA2* mutation carriers [60]. The hypothesis is that combining a tumor restricted constitutive defect in homologous recombination with drug-induced inhibition in base excision and single strand break repair pathways would lead to synthetic lethality restricted to tumor cells without impact on normal tissues. Indeed, inhibition of poly-ADP ribose polymerase (PARP), a key enzyme in base excision repair, causes highly selective cell killing in cells that have lost functional *BRCA1* or *BRCA2* [61, 62]. Sensitivity to PARP inhibition has been demonstrated in tumor cell lines deficient in *BRCA1* [63] and *BRCA2* [64] function and in vivo in conditional mouse models [65] and *BRCA1* defective spontaneous tumor models [66].

The preclinical results with PARP inhibitors have led to the development of several clinical trials that are exploring this compound in advanced breast cancer. A single agent, first in human, phase I study of a potent, orally active PARP inhibitor, olaparib (AZD2281) in patients with advanced cancer showed linear pharmacokinetics, and a favorable toxicity profile with mild nausea and fatigue [67]. Twenty-two of the 60 patients in the study were carriers of a *BRCA1* or *BRCA2* mutation: objective antitumor activity was reported only in mutation carriers (all of whom had breast, ovarian or prostate cancer and had received multiple treatment regimens). Proof of concept phase II clinical trials in *BRCA1* and *BRCA2* carriers with advanced ovarian cancer or advanced breast cancer are presently underway.

In addition to the concept that germline mutations in *BRCA1* or *BRCA2* may help guide therapy in breast cancer, there has also been much interest on other mechanisms for the loss of *BRCA1* or *BRCA2* function that may exist in sporadic breast cancers. The loss of function of genes associated with the DNA damage response pathways predisposes to breast cancer with mutations in *BRCA1*, *BRCA2*, *CHEK2*, and *PALB2*, all significantly elevating risk [68]. The overlap between *BRCA1*-mutated cancers and sporadic cancers with basal-like features is striking [69, 70], and a number of studies suggest that dysregulation of the *BRCA1* function via a variety of different mechanisms may be a frequent feature of significant subgroups within basal-like breast cancers [70–73].

The current recommendations for the screening of women at risk for HBOC is based on the best available evidence and is expected to change as more specific features of *BRCA1*- and *BRCA2*-related disease become available. Mammography is the universally accepted standard of care for breast cancer screening in women 40 years of age and older. However, breast cancers in mutation carriers frequently occur at a younger age. The data available on the efficacy of mammography as a screening modality in *BRCA1* or *BRCA2* carriers indicate that tumors are commonly only detected at a high clinical stage and are often present as interval cancers [74]. This is likely to be due to the combination of early onset cancer in a denser breast parenchyma, higher proliferative rate and the broad pushing morphology of *BRCA1*-associated cancers. This has led to six international trials to assess breast MRI in addition to mammographic screening in high-risk women and five of these studies have undergone a combined analysis [75]. The data showed that MRI has significantly better sensitivity (pooled data 81%) than mammography alone (40%), but this comes at the cost of reduced specificity and a higher false positive rate. National and international guidelines now recommend MRI screening in addition to mammographic screening for *BRCA1* and *BRCA2* carriers. The National Comprehensive Cancer Network Guidelines (NCCN), for example, recommend that women should, in addition to regular monthly BSE starting at age 18 and clinical breast exam semiannually starting at age 25, begin having annual mammograms and breast MRI screening at age 25 or on an individualized timetable based on the earliest age of cancer onset in family members [76–79].

Male *BRCA* mutation carriers are advised to perform regular monthly BSE, semiannual clinical breast examinations, and work-up of any suspicious breast lesions is recommended. The NCCN also recommend that a baseline mammogram be considered, with an annual mammogram if gynecomastia or parenchymal/glandular breast density is identified on baseline study [79]. The NCCN guidelines recommend that male BRCA mutation carriers should begin prostate cancer screening at age 50, or earlier, based on the youngest age of diagnosis in the family, with others suggesting that *BRCA* carriers should begin screening for prostate cancer at age 40 [29, 79].

Surgical management of HBOC is complex and is covered in Chap. 4. Risk-reduction mastectomy is an appropriate consideration for women at the highest hereditary risk for breast cancer. Studies have shown a 90–95% reduction in breast cancer risk following prophylactic mastectomy [50, 74, 80, 81]. Discussion of the benefits and risks of mastectomy should include a review of the degree of protection, reconstruction options, and potential psychological impact. Risk-reducing bilateral salpingo-oophorectomy (RRBSO), ideally between the ages of 35 and 40 years, or on completion of child bearing, is recommended for ovarian cancer management in *BRCA* carriers. Two recent studies support the role of risk reducing salpingo-oophorectomy: the hazard ratio for ovarian cancer for women who underwent prophylactic surgery compared to those who chose close surveillance was 0.15 and 0.04, respectively [26, 27]. Women should be informed about the potential for the subsequent development of peritoneal carcinomatosis, which has been reported up to 15 years following RRBSO [34, 82]. Individuals who do not elect risk-reducing surgery should undergo concurrent transvaginal ultrasound and CA-125 every 6 months beginning at 35 years of age, or 5–10 years younger than the first ovarian cancer diagnosis in the family [83]. Combination oral contraceptives containing estrogen and progestin result in a protective effect against ovarian cancer in some studies, although one study did not find this effect [84–86]. Particularly in *BRCA1* carriers, there remains the concern of a small increased risk of breast cancer due to oral contraceptives in this group [86]. However, the data are inconsistent and a large multinational case-control study including 1,156 breast cancer cases diagnosed under the age 40 (of which 47 were *BRCA1* carriers and 35 *BRCA2* carriers) as well as 815 controls, did not demonstrate an increased risk of OCP-associated breast cancer [87]. Given the excess mortality associated with ovarian cancer compared with breast cancer, a reasonable risk reduction strategy is OCP use before childbearing, and salpingo-oophorectomy once childbearing is complete.

The evidence for the use of tamoxifen as a chemopreventative agent in *BRCA* carriers is limited. A small number of *BRCA1* and *BRCA2* carriers were identified in the NSABP-P1 prevention trial that randomized women to tamoxifen versus placebo [88]. Although the point estimate for the relative risk of breast cancer suggested some benefit to tamoxifen in the 11 identified *BRCA2* carriers in the study (RR 0.38; 95% CI 0.06–1.56) but not in the eight *BRCA2* carriers studied (RR 1.67; 95% CI 0.32–10.70), this result was not statistically significant and cannot be used to inform therapy. The strongest argument for the consideration of tamoxifen comes from studies of *BRCA* carriers with breast cancer, where tamoxifen has been shown to reduce the risk of contralateral breast cancers [89, 90]. A study measuring 10 and 15 year risk of contralateral breast cancer in *BRCA1* and *BRCA2* carriers found that in mutation carriers taking tamoxifen there was a 69% reduction in contralateral breast cancer risk in comparison to mutation carriers who were not treated with tamoxifen (HR 0.31, *P* = 0.5) [46]. Thus, this encouraging retrospective data should be discussed with carriers who do not wish to undergo prophylactic risk reducing bilateral mastectomy.

Li–Fraumeni Syndrome

Clinical Features and Genetics

LFS is a rare cancer predisposition syndrome that accounts for approximately 1% of hereditary breast cancer [91]. Germline mutations in the well-known tumor suppressor gene *p53* are the primary cause of LFS. Classic LFS is defined as three first-degree relatives with component tumors diagnosed before the age of 45 years: soft tissue and osteosarcomas, breast cancer, brain tumors, adrenal cortical carcinoma (ACC), and leukemia [92]. Subsequently, many additional tumors have been observed to occur with increased frequency in LFS, including gastric, pancreatic, and other pediatric cancers [93–96].

The cancer risk associated with LFS has been studied extensively. A study of LFS relatives in 159 extended families found the risk for developing cancer among carriers was 12, 35, 52, and 80% by 20, 30 ,40, and 50 years of age, respectively [97]. In regards to breast cancer risk, a woman with LFS has a breast cancer risk of 56% by age 45 and greater than 90% by age 70, with most diagnoses of breast cancer occurring under the age of 40 [96, 98, 99].

Li and Fraumeni and colleagues developed the first clinical diagnostic criteria for LFS, based on their study of 24 LFS kindreds, and these criteria have come to be known as the classic or strictest diagnostic criteria [92]. In an attempt to determine who to test for germline mutations associated with LFS, other groups loosened the strict LFS criteria, developing criteria for Li-Fraumeni-like (LFL) syndrome [100]. LFL is a proband with any childhood cancer or sarcoma, brain cancer, or ACC diagnosed by the age of 45, who has a first-degree or second-degree family member a typical LFS cancer at any age, and another first-degree or second-degree family member with cancer diagnosed before the age of 60. Another definition of LFL [101] was described as two first- or second-degree relatives with LFS-related tumor diagnosed at any age. Chompret and colleagues [98] recommended that testing for *p53* mutations should be considered in families who meet the following criteria: a proband affected by sarcoma, brain tumor, breast cancer, or ACC before 36 years of age, with at least one first- or second-degree relative with cancer (other than breast if the proband has breast cancer)

Table 3.4 Classic and Chompret criteria for Li–Fraumeni syndrome[a]

Classic Li–Fraumeni syndrome [92]
- Proband with sarcoma diagnosed ≤45 years, and
- First-degree relative with any cancer diagnosed ≤45 years, and
- Another first- or second-degree relative in the same lineage diagnosed ≤45 years with any cancer or a sarcoma at any age

Chompret criteria [98]
- One first- or second-degree relative with cancer diagnosed before the age of 46
- Multiple primary tumors in the proband, regardless of family history

[a]In a cohort of 525 patients undergoing testing for *p53* germline mutations, 95% of patients (71 of 75) with a mutation met either classic or Chompret criteria [102]

before age 46 years of age, or, a relative with multiple primary tumors at any age. The largest single report of diagnostic testing for germline *p53* mutations in 525 consecutive patients whose blood samples were submitted for diagnostic testing was published in 2009 [102]. Mutations were identified in 17% of the 525 patients submitted for testing: all families with a *p53* mutation had at least one family member with a sarcoma, breast, brain, or adrenocortical carcinoma, every individual with a choroid plexus tumor (8/8) and 14 of 21 individuals with a childhood ACC had a mutation regardless of family history. Based on reported personal and family history, 95% of patients with a mutation met either classic LFS or Chompret criteria (Table 3.4).

Clinical Management

Management of individuals at risk for LFS is difficult because of the diverse array of tumors and the fact that the rarity of the syndrome has made studies of intensified surveillance logistically difficult. Current breast screening guidelines [79] recommend training and education in breast self-exam and regular monthly breast self-exam starting at age 18 years of age, semiannual clinical breast exam starting at age 20–25 years of age or 5–10 years before the earliest known breast cancer in the family (whichever is earliest), annual mammogram and breast MRI screening should start at age 20–25 years of age, or individualized based on the earliest age of onset in family. Options for risk-reducing mastectomy should be discussed on a case by case basis and include counseling on the degree of protection, degree of cancer risk, and reconstruction options. Many of the other cancers associated with *p53* do not lend themselves to early detection. Screening may be considered for cancer survivors with LFS and a good prognosis from their primary tumors with annual comprehensive physical exam with a high index of suspicion for rare cancers and second malignancies and consider colonoscopy every 2–5 years starting no later than 25 years of age. Pediatricians should be apprised of the risk of childhood cancers in affected families.

Cowden Syndrome

Clinical Features and Genetics

CS, also known as multiple hamartoma syndrome, is characterized by the formation of multiple hamartomas that may develop in any organ, with a high risk of benign and malignant tumors of the thyroid, breast, and endometrium. Consensus diagnostic criteria for CS establish three diagnostic categories [79], with pathognomonic criteria including Adult Lhermitte-Duclos disease (cerebellar tumors), facial trichilemmomas, acral keratoses, and papillomatous papules. Major and minor criteria may also be considered, including benign lesions of the breast and other organs. (Table 3.5)

Table 3.5 Cowden syndrome diagnostic criteria

Pathognomonic criteria
- Adult Lhermitte-Duclos disease (LDD) (cerebellar tumors)
- Mucocutaneous lesions
  - Trichilemmomas, facial
  - Acral keratoses
  - Papillomatous papules

Major criteria
- Breast cancer
- Non-medullary thyroid carcinoma
- Macrocephaly (megalocephaly) (i.e., ≥ 97th percentile)
- Endometrial carcinoma

Minor criteria
- Other thyroid disease (e.g., adenoma, multinodular goiter)
- Mental retardation (IQ≤75)
- Gastrointestinal hamartomas
- Fibrocystic disease of the breast
- Lipomas
- Fibromas
- Genitourinary tumors (especially renal cell carcinoma)
- Genitourinary structural manifestations
- Uterine fibroids

Operational diagnosis in an individual
1. Any single pathognomonic criterion:
   - Mucocutaneous lesions alone if there are:
     - Six or more facial papules, of which three or more must be trichilemmoma, or
     - Cutaneous facial papules and oral mucosal papillomatosis, or
     - Oral mucosal papillomatosis and acral keratoses, or
     - Six or more palmoplantar keratoses
2. Two or more major criteria (one must be macrocephaly) or
3. One major and ≥ three minor criteria or
4. ≥ Four minor criteria

Operational diagnosis for individuals in a family where one relative is diagnostic for Cowden syndrome. The individual must have one or more of the following:
- A pathognomonic criterion
- Any one major criteria with or without minor criteria
- Two minor criteria
- History of Bannayan-Riley-Ruvalcaba syndrome

Source: National Comprehensive Cancer Network 2009 [79]

Women with CS have up to a 76% risk for benign breast disease, such as fibroadenomas and fibrocystic breast disease, and a 25–50% lifetime risk for breast cancer [103–105]. An increased risk of early-onset male breast cancer has also been identified in mutation carriers [106].

The gene for CS, *PTEN*, a tumor suppressor gene, has been mapped to 10q22-23 [107]. *PTEN* acts as a tumor suppressor by mediating cell cycle arrest and/or apoptosis [108]. Mutations in the *PTEN* gene are also associated with Bannayan-Riley-Ruvalcaba syndrome, Proteus (and Proteus-like) syndrome. Full sequencing and molecular testing by southern blot are available clinically and on a research basis respectively. A *PTEN* mutation can be detected in about 80% of patients who meet the strict operational diagnostic criteria for CS [109].

Clinical Management

Women who have CS should be screened for breast cancer, with regular monthly breast self examination beginning at age 18 years, clinical breast examinations beginning at age 25 years or 5–10 years earlier than the earliest known breast cancer in the family, and annual mammography and breast MRI beginning at age 30–35 years, or 5–10 years earlier than the earliest onset breast cancer diagnosis in the family (whichever is earlier) [79]. The American Cancer Society recommends annual breast MRI for individuals with CS and their first-degree relatives [110]. Options for prophylactic mastectomy should be discussed on a case by case basis. Endometrial carcinoma screening with blind endometrial biopsies should be performed annually in premenopausal women starting at age 35–40 years (or 5 years before the earliest endometrial cancer diagnosis in the family), and annual endometrial ultrasonography in postmenopausal women [79]. A comprehensive annual physical examination starting at age 18 years with screening for skin and thyroid lesions, including a baseline thyroid ultrasound, is recommended for men and women with CS. Annual dermatological examination should also be considered. An annual urinalysis, with consideration for annual urine cytology and renal ultrasound, should be performed in both men and women if there is a family history of renal carcinoma.

Hereditary Diffuse Gastric Carcinoma

HDGC is the autosomal dominant susceptibility for diffuse gastric cancer. Chapter 8 is devoted to this topic. The common familial histology is a poorly differentiated diffuse gastric adenocarcinoma often with signet ring histology [111]. Penetrance of the syndrome is estimated to be at 60–80%, with the average age of onset at 38 years (range, 14–69 years). Women have an increased risk for breast cancer, especially lobular carcinoma, and early-onset colon cancers have been reported [112, 113]. The e-cadherin gene (*CDH1*) is a calcium-dependent cell–cell adhesion molecule expressed in junctions between epithelial cells [114], and is the only gene known to be associated with HDGC. Mutations in *CDH-1* are found in up to 48% of diffuse gastric cancer kindreds [115].

The 5-year survival rate for diffuse gastric cancer is about 10%. Although it has been proposed that individuals who have a *CDH1* mutation undergo routine surveillance for gastric cancer, the optimal management of individuals at risk is uncertain because of the unproven value of surveillance regimens and prophylactic gastrectomy has become part of the management of this syndrome. Postgastrectomy screening and follow-up should include breast and colon cancer screening. Although there are no defined screening guidelines, based on the lifetime risk of approximately 40% of developing breast cancer, referral of women with a *CDH1* mutation to a high-risk breast cancer screening program is appropriate, and breast cancer screening should include a clinical breast examination every 6 months, annual mammography and annual breast MRI.

Summary

Cancer genetics has become an integral subspecialty of the practice of preventative medicine and oncology. The discovery of high-risk cancer susceptibility genes has translated into the need for specialized care for individuals who inherit a predisposition to cancer. This care begins with the identification of individuals at high-risk and proceeds to expert education and genetic counseling regarding the implication of the risk of genetic cancer, culminating in the heightened surveillance and medical management that is often required for high-risk individuals and possibly their family members. Ultimately, the goal is the appropriate identification and care of high-risk individuals who can benefit from specialized psychosocial and medical support.

References

1. Easton DF, Pooley KA, Dunning AM et al (2007) Genome-wide association study identifies novel breast cancer susceptibility loci. Nature 447(7148):1087–1093
2. Ford D, Easton DF, Stratton M et al (1998) Genetic heterogeneity and penetrance analysis of the BRCA1 and BRCA2 genes in breast cancer families. The Breast Cancer Linkage Consortium. Am J Hum Genet 62(3):676–689

3. Gudmundsdottir K, Ashworth A (2006) The roles of BRCA1 and BRCA2 and associated proteins in the maintenance of genomic stability. Oncogene 25(43):5864–5874

4. Chappuis PO, Nethercot V, Foulkes WD (2000) Clinico-pathological characteristics of BRCA1- and BRCA2-related breast cancer. Semin Surg Oncol 18(4):287–295

5. Phillips KA, Andrulis IL, Goodwin PJ (1999) Breast carcinomas arising in carriers of mutations in BRCA1 or BRCA2: are they prognostically different? J Clin Oncol 17(11):3653–3663

6. Bane AL, Beck JC, Bleiweiss I et al (2007) BRCA2 mutation-associated breast cancers exhibit a distinguishing phenotype based on morphology and molecular profiles from tissue microarrays. Am J Surg Pathol 31(1):121–128

7. Turner NC, Reis-Filho JS (2006) Basal-like breast cancer and the BRCA1 phenotype. Oncogene 25(43):5846–5853

8. Eisinger F, Nogues C, Birnbaum D, Jacquemier J, Sobol H (1998) BRCA1 and medullary breast cancer. JAMA 280(14):1227–1228

9. Hosey AM, Gorski JJ, Murray MM et al (2007) Molecular basis for estrogen receptor alpha deficiency in BRCA1-linked breast cancer. J Natl Cancer Inst 99(22):1683–1694

10. Lakhani SR, Reis-Filho JS, Fulford L et al (2005) Prediction of BRCA1 status in patients with breast cancer using estrogen receptor and basal phenotype. Clin Cancer Res 11(14):5175–5180

11. Miki Y, Swensen J, Shattuck-Eidens D et al (1994) A strong candidate for the breast and ovarian cancer susceptibility gene BRCA1. Science 266(5182):66–71

12. Wooster R, Bignell G, Lancaster J et al (1995) Identification of the breast cancer susceptibility gene BRCA2. Nature 378(6559):789–792

13. Wooster R, Neuhausen SL, Mangion J et al (1994) Localization of a breast cancer susceptibility gene, BRCA2, to chromosome 13q12-13. Science 265(5181):2088–2090

14. Walsh T, Casadei S, Coats KH et al (2006) Spectrum of mutations in BRCA1, BRCA2, CHEK2, and TP53 in families at high risk of breast cancer. JAMA 295(12):1379–1388

15. Nagy R, Sweet K, Eng C (2004) Highly penetrant hereditary cancer syndromes. Oncogene 23(38):6445–6470

16. Easton DF, Deffenbaugh AM, Pruss D et al (2007) A systematic genetic assessment of 1, 433 sequence variants of unknown clinical significance in the BRCA1 and BRCA2 breast cancer-predisposition genes. Am J Hum Genet 81(5):873–883

17. Xia B, Sheng Q, Nakanishi K et al (2006) Control of BRCA2 cellular and clinical functions by a nuclear partner, PALB2. Mol Cell 22(6):719–729

18. Struewing JP, Hartge P, Wacholder S et al (1997) The risk of cancer associated with specific mutations of BRCA1 and BRCA2 among Ashkenazi Jews. N Engl J Med 336(20):1401–1408

19. Kauff ND, Perez-Segura P, Robson ME et al (2002) Incidence of non-founder BRCA1 and BRCA2 mutations in high risk Ashkenazi breast and ovarian cancer families. J Med Genet 39(8):611–614

20. Thorlacius S, Olafsdottir G, Tryggvadottir L et al (1996) A single BRCA2 mutation in male and female breast cancer families from Iceland with varied cancer phenotypes. Nat Genet 13(1):117–119

21. Unger MA, Nathanson KL, Calzone K et al (2000) Screening for genomic rearrangements in families with breast and ovarian cancer identifies BRCA1 mutations previously missed by conformation-sensitive gel electrophoresis or sequencing. Am J Hum Genet 67(4):841–850

22. Antoniou A, Pharoah PD, Narod S et al (2003) Average risks of breast and ovarian cancer associated with BRCA1 or BRCA2 mutations detected in case Series unselected for family history: a combined analysis of 22 studies. Am J Hum Genet 72(5):1117–1130

23. King MC, Marks JH, Mandell JB (2003) Breast and ovarian cancer risks due to inherited mutations in BRCA1 and BRCA2. Science 302(5645):643–646

24. Risch HA, McLaughlin JR, Cole DE et al (2001) Prevalence and penetrance of germline BRCA1 and BRCA2 mutations in a population series of 649 women with ovarian cancer. Am J Hum Genet 68(3):700–710

25. Thompson D, Easton D (2001) Variation in cancer risks, by mutation position, in BRCA2 mutation carriers. Am J Hum Genet 68(2):410–419

26. Rebbeck TR, Lynch HT, Neuhausen SL et al (2002) Prophylactic oophorectomy in carriers of BRCA1 or BRCA2 mutations. N Engl J Med 346(21):1616–1622

27. Kauff ND, Satagopan JM, Robson ME et al (2002) Risk-reducing salpingo-oophorectomy in women with a BRCA1 or BRCA2 mutation. N Engl J Med 346(21):1609–1615

28. Easton D, Thompson D, McGuffog L et al (1999) Cancer risks in BRCA2 mutation carriers. The Breast Cancer Linkage Consortium. J Natl Cancer Inst 91(15):1310–1316

29. Liede A, Karlan BY, Narod SA (2004) Cancer risks for male carriers of germline mutations in BRCA1 or BRCA2: a review of the literature. J Clin Oncol 22(4):735–742

30. Thompson D, Easton DF (2002) Cancer Incidence in BRCA1 mutation carriers. J Natl Cancer Inst 94(18):1358–1365

31. van Asperen CJ, Brohet RM, Meijers-Heijboer EJ et al (2005) Cancer risks in BRCA2 families: estimates for sites other than breast and ovary. J Med Genet 42(9):711–719

32. Boyd J, Sonoda Y, Federici MG et al (2000) Clinicopathologic features of BRCA-linked and sporadic ovarian cancer. JAMA 283(17):2260–2265

33. Lakhani SR, Manek S, Penault-Llorca F et al (2004) Pathology of ovarian cancers in BRCA1 and BRCA2 carriers. Clin Cancer Res 10(7):2473–2481

34. Levine DA, Argenta PA, Yee CJ et al (2003) Fallopian tube and primary peritoneal carcinomas associated with BRCA mutations. J Clin Oncol 21(22):4222–4227

35. Cass I, Baldwin RL, Varkey T, Moslehi R, Narod SA, Karlan BY (2003) Improved survival in women with BRCA-associated ovarian carcinoma. Cancer 97(9):2187–2195

36. Smith P, McGuffog L, Easton DF et al (2006) A genome wide linkage search for breast cancer susceptibility genes. Genes Chromosomes Cancer 45(7):646–655

37. Hunter DJ, Kraft P, Jacobs KB et al (2007) A genome-wide association study identifies alleles in FGFR2 associated with risk of sporadic postmenopausal breast cancer. Nat Genet 39(7):870–874

38. Stacey SN, Manolescu A, Sulem P et al (2007) Common variants on chromosomes 2q35 and 16q12 confer susceptibility to estrogen receptor-positive breast cancer. Nat Genet 39(7):865–869

39. Frank B, Wiestler M, Kropp S et al (2008) Association of a common AKAP9 variant with breast cancer risk: a collaborative analysis. J Natl Cancer Inst 100(6):437–442

40. Gold B, Kirchhoff T, Stefanov S et al (2008) Genome-wide association study provides evidence for a breast cancer risk locus at 6q22.33. Proc Natl Acad Sci U S A 105(11):4340–4345

41. Nevanlinna H, Bartek J (2006) The CHEK2 gene and inherited breast cancer susceptibility. Oncogene 25(43):5912–5919

42. Erkko H, Xia B, Nikkila J et al (2007) A recurrent mutation in PALB2 in Finnish cancer families. Nature 446(7133):316–319

43. Foulkes WD, Ghadirian P, Akbari MR et al (2007) Identification of a novel truncating PALB2 mutation and analysis of its contribution to early-onset breast cancer in French-Canadian women. Breast Cancer Res 9(6):R83

44. Liebens FP, Carly B, Pastijn A, Rozenberg S (2007) Management of BRCA1/2 associated breast cancer: a systematic qualitative review of the state of knowledge in 2006. Eur J Cancer 43(2):238–257

45. Metcalfe K, Lynch HT, Ghadirian P et al (2004) Contralateral breast cancer in BRCA1 and BRCA2 mutation carriers. J Clin Oncol 22(12):2328–2335

46. Pierce LJ, Levin AM, Rebbeck TR et al (2006) Ten-year multi-institutional results of breast-conserving surgery and radiotherapy

in BRCA1/2-associated stage I/II breast cancer. J Clin Oncol 24(16):2437–2443

47. Moller P, Evans DG, Reis MM et al (2007) Surveillance for familial breast cancer: Differences in outcome according to BRCA mutation status. Int J Cancer 121(5):1017–1020

48. Rennert G, Bisland-Naggan S, Barnett-Griness O et al (2007) Clinical outcomes of breast cancer in carriers of BRCA1 and BRCA2 mutations. N Engl J Med 357(2):115–123

49. Foulkes WD, Metcalfe K, Hanna W et al (2003) Disruption of the expected positive correlation between breast tumor size and lymph node status in BRCA1-related breast carcinoma. Cancer 98(8):1569–1577

50. Robson M, Svahn T, McCormick B et al (2005) Appropriateness of breast-conserving treatment of breast carcinoma in women with germline mutations in BRCA1 or BRCA2: a clinic-based series. Cancer 103(1):44–51

51. Rodriguez-Pinilla SM, Sarrio D, Honrado E et al (2006) Prognostic significance of basal-like phenotype and fascin expression in node-negative invasive breast carcinomas. Clin Cancer Res 12(5):1533–1539

52. Moynahan ME, Cui TY, Jasin M (2001) Homology-directed dna repair, mitomycin-c resistance, and chromosome stability is restored with correction of a Brca1 mutation. Cancer Res 61(12):4842–4850

53. Tutt A, Bertwistle D, Valentine J et al (2001) Mutation in Brca2 stimulates error-prone homology-directed repair of DNA double-strand breaks occurring between repeated sequences. EMBO J 20(17):4704–4716

54. Bhattacharyya A, Ear US, Koller BH, Weichselbaum RR, Bishop DK (2000) The breast cancer susceptibility gene BRCA1 is required for subnuclear assembly of Rad51 and survival following treatment with the DNA cross-linking agent cisplatin. J Biol Chem 275(31):23899–23903

55. Howlett NG, Taniguchi T, Olson S et al (2002) Biallelic inactivation of BRCA2 in Fanconi anemia. Science 297(5581):606–609

56. Kennedy RD, Quinn JE, Mullan PB, Johnston PG, Harkin DP (2004) The role of BRCA1 in the cellular response to chemotherapy. J Natl Cancer Inst 96(22):1659–1668

57. Byrski T, Gronwald J, Huzarski T et al (2008) Response to neoadjuvant chemotherapy in women with BRCA1-positive breast cancers. Breast Cancer Res Treat 108(2):289–296

58. Zhou C, Smith JL, Liu J (2003) Role of BRCA1 in cellular resistance to paclitaxel and ionizing radiation in an ovarian cancer cell line carrying a defective BRCA1. Oncogene 22(16):2396–2404

59. Venkitaraman AR (2002) Cancer susceptibility and the functions of BRCA1 and BRCA2. Cell 108(2):171–182

60. Ashworth A (2008) A synthetic lethal therapeutic approach: poly(ADP) ribose polymerase inhibitors for the treatment of cancers deficient in DNA double-strand break repair. J Clin Oncol 26(22):3785–3790

61. Farmer H, McCabe N, Lord CJ et al (2005) Targeting the DNA repair defect in BRCA mutant cells as a therapeutic strategy. Nature 434(7035):917–921

62. Bryant HE, Schultz N, Thomas HD et al (2005) Specific killing of BRCA2-deficient tumours with inhibitors of poly(ADP-ribose) polymerase. Nature 434(7035):913–917

63. McCabe N, Turner NC, Lord CJ et al (2006) Deficiency in the repair of DNA damage by homologous recombination and sensitivity to poly(ADP-ribose) polymerase inhibition. Cancer Res 66(16):8109–8115

64. McCabe N, Lord CJ, Tutt AN, Martin NM, Smith GC, Ashworth A (2005) BRCA2-deficient CAPAN-1 cells are extremely sensitive to the inhibition of Poly (ADP-Ribose) polymerase: an issue of potency. Cancer Biol Ther 4(9):934–936

65. Hay T, Jenkins H, Sansom OJ, Martin NM, Smith GC, Clarke AR (2005) Efficient deletion of normal Brca2-deficient intestinal epithelium by poly(ADP-ribose) polymerase inhibition models potential prophylactic therapy. Cancer Res 65(22):10145–10148

66. Rottenberg S, Nygren AO, Pajic M et al (2007) Selective induction of chemotherapy resistance of mammary tumors in a conditional mouse model for hereditary breast cancer. Proc Natl Acad Sci U S A 104(29):12117–12122

67. Fong PC, Boss DS, Yap TA et al (2009) Inhibition of poly(ADP-Ribose) polymerase in tumors from BRCA mutation carriers. N Engl J Med 361(2):123–134

68. Johnson N, Fletcher O, Palles C et al (2007) Counting potentially functional variants in BRCA1, BRCA2 and ATM predicts breast cancer susceptibility. Hum Mol Genet 16(9):1051–1057

69. Sorlie T, Tibshirani R, Parker J et al (2003) Repeated observation of breast tumor subtypes in independent gene expression data sets. Proc Natl Acad Sci U S A 100(14):8418–8423

70. Turner NC, Reis-Filho JS, Russell AM et al (2007) BRCA1 dysfunction in sporadic basal-like breast cancer. Oncogene 26(14):2126–2132

71. Matros E, Wang ZC, Lodeiro G, Miron A, Iglehart JD, Richardson AL (2005) BRCA1 promoter methylation in sporadic breast tumors: relationship to gene expression profiles. Breast Cancer Res Treat 91(2):179–186

72. Abd El-Rehim DM, Ball G, Pinder SE et al (2005) High-throughput protein expression analysis using tissue microarray technology of a large well-characterised series identifies biologically distinct classes of breast cancer confirming recent cDNA expression analyses. Int J Cancer 116(3):340–350

73. Richardson AL, Wang ZC, De Nicolo A et al (2006) X chromosomal abnormalities in basal-like human breast cancer. Cancer Cell 9(2):121–132

74. Hartmann LC, Sellers TA, Schaid DJ et al (2001) Efficacy of bilateral prophylactic mastectomy in BRCA1 and BRCA2 gene mutation carriers. J Natl Cancer Inst 93(21):1633–1637

75. Sardanelli F, Podo F, D'Agnolo G et al (2007) Multicenter comparative multimodality surveillance of women at genetic-familial high risk for breast cancer (HIBCRIT study): interim results. Radiology 242(3):698–715

76. Kriege M, Brekelmans CT, Boetes C et al (2004) Efficacy of MRI and mammography for breast-cancer screening in women with a familial or genetic predisposition. N Engl J Med 351(5):427–437

77. Warner E, Plewes DB, Hill KA et al (2004) Surveillance of BRCA1 and BRCA2 mutation carriers with magnetic resonance imaging, ultrasound, mammography, and clinical breast examination. JAMA 292(11):1317–1325

78. Stoutjesdijk MJ, Boetes C, Jager GJ et al (2001) Magnetic resonance imaging and mammography in women with a hereditary risk of breast cancer. J Natl Cancer Inst 93(14):1095–1102

79. NCCN (2009) NCCN Clinical Practice Guidelines in oncology: high-risk assesment: breast and ovarian. V.1.2009

80. Rebbeck TR, Friebel T, Lynch HT et al (2004) Bilateral prophylactic mastectomy reduces breast cancer risk in BRCA1 and BRCA2 mutation carriers: the PROSE Study Group. J Clin Oncol 22(6):1055–1062

81. Meijers-Heijboer H, van Geel B, van Putten WL et al (2001) Breast cancer after prophylactic bilateral mastectomy in women with a BRCA1 or BRCA2 mutation. N Engl J Med 345(3):159–164

82. Piver MS, Jishi MF, Tsukada Y, Nava G (1993) Primary peritoneal carcinoma after prophylactic oophorectomy in women with a family history of ovarian cancer. A report of the Gilda Radner Familial Ovarian Cancer Registry. Cancer 71(9):2751–2755

83. Burke W, Daly M, Garber J et al (1997) Recommendations for follow-up care of individuals with an inherited predisposition to cancer. II. BRCA1 and BRCA2. Cancer Genetics Studies Consortium. JAMA 277(12):997–1003

84. Modan B, Hartge P, Hirsh-Yechezkel G et al (2001) Parity, oral contraceptives, and the risk of ovarian cancer among carriers and

noncarriers of a BRCA1 or BRCA2 mutation. N Engl J Med 345(4):235–240

85. Narod SA, Risch H, Moslehi R et al (1998) Oral contraceptives and the risk of hereditary ovarian cancer. Hereditary Ovarian Cancer Clinical Study Group. N Engl J Med 339(7):424–428

86. Narod SA, Dube MP, Klijn J et al (2002) Oral contraceptives and the risk of breast cancer in BRCA1 and BRCA2 mutation carriers. J Natl Cancer Inst 94(23):1773–1779

87. Milne RL, Knight JA, John EM et al (2005) Oral contraceptive use and risk of early-onset breast cancer in carriers and noncarriers of BRCA1 and BRCA2 mutations. Cancer Epidemiol Biomarkers Prev 14(2):350–356

88. King MC, Wieand S, Hale K et al (2001) Tamoxifen and breast cancer incidence among women with inherited mutations in BRCA1 and BRCA2: National Surgical Adjuvant Breast and Bowel Project (NSABP-P1) Breast Cancer Prevention Trial. JAMA 286(18):2251–2256

89. Narod SA, Brunet JS, Ghadirian P et al (2000) Tamoxifen and risk of contralateral breast cancer in BRCA1 and BRCA2 mutation carriers: a case-control study. Hereditary Breast Cancer Clinical Study Group. Lancet 356(9245):1876–1881

90. Gronwald J, Tung N, Foulkes WD et al (2006) Tamoxifen and contralateral breast cancer in BRCA1 and BRCA2 carriers: an update. Int J Cancer 118(9):2281–2284

91. Sidransky D, Tokino T, Helzlsouer K et al (1992) Inherited p53 gene mutations in breast cancer. Cancer Res 52(10):2984–2986

92. Li FP, Fraumeni JF Jr, Mulvihill JJ et al (1988) A cancer family syndrome in twenty-four kindreds. Cancer Res 48(18): 5358–5362

93. Nichols KE, Malkin D, Garber JE, Fraumeni JF Jr, Li FP (2001) Germ-line p53 mutations predispose to a wide spectrum of early-onset cancers. Cancer Epidemiol Biomarkers Prev 10(2):83–87

94. Hartley AL, Birch JM, Marsden HB, Harris M (1987) Malignant melanoma in families of children with osteosarcoma, chondrosarcoma, and adrenal cortical carcinoma. J Med Genet 24(11): 664–668

95. Jay M, McCartney AC (1993) Familial malignant melanoma of the uvea and p53: a Victorian detective story. Surv Ophthalmol 37(6):457–462

96. Birch JM, Alston RD, McNally RJ et al (2001) Relative frequency and morphology of cancers in carriers of germline TP53 mutations. Oncogene 20(34):4621–4628

97. Hwang SJ, Lozano G, Amos CI, Strong LC (2003) Germline p53 mutations in a cohort with childhood sarcoma: sex differences in cancer risk. Am J Hum Genet 72(4):975–983

98. Chompret A, Brugieres L, Ronsin M et al (2000) P53 germline mutations in childhood cancers and cancer risk for carrier individuals. Br J Cancer 82(12):1932–1937

99. Le Bihan C, Bonaiti-Pellie C (1994) A method for estimating cancer risk in p53 mutation carriers. Cancer Detect Prev 18(3): 171–178

100. Birch JM, Hartley AL, Tricker KJ et al (1994) Prevalence and diversity of constitutional mutations in the p53 gene among 21 Li-Fraumeni families. Cancer Res 54(5):1298–1304

101. Eeles RA (1995) Germline mutations in the TP53 gene. Cancer Surv 25:101–124

102. Gonzalez KD, Noltner KA, Buzin CH et al (2009) Beyond Li Fraumeni Syndrome: Clinical Characteristics of Families With p53 Germline Mutations. J Clin Oncol 27(8):1250–1256

103. Starink TM, van der Veen JP, Arwert F et al (1986) The Cowden syndrome: a clinical and genetic study in 21 patients. Clin Genet 29(3):222–233

104. Brownstein MH, Wolf M, Bikowski JB (1978) Cowden's disease: a cutaneous marker of breast cancer. Cancer 41(6):2393–2398

105. Eng C (2003) PTEN: one gene, many syndromes. Hum Mutat 22(3):183–198

106. Fackenthal JD, Marsh DJ, Richardson AL et al (2001) Male breast cancer in Cowden syndrome patients with germline PTEN mutations. J Med Genet 38(3):159–164

107. Li J, Yen C, Liaw D et al (1997) PTEN, a putative protein tyrosine phosphatase gene mutated in human brain, breast, and prostate cancer. Science 275(5308):1943–1947

108. Eng C (2002) Role of PTEN, a lipid phosphatase upstream effector of protein kinase B, in epithelial thyroid carcinogenesis. Ann N Y Acad Sci 968:213–221

109. Marsh DJ, Kum JB, Lunetta KL et al (1999) PTEN mutation spectrum and genotype-phenotype correlations in Bannayan-Riley-Ruvalcaba syndrome suggest a single entity with Cowden syndrome. Hum Mol Genet 8(8):1461–1472

110. Saslow D, Castle PE, Cox JT et al (2007) American Cancer Society Guideline for human papillomavirus (HPV) vaccine use to prevent cervical cancer and its precursors. CA Cancer J Clin 57(1):7–28

111. Charlton A, Blair V, Shaw D, Parry S, Guilford P, Martin IG (2004) Hereditary diffuse gastric cancer: predominance of multiple foci of signet ring cell carcinoma in distal stomach and transitional zone. Gut 53(6):814–820

112. Guilford PJ, Hopkins JB, Grady WM et al (1999) E-cadherin germline mutations define an inherited cancer syndrome dominated by diffuse gastric cancer. Hum Mutat 14(3):249–255

113. Pharoah PD, Guilford P, Caldas C (2001) Incidence of gastric cancer and breast cancer in CDH1 (E-cadherin) mutation carriers from hereditary diffuse gastric cancer families. Gastroenterology 121(6):1348–1353

114. Graziano F, Humar B, Guilford P (2003) The role of the E-cadherin gene (CDH1) in diffuse gastric cancer susceptibility: from the laboratory to clinical practice. Ann Oncol 14(12): 1705–1713

115. Brooks-Wilson AR, Kaurah P, Suriano G et al (2004) Germline E-cadherin mutations in hereditary diffuse gastric cancer: assessment of 42 new families and review of genetic screening criteria. J Med Genet 41(7):508–517

116. Gene tests. GeneTests 2009; available at www.ncbi.nlm.nih.gov/sites/GeneTests/?db = GeneTests

Chapter 4
Surgical Management of Hereditary Breast and Ovarian Cancer

Michelle C. Specht, Marcela G. del Carmen, and Barbara L. Smith

Keywords Breast cancer • Ovarian cancer • Mastectomy • Reconstructive surgery • Prophylactic surgery • Salpingo-oophorectomy • Breast cancer screening

Introduction

Hereditary breast cancer may result from germline mutations in one of several genes. Different genes confer different levels of risk for the development of breast cancer, and may also confer a significantly increased risk of cancer in other organ sites. For example, mutations and the BRCA1 and BRCA2 genes, the most common cause of hereditary breast cancer, also markedly increase the risk of ovarian cancer.

Patients at significantly elevated risk of breast cancer may elect prophylactic bilateral mastectomies for risk reduction. Patients who are found to have a gene mutation in conjunction with a new breast cancer diagnosis may choose therapeutic mastectomy for the cancer-bearing breast and prophylactic contralateral mastectomy for risk reduction. Prophylactic mastectomy has been shown to markedly decrease the risk of developing breast cancer, and to reduce worry about breast cancer, but is also associated with significant physical and psychological changes. The pros and cons of risk-reducing prophylactic mastectomy are evaluated for each patient, with decisions made in a collaborative manner with input from the patient, her family members, and her physicians.

Surgical management of hereditary breast cancer and surgery for risk reduction is reviewed in this chapter. Screening and medical management of hereditary breast and ovarian cancer is discussed in Chap. 3.

BRCA1 and BRCA2 Mutations

BRCA1 germline mutations confer an estimated 50–80% cumulative breast cancer risk and a 35–50% lifetime ovarian cancer risk; for BRCA2 germline mutations, cumulative breast cancer risk is estimated to be 40–70% and ovarian cancer risk 13–25% [1–4].

Efficacy of Bilateral Prophylactic Mastectomy in BRCA Gene Mutation Carriers

Prophylactic mastectomy reduces breast cancer risk in BRCA mutation carriers by 90–95% [5–7], with additional reduction in breast cancer risk seen with the surgical menopause associated with prophylactic oophorectomy. BRCA mutation carriers may elect risk reduction through bilateral prophylactic mastectomy, bilateral prophylactic salpingo-oophorectomy or both.

In a cohort of 483 BRCA gene mutation carriers, breast cancer was diagnosed in two (1.9%) of 105 women who had bilateral prophylactic mastectomy and in 184 (48.7%) of 378 matched controls who did not undergo the procedure, at a mean follow-up of 6.4 years [6]. Bilateral prophylactic mastectomy reduced the risk of breast cancer by approximately 95% in women with prior or concurrent bilateral prophylactic oophorectomy and by approximately 90% in women with intact ovaries.

Genetic testing was performed retrospectively in women who underwent prophylactic mastectomy for a positive family history of breast cancer [5]. None among 26 patients with a BRCA1 or 2 mutation developed breast cancer after prophylactic mastectomy, a risk reduction of 89.5–100% relative to predicted incidence in mutation carriers.

In another cohort of 139 BRCA 1 or 2 mutation carriers, none among 76 women who underwent bilateral prophylactic mastectomy developed breast cancer at 3 years median follow-up, compared with 8 breast cancers in 63 patients who chose surveillance alone [7] (Table 4.1).

B.L. Smith (✉)
Massachusetts General Hospital Cancer Center,
Harvard Medical School, Boston, MA, USA

Table 4.1 Efficacy of bilateral prophylactic mastectomy (BPM) for breast cancer risk reduction in BRCA1/2 mutation carriers

Author	Breast cancer incidence	Follow-up
Hartman [5]	BPM group, 0/26	13.4 years
	Expected based on two models, 6–9	
Meijers-Heijboer [7]	BPM group, 0/76	3 years
	Surveillance group, 8/63	
Rebbeck [6]	BPM, 2/105 (1.9%)	6.4 years
	Surveillance group, 184/378 (48.7%)	

Table 4.2 Clinical characteristics of patients opting for bilateral prophylactic mastectomy

History of breast cancer
Lower stage of breast cancer (0 or 1)
History of breast biopsy
Family history of ovarian cancer
Age < 60 years
Use of another risk-reducing surgery

Risk-reducing bilateral salpingo-oophorectomy reduces the risk of breast cancer in BRCA gene mutation carriers by approximately 50% and may be an appealing option for carriers who do not wish to undergo prophylactic mastectomy. After mean follow-up of 8.8 years, only 21% (21 of 99) of BRCA mutation carriers who underwent bilateral prophylactic oophorectomy developed breast cancer, as compared with 42% (60 of 142) of carriers in the control group with intact ovaries (hazard ratio, 0.47; 95% confidence interval, 0.29–0.77) [8].

Decision-Making: High-Risk Screening Versus Prophylactic Mastectomy

Women with BRCA gene mutations can manage their breast cancer risk with high-risk screening (MRI, mammography and physical examination) with or without addition of tamoxifen chemoprevention (see Chap. 3), or may consider risk-reducing prophylactic mastectomy and or bilateral salpingo-oophorectomy.

Genetic counseling can assist patients in making decisions about surveillance versus risk-reducing surgery. These consultations include detailed discussions of cancer family history, cancer risks, and risk-reducing strategies. Patients report that these detailed discussions influence their decision making, including decisions about prophylactic mastectomy [9].

In a review of 554 women who underwent genetic testing, 36% with a mutation chose bilateral risk-reducing mastectomy [10]. Many mutation carriers are reluctant to consider bilateral prophylactic mastectomy due to concerns about altered body image, impact on sexuality, and decrease in quality of life.

In another series of 272 carriers, 23% of women chose bilateral prophylactic mastectomy [11]. Those who chose risk-reducing surgery underwent surgery about 4 months after a positive genetic test. Predictors of bilateral prophylactic mastectomy included age under 60 years, previous breast cancer and election of bilateral prophylactic salpingo-oophrectomy (Table 4.2).

Prophylactic mastectomy has been cited by carriers as the most effective means to decrease the risk of breast cancer and worry of breast cancer [12]. In an analysis of 554 women who presented for genetic testing, women most likely to choose prophylactic mastectomy were those with a history of breast cancer, particularly lower-stage disease. Patients with a history of ovarian cancer were more likely to choose surveillance than prophylactic mastectomy. Ethnicity, marital status, and parity were not associated with the selection of risk-reducing surgery [10].

Patient Satisfaction After Prophylactic Mastectomy

The majority of women who choose bilateral prophylactic mastectomy are satisfied with their decision. Nearly all report significant reduction in worry about breast cancer risk, but most also note a negative impact on body image and/or sexuality.

At mean follow-up of 14.5 years after prophylactic mastectomy Frost et al. [13] reported that 70% were satisfied with the procedure, 11% were neutral, and 19% were dissatisfied. Seventy-four percent reported a diminished level of emotional concern about developing breast cancer. The majority of women reported no change/favorable effects in levels of emotional stability (68%/23%), level of stress (58%/28%), self-esteem (69%/13%), sexual relationships (73%/4%), and feelings of femininity (67%/8%). Forty-eight percent reported no change in their level of satisfaction with body appearance; 16% reported favorable effects. However, 9, 14, 18, 23, 25, and 36% reported negative effects in these 6 variables, respectively.

In another study, 84% of women who underwent prophylactic bilateral mastectomy were satisfied with their decision for surgery [14] and 61% reported a high degree of contentment with their quality of life, a figure similar to that reported by high-risk women who did not undergo prophylactic surgery. Women who chose prophylactic mastectomy also reported decreased anxiety about cancer risk, and reported satisfaction with body image and sex life similar to women who did not undergo surgery.

As might be expected, satisfaction with prophylactic mastectomy is related to operative complications, ongoing physical complaints and limitations in daily life. Dissatisfaction with prophylactic surgery has also been related to psychiatric history, level of cancer related distress prior to surgery, and having children under the age of 15. Lack of family support and changes in relationships with family also contributed to distress after prophylactic mastectomy [15].

Prophylactic Mastectomy for Other Hereditary Breast Cancer Syndromes

Although BRCA gene mutations are the most frequent cause of hereditary breast cancer, germline mutations in several other genes, including p53, PTEN, and CDH1, are also associated with elevated breast cancer risk. The magnitude of risk reduction achieved with prophylactic mastectomy and psychological concerns about risk and risk-reducing surgery for these mutation carriers are thought to be similar to those seen in women with BRCA gene mutations. However, patients with mutations in other hereditary breast cancer genes are also at increased risk for a number of types of cancer, making the value of prophylactic mastectomy more controversial than for BRCA gene mutation carriers. Decisions about prophylactic mastectomy are therefore made based on an individual patient's circumstances and preferences.

p53 Mutation Carriers: Li Fraumeni Syndrome

Germline mutations in the p53 tumor suppressor gene (Li-Fraumeni Syndrome) result in increased risk of many malignancies, including soft tissue and osteosarcomas, brain tumors, adrenal cortical carcinoma, leukemia [16] and account for approximately 1% of hereditary breast cancers [17]. Women with germline p53 mutations are estimated to have a 56% risk of breast cancer by age 45 and greater than 90% risk by age 70 [18–20].

Prophylactic bilateral mastectomy is unlikely to reduce overall cancer mortality for women with germline p53 mutations, due to the multiplicity of cancer types caused by p53 mutations. Some patients may choose bilateral mastectomies at the time of a breast cancer diagnosis for both treatment and prevention, but breast-conserving surgery followed by careful surveillance also remains an option.

PTEN Mutation Carriers: Cowden's Syndrome

Cowden's disease, the multiple hamartoma syndrome, is caused by a mutation in the PTEN tumor suppressor gene. PTEN mutation carriers are at increased risk for benign and malignant tumors of the breast, thyroid, and endometrium. The cumulative risk of breast cancer in PTEN mutation carriers is estimated to be 25–50% [21, 22]. High-risk screening with mammography and MRI is recommended and prophylactic mastectomy may be considered.

CDH1 Mutation Carriers: Hereditary Diffuse Gastric Carcinoma Syndrome

The e-cadherin gene (CDH1) is a calcium-dependent cell–cell adhesion molecule. CDH1 mutations confer markedly increased risk of diffuse gastric carcinoma and increased risk of lobular carcinoma in women. For females with germline mutations in CDH1, the cumulative risk of breast cancer is estimated to be 39% [23]. However, this risk must be evaluated in the context of an estimated cumulative risk of gastric cancer by age 80 years of 83% seen in women with CDH1 mutations. CDH1 mutation carriers are considered for prophylactic total gastrectomy and high-risk breast screening, including mammography and breast MRI, is recommended [24]. Prophylactic bilateral mastectomy or contralateral prophylactic mastectomy after a breast cancer diagnosis may be considered given the challenge of early detection of lobular carcinoma.

Technical Considerations in Prophylactic Mastectomy

Complete removal of breast tissue is not possible in prophylactic mastectomy. No distinct boundary separates breast tissue from adjacent adipose tissue, and it has been demonstrated that breast structures may extend into pectoralis muscle and along Cooper's ligaments into subcutaneous fat [25, 26]. Prophylactic mastectomy should be carried out in thin but fairly consistent and nearly avascular fibrous plane that exists between breast parenchyma and subcutaneous fat to maximize the removal of at-risk breast tissue while leaving the blood supply to the skin intact.

Skin flaps are raised superiorly to the clavicle, medially to the sternum, inferiorly to the inframammary fold and laterally to the border of the latissimus dorsi muscle. Vessels in the skin flap are carefully preserved to maintain flap perfusion. The breast is then removed from the underlying pectoralis muscle taking pectoral muscle fascia with the breast specimen, creating a well-defined deep margin. All axillary breast tissues superficial to the fascia of the axillary fat pad should be included in the mastectomy specimen. After the breast has been removed, the skin flaps are inspected and any remaining visible breast tissue excised.

Mastectomy Options

The extent of breast tissue removed during a prophylactic mastectomy should be the same as in a therapeutic mastectomy for cancer. The extent of skin removed will depend on reconstruction plans. A simple or total mastectomy includes complete removal of the breast, nipple, and areola and is used for patients who do not undergo immediate reconstruction. Commercially available breast prostheses are available for patients to wear after total mastectomy. Skin-sparing and nipple-sparing mastectomy approaches are considered for women undergoing immediate reconstruction.

Skin-Sparing Mastectomy

Skin-sparing mastectomy removes the nipple and areola while leaving all other skin for use in the reconstruction. Several mature studies confirm that local recurrence rates after skin-sparing mastectomy for breast cancer are equivalent to those seen after simple mastectomy without reconstruction [27–33]. Skin-sparing approaches are appropriate for patients undergoing prophylactic mastectomy and immediate reconstruction and markedly improve cosmetic outcome for both implant/expander and autologous tissue reconstructions. Nipple and areola reconstruction is performed as a second procedure after healing to allow proper positioning of the nipple on the new breast mound.

Studies have demonstrated high-level patient satisfaction with skin-sparing mastectomy and immediate reconstruction [34]. Risks of skin-sparing mastectomy include infection, bleeding, and necrosis of the skin flaps.

Nipple-Sparing Mastectomy

The efficacy of skin-sparing mastectomy in achieving local control has led to reconsideration of nipple-sparing mastectomy in prophylactic mastectomy and for selected patients with early stage breast cancer [35]. In nipple-sparing mastectomy all skin, including the nipple and areola, is left in place, with the mastectomy performed through an incision that is closed primarily (Fig. 4.1). Preservation of the nipple–areola complex provides improved cosmesis but does not preserve nipple sensation.

It should be noted that nipple-sparing subcutaneous mastectomy was performed in more than 90% of prophylactic mastectomies in the landmark Mayo Clinic prophylactic mastectomy of Hartmann et al. [5]. At least 90% reduction in breast cancer risk was seen despite retention of subareolar breast tissue.

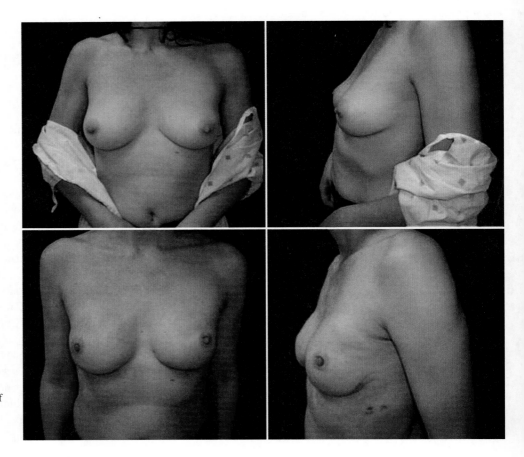

Fig. 4.1 Bilateral nipple-sparing mastectomy with single-stage silicone implant reconstruction. Upper images are anterior and lateral views prior to surgery. Lower images are anterior and lateral views after bilateral nipple-sparing mastectomies and single-stage silicone implant reconstructions. (Photo courtesy of Dr. Amy Colwell, Division of Plastic Surgery, Massachusetts General Hospital)

Current nipple-sparing techniques differ from prior subcutaneous mastectomy approaches that left a thick flap of tissue under the nipple and areola. Nipple-sparing mastectomy techniques now create standard thin skin flaps and remove all visible breast tissues under the nipple and areola, often including excision of duct tissue from within the nipple papilla [36–38]. Early follow-up of nipple-sparing mastectomy in selected patients have shown acceptable rates of nipple necrosis [39–42]. Risk of nipple involvement by tumor is extremely low in women undergoing prophylactic mastectomy; Brachtel et al. found no evidence of nipple duct involvement by tumor in 84 prophylactic mastectomy specimens [43].

Nipple–areola complex tumor recurrence is rare after nipple-sparing prophylactic mastectomy. In a multi-institutional study of 55 patients who underwent nipple-sparing mastectomy with immediate reconstruction for risk reduction, two women developed breast cancer at a median follow-up of 24 months. Neither recurrence involved the nipple areola complex [42].

Patients considering nipple-sparing mastectomy should have pre-operative mammography with magnification views of the subareolar area to rule out microcalcifications extending into the nipple. Some centers advocate routine use of breast MRI to select patients for nipple-sparing mastectomy [44].

Complications of the nipple-sparing mastectomy include infection, bleeding, necrosis of the skin flaps and potential nipple loss due to necrosis. In one series, smokers had the highest nipple areola complex necrosis rate at 60% compared to approximately 20% in nonsmokers [44].

Satisfaction with Reconstruction After Prophylactic Mastectomy

A retrospective review of 114 mutation carriers who underwent bilateral prophylactic mastectomy with immediate reconstruction demonstrated a 60% satisfaction rate with the reconstruction 3 years after surgery. Higher satisfaction rates were seen in patients who felt they were well informed about the procedure prior to surgery and in patients with fewer post-operative complications [45].

Sentinel Lymph Node Biopsy in the Setting of Risk-Reducing Mastectomy

Sentinel lymph node biopsy is used selectively in patients undergoing prophylactic mastectomy to avoid axillary dissection if invasive malignancy is identified in the mastectomy specimen. Occult breast cancers are detected in 5 and 8% of prophylactic mastectomy specimens, and axillary lymph node dissection would usually be required if sentinel lymph node biopsy had not been performed at the time of mastectomy.

Use of pre-operative MRI has been considered as an alternative to sentinel node biopsy. Recent studies have demonstrated that the use of pre-operative breast MRI in patients undergoing bilateral prophylactic surgery can identify occult invasive breast cancers [46, 47]. An algorithm for selective use of sentinel lymph node biopsy in patients undergoing prophylactic mastectomy is presented in Fig. 4.2.

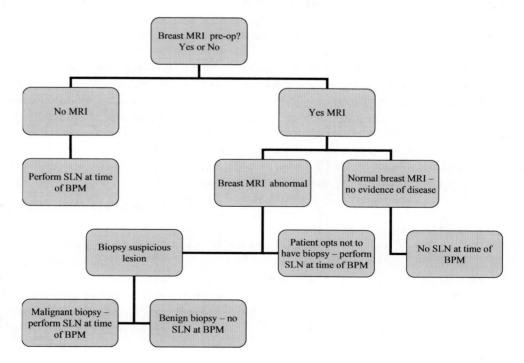

Fig. 4.2 Decision tree for the use of sentinel lymph node biopsy in patients undergoing prophylactic mastectomy (SLN: sentinel lymph node biopsy; BPM: bilateral prophylactic mastectomy)

Sentinel node mapping for a prophylactic mastectomy is the same as for mapping in cancer patients. Technetium sulfur colloid, methylene blue dye or isosulfan blue dye is injected in the subareolar area, and nodes taking up the dye excised for histopathological analysis. The sentinel node may be excised through the mastectomy or through a separate axillary incision. Addition of sentinel lymph node biopsy adds little to the morbidity or complication rate of a mastectomy.

Breast Cancer Screening After Prophylactic Mastectomy

After bilateral prophylactic mastectomy, a physical exam including careful manual palpation of the chest wall should be performed on an annual basis. The goal of the exam is to detect any palpable lesions in the skin of the chest wall or axilla that may represent breast cancer. Imaging with mammography, ultrasound or breast MRI is not recommended after prophylactic mastectomy. BRCA mutation carriers should also continue high-risk ovarian cancer screening.

Surgical Management of BRCA 1 or 2 Carriers with a New Cancer Diagnosis

For some patients, a BRCA gene mutation is identified by genetic testing performed after a new diagnosis of breast cancer. Treatment decisions for such women must address the management of the current cancer and also address the management of future breast cancer risk. Patients and their physicians may consider bilateral mastectomies to provide both treatment and prevention, or breast conserving therapy with high-risk screening, risk-reducing bilateral salpingo-oophorectomy and tamoxifen chemoprevention.

Current breast cancer treatments are equally effective against tumors in BRCA mutation carriers as for sporadic tumors. Pierce et al found no difference in outcome following breast conserving therapy in 71 BRCA1/2 mutation carriers with stage I or II breast cancer compared with 213 women with sporadic breast cancer. Five-year actuarial overall survival, relapse-free survival, and rates of tumor control in the treated breast for the patients in the genetic cohort were 86, 78, and 98%, respectively, compared with 91, 80, and 96%, respectively, for the sporadic cohort ($P =$NS) [48].

Mutation carriers are, however, at substantial risk for new ipsilateral and contralateral primary cancers [49–53] and may opt for bilateral mastectomy for both treatment and prevention when diagnosed with early stage breast cancer.

In 491 BRCA1 and BRCA2 carriers diagnosed with breast cancer, actuarial risk of contralateral breast cancer at 10 years was 29.5% [54]. For women who did not have an oophorectomy or take tamoxifen, the 10-year risk of contralateral cancer was 43.4% for BRCA1 carriers and 34.6% for BRCA2 carriers.

Pierce et al. compared outcomes after breast-conserving therapy in160 BRCA mutation carriers and 445 sporadic breast cancer controls [49]. After 15 years' follow-up, 39% of BRCA carriers had developed contralateral breast cancer, compared with 7% of controls. Rates of in breast recurrence were higher compared with controls in mutation carriers who had not undergone a bilateral prophylactic salpingo-oophorectomy.

Among 87 BRCA gene mutation carriers who underwent breast conserving therapy for 95 invasive breast tumors 5-year and 10-year probabilities of metachronous ipsilateral breast carcinoma were 11.2 and 13.6%, respectively, similar to rates seen after breast conservation for sporadic cancers. The 5-year and 10-year probabilities of metachronous contralateral breast carcinoma after the treatment of the index tumor were 11.9 and 37.6% [53].

The radiation required for breast conserving therapy can limit reconstruction options for patients who develop an ipsilateral recurrence or new primary breast cancer. Although single stage implant or expander reconstructions are sometimes possible, complication rates and implant loss rates are increased and the cosmetic outcome is less favorable after radiation. Autologous tissue reconstructions are usually preferred in previously irradiated tissue, but still have substantial complication rates. A 30% peri-operative complication rate was seen in 58 patients who underwent mastectomy and latissimus dorsi/implant reconstruction for recurrent breast cancer in a previously irradiated breast [55]. Cosmetic outcome at 4-year follow-up was good to excellent cosmetic in only 70% of patients.

Given their risk of future ipsilateral and contralateral breast cancers, some gene mutation carriers may elect bilateral mastectomies with implant or expander reconstruction at the time of initial cancer diagnosis rather than the risk of bilateral autologous tissue reconstruction for recurrent breast cancer.

Hereditary Ovarian Cancer

Ovarian cancer is the leading cause of death due to a gynecologic malignancy and is the fourth most common cause of cancer death in the United States. Approximately 21,550 women will be diagnosed with epithelial ovarian cancer in the United States in 2009, with an estimated 14,600 deaths [56]. The high mortality associated with ovarian cancer is due at least in part to the high incidence of metastatic disease at initial presentation. In contrast to breast cancer, there are no effective screening methods that permit early detection of ovarian cancer.

Approximately 10% of epithelial ovarian cancer cases are the result of a familial or inherited syndrome. Three familial ovarian cancer syndromes have been described: (1) Breast–ovarian cancer syndrome; (2) Site-specific ovarian cancer syndrome, and; (3) Lynch/hereditary non-polyposis colorectal cancer (HNPCC) syndrome [57].

Table 4.3 Efficacy of bilateral prophylactic oophorectomy

Author	Follow-up	Breast cancer incidence	Ovarian cancer incidence
Rebbeck [8]	8.8 years	BPO+, 21/99 (21.2%) BPO−, 60/142 (43.2%)	BPO+, 2/259 (0.8%) BPO−, 58/292 (19.9%)
Kauff [66]	24.2 months	BPO+, 3/98 (3%) BPO−, 8/72 (11%)	BPO+, 1/98 (1%) BPO−, 5/72 (7%)
Finch [70]	3.5 years	Not reported	BPO+, 7/1045 (0.6%) BPO−, 32/783 (4%)
Kauff [68]	3 years	BPO+, 19/303 (6.3%) BPO−, 28/294 (9.5%)	BPO+, 3/509 (0.5%) BPO−, 12/283 (4.2%)

BPO, bilateral prophylactic oophorectomy

Bilateral Prophylactic Salpingo-Oophrectomy for BRCA Carriers

Women with the breast–ovarian cancer syndrome carry germline mutations in one of the breast cancer susceptibility genes, BRCA1 or BRCA2. BRCA gene mutation carriers have an approximately tenfold greater risk of developing ovarian cancer than of a woman without a mutation [58–61]. The estimated lifetime risk of developing ovarian cancer for a BRCA1 mutation carrier is 35–50% and 15–25% for a BRCA2 mutation carrier [58–61]. Women with a BRCA mutation also have an increased risk of developing fallopian tube and peritoneal cancer, with an estimated 0.6% lifetime risk of primary fallopian tube cancer and 1.3% lifetime risk of primary peritoneal cancer [62].

For women with Lynch syndrome, the estimated lifetime risk of ovarian and endometrial cancer is 13 and 60%, respectively [63]. Given the increased risk of developing ovarian and fallopian tube cancer among women with these syndromes, as well as the limited efficacy of current technology for achieving early detection, bilateral salpingo-oophorectomy (BSO) is an appropriate strategy for risk reduction.

Efficacy of Risk-Reducing Bilateral Salpingo-Oophorectomy

Several studies have demonstrated the efficacy of risk-reducing BSO in lowering the risk of ovarian, fallopian tube, peritoneal, and breast cancer [8, 63–69] (Table 4.3). In a prospective study including, 1,828 women with a BRCA1 or BRCA2 mutation and no clinical evidence of ovarian, fallopian tube, or peritoneal cancer, BSO resulted in an 80% reduction in ovarian cancer risk (mean follow-up of 3.5 years, hazard ratio 0.20; 95% CI 0.07–0.58) [70]. Another prospective of women with a BRCA1 or BRCA2 mutation showed that women who underwent risk-reducing BSO had a lower ovarian cancer-specific mortality (hazard ratio 0.05, 95% CI 0.01–0.46) and overall mortality (hazard ratio 0.24, 95% CI 0.08–0.71) compared to women who did not undergo BSO [71].

Studies of women with a BRCA1 or BRCA2 mutation have identified occult fallopian tube cancers at the time of prophylactic surgery, supporting the role of removal of both fallopian tubes in risk-reducing surgery. In a study of 483 women with a BRCA1 mutation, a 120-fold increased risk of a primary fallopian tube cancer was seen, compared to population-based estimates [72]. In another series of 159 women with a BRCA mutation, seven occult cancers were reported (3 involving both ovaries and fallopian tubes; 3 involving only the fallopian tubes, and 1 involving only the ovary) [73].

Women with a hereditary predisposition for ovarian/fallopian tube cancer remain at risk of developing a primary peritoneal cancer after risk-reducing BSO. Primary peritoneal cancer diffusely involves the peritoneal surfaces lining the abdomen and pelvis, clinically behaving like stage III ovarian cancer [74, 75]. In a review of 846 patients from five studies, the risk of a primary peritoneal cancer was reported to be 1.7% following risk-reducing BSO [76]. In a prospective study of 1,045 BRCA mutation carriers, the cumulative incidence of primary peritoneal cancer was 4.4% over 20 years' follow-up after risk-reducing BSO [70]. Women with a BRCA1 mutation may have a higher risk of a peritoneal malignancy than those with a BRCA2 mutation.

As discussed earlier, risk-reducing BSO also reduces the risk of breast cancer by approximately 50% in premenopausal women with BRCA gene mutations [8, 68].

Risk-Reducing Ovarian Cancer Surgery

The risk of detecting an occult gynecologic malignancy at the time of risk-reducing surgery is in the 4–8% range [73, 76–78]. The tumor may be obvious at the time of surgery or noted on final histopathology. This possibility of encountering malignancy at risk-reducing surgery must be discussed with the patient pre-operatively and consent obtained for a full staging procedure should occult malignancy of the ovary or fallopian tubes be discovered at the time of risk-reducing surgery.

The preferred surgical procedure for risk reduction is a laparoscopic BSO. A hysterectomy is generally not indicated as part of risk-reducing surgery for ovarian risk. Laparoscopic removal of both ovaries and fallopian tubes is favored given the low risk of morbidity. The abdomen and the pelvis should be methodically inspected. Careful attention should be given to the hemidiaphragms, the omentum, paracolic gutters, appendix, bowel, cul-de-sac, uterus, fallopian tubes, and ovaries. The surgery should include a peritoneal lavage, and biopsy of any suspicious areas [79, 80]. It is imperative to remove all ovarian tissue and as much of the fallopian tubes as possible. We recommend transecting the ovarian artery and vein at the pelvic brim to assure removal of all ovarian tissue. In order to carry this out safely, identification of the ureter and isolation the infudibulopelvic ligament from other structures prior to transaction is recommended.

As much of the fallopian tube as possible should be resected. Complete resection of the cornual end of the fallopian tube is not possible, especially through a laparoscopic approach. To date, there have been no reported cases of fallopian tube malignancies arising from the cornual end of the fallopian tube [81]. Given the risk of occult malignancy, pathologic analysis of excised specimens should include serial sectioning of both ovaries and fallopian tubes in their entirety [77].

Timing of Risk-Reducing BSO

The mean age at diagnosis for hereditary ovarian cancer is 48–51 years of age [75]. Although the surgical risks of laparoscopic BSO are small, the timing of the surgery needs to be carefully weighed against the patient's desire to maintain fertility and against other considerations such as premature menopause. Evidence suggests that the benefit of risk-reducing BSO decreases with age [67, 75]. It is generally recommended that BSO surgery take place as soon as a woman completes childbearing or no later than age 35. This recommendation is based on the fact that annual risk of developing ovarian cancer in women with a BRCA1 mutation becomes significant starting at age 35. For women with a BRCA2 mutation, ovarian cancer risk becomes more significant at approximately age 45. Women with the BRCA2 mutation who delay risk-reducing surgery until their forties may not gain the benefit BSO confers on risk reduction for breast cancer [82].

Concurrent Hysterectomy

Hysterectomy at the time of risk-reducing BSO is generally not recommended as it adds surgical risk but provides no significant survival benefit. Risk-reducing hysterectomy should, however, be considered in a subset of women. Women with a Lynch/HNPCC mutation have an increased risk of developing both endometrial and ovarian cancer and should undergo both hysterectomy and BSO when risk-reducing surgery is performed [83].

Women planning to take tamoxifen, for breast cancer prevention should also consider hysterectomy at the time of risk-reducing BSO as tamoxifen use is associated with an increased risk of endometrial cancer [75]. Women considering unopposed estrogen replacement therapy after risk-reducing BSO should also consider a hysterectomy as unopposed estrogen use is also associated with an increased risk of endometrial cancer.

Data on the association of endometrial cancer with the BRCA mutation is controversial. While some studies have documented an increased risk of serous endometrial cancer in women with BRCA mutations, others have refuted it [84–87]. Since the data is inconclusive and the risk of serous endometrial cancer in these women seems to be low, risk-reducing BSO without concurrent hysterectomy is favored for women with a BRCA1 or BRCA2 mutation [88]. It is important to highlight the fact that the risk that a woman undergoing risk-reducing BSO will require hysterectomy at a later date is small. In a series of 44 women undergoing risk-reducing BSO, only four subsequently underwent hysterectomy [89].

In summary, women with a hereditary predisposition for ovarian, fallopian tube and peritoneal cancer should be offered risk-reducing surgery, preferably a laparoscopic BSO, as soon as they have completed childbearing or by age 35. A concurrent hysterectomy is generally not recommended except for women with special circumstances for whom the benefit of the procedure outweighs the added surgical risks.

References

1. Ford D, Easton DF, Stratton M et al (1998) Genetic heterogeneity and penetrance analysis of the BRCA1 and BRCA2 genes in breast cancer families. Am J Hum Genet 62:676–689
2. Antoniou A, Pharoah PD, Narod S et al (2003) Average risks of breast and ovarian cancer associated with BRCA1 or BRCA2 mutations detected in case series unselected for family history: a combined analysis of 22 studies. Am J Hum Genet 72:1117–1130
3. King MC, Marks JH, Mandell JB (2003) Breast and ovarian cancer risks due to inherited mutations in BRCA1 and BRCA2. Science 302:643–646
4. Chen S, Iverson ES, Friebel T et al (2006) Characterization of BRCA1 and BRCA2 mutations in a large United States sample. J Clin Oncol 24:863–871

5. Hartmann LC, Sellers TA, Schaid DJ et al (2001) Efficacy of bilateral prophylactic mastectomy in women with a family history of breast cancer. J Natl Canc Inst 93:1633–1637

6. Rebbeck TR, Friebel T, Lynch HT et al (2004) Bilateral prophylactic mastectomy reduces breast cancer risk in BRCA1 and BRCA2 mutation carriers: the PROSE Study Group. J Clin Oncol 22:1055–1062

7. Meijers-Heijboer H, van Geel B, van Putten WL et al (2001) Breast cancer after prophylactic mastectomy in women with a BRCA 1 or 2 mutation. N Engl J Med 354:159–164

8. Rebbeck TR et al (2002) The Prevention and Observation of Surgical End Points Study Group: prophylactic oophorectomy in carriers of BRCA 1 or BRCA2 mutations. N Eng J Med 346:1616–1622

9. Ray J, Loescher L, Brewer M (2005) Risk-reduction surgery decisions in high-risk women seen for genetic counseling. J Genet Couns 14:473–484

10. Uyei A, Peterson SK, Erlichman J et al (2006) Association between clinical characteristics and risk-reduction interventions in women who underwent BRCA1 and BRCA2 testing. Cancer 107:2745–2751

11. Beattie MS, Crawford B, Lin F et al (2009) Uptake, time course and predictors of risk-reducing surgeries in BRCA carriers. Genet Test Mol Biosmarkers 13:51–56

12. Litton JK, Westin SN, Ready K et al (2009) Perception of screening and risk reduction surgeries in patients tested for a BRCA deleterious mutation. Cancer 115:1598–1604

13. Frost MH, Schaid DJ, Sellers TA et al (2000) Long-term satisfaction and psychological and social function following bilateral prophylactic mastectomy. JAMA 284:319–324

14. Geiger AM, Nekhlyudov L, Herrinton LJ et al (2006) Quality of life after bilateral prophylactic mastectomy. Ann Surg Oncol 14:686–694

15. Van Oostrom I, Meijers-Heijboer H, Lodder LN et al (2003) Long-term psychologic impact of carrying a BRCA1/2 mutation and prophylactic surgery: a 5-year follow-up study. J Clin Oncol 21:3867–3874

16. Li FP, Fraumeni JF Jr, Mulvihill JJ et al (1988) A cancer family syndrome in twenty-four kindreds. Cancer Res 48:5358–5362

17. Sidransky D, Tokino T, Helzlsouer K et al (1992) Inherited p53 gene mutations in breast cancer. Cancer Res 52:2984–2986

18. Birch JM, Alston RD, McNally RJ et al (2001) Relative frequency and morphology of cancers in carriers of germline TP53 mutations. Oncogene 20:4621–4628

19. Chompret A, Brugieres L, Ronsin M et al (2000) P53 germline mutations in childhood cancers and cancer risk for carrier individuals. Br J Cancer 82:1932–1937

20. Le Bihan C, Bonaiti-Pellie C (1994) A method for estimating cancer risk in p53 mutation carriers. Cancer Detect Prev 18:171–178

21. Eng C (2003) PTEN: one gene, many syndromes. Hum Mutat 22:183–198

22. Starink TM, van der Veen JP, Arwert F et al (1986) The Cowden syndrome: a clinical and genetic study in 21 patients. Clin Genet 29:222–233

23. Pharoah P, Guilford P, Caldas C et al (2001) Incidence of gastric cancer and breast cancer in CDH1 (E-cadherin) mutation carriers from hereditary diffuse gastric cancer families. Gastroenterology 121:1348–1353

24. Norton JA, Ham CM, Van Dam J et al (2007) CDH1 truncating mutations in the E-cadherin gene an indication for total gastrectomy to treat hereditary diffuse gastric cancer. Ann Surg 245:873–879

25. Beer GM, Varga Z, Budi S, Seifert B, Meyer VE (2002) Incidence of the superficial fascia and its relevance in skin-sparing mastectomy. Cancer 94:1619–1625

26. Ho CM, Mak CK, Lau Y, Cheung WY, Chan MC, Hung WK (2003) Skin involvement in invasive breast carcinoma: safety of skin-sparing mastectomy. Ann Surg Oncol 10:102–107

27. Carlson GW, Styblo TM, Lyles RH, Jones G, Murray DR, Staley CA et al (2003) The use of skin sparing mastectomy in the treatment of breast cancer: The Emory experience. Surg Oncol 12:265–269

28. Gerber B, Krause A, Reimer T, Muller H, Kuchenmeister I, Makovitzky J et al (2003) Skin-sparing mastectomy with conservation of the nipple-areola complex and autologous reconstruction is an oncologically safe procedure. Ann Surg 238:120–127

29. Greenway RM, Schlossberg L, Dooley WC (2005) Fifteen-year series of skin-sparing mastectomy for stage 0 to 2 breast cancer. Am J Surg 190:918–922

30. Kroll SS, Khoo A, Singletary SE, Ames FC, Wang BG, Reece GP et al (1999) Local recurrence risk after skin-sparing and conventional mastectomy: a 6-year follow-up. Plast Reconstr Surg 104:421–425

31. Spiegel AJ, Butler CE (2003) Recurrence following treatment of ductal carcinoma in situ with skin-sparing mastectomy and immediate breast reconstruction. Plast Reconstr Surg 111:706–711

32. Drucker-Zertuche M, Robles-Vidal C (2007) A 7-year experience with immediate breast reconstruction after skin sparing mastectomy for cancer. Eur J Surg Oncol 33:140–146

33. Carlson GW, Page A, Johnson E et al (2007) Local recurrence of ductal carcinoma in situ after skin-sparing mastectomy. J Am Coll Surg 204:1074–1080

34. Salhab M, Al Sarakbi W, Joseph A et al (2006) Skin-sparing mastectomy and immediate breast reconstruction: patient satisfaction and clinical outcomes. In J Clin Oncol 11:51–54

35. Chung A, Sacchini V (2008) Nipple-sparing mastectomy: where are we now? Surg Oncol 17:261–266

36. Rusby JE, Kirstein LJ, Brachtel EF, Taghian AG, Michaelson JS, Koerner FC, Smith BL et al (2008) Nipple sparing mastectomy: lessons from ex-vivo procedures. Breast J 14:464–470

37. Crowe JP Jr, Kim JA, Yetman R, Banbury J, Patrick RJ, Baynes D (2004) Nipple-sparing mastectomy: technique and results of 54 procedures. Arch Surg 139:148–150

38. Crowe JP, Patrick RJ, Yetman RJ, Djohan R (2008) Nipple-sparing mastectomy update: one hundred forty-nine procedures and clinical outcomes. Arch Surg 143:1106–1110

39. Stolier AJ, Sullivan SK, Dellacroce FJ (2008) Technical considerations in nipple-sparing mastectomy: 82 consecutive cases without necrosis. Ann Surg Oncol 15:1341–1347

40. Caruso F, Ferrara M, Castiglione G, Trombetta G, De Meo L, Catanuto G et al (2006) Nipple sparing subcutaneous mastectomy: sixty-six months follow-up. Eur J Surg Oncol 32:937–940

41. Petit JY, Veronesi U, Orecchia R, Luini A, Rey P, Intra M et al (2006) Nipple-sparing mastectomy in association with intra operative radiotherapy (ELIOT): a new type of mastectomy for breast cancer treatment. Breast Cancer Res Treat 96:47–51

42. Sacchini V, Pinotti JA, Barros AS et al (2006) Nipple-sparing mastectomy for breast cancer and risk reduction: oncologic or technical problem? J Am Coll Surg 203:704–714

43. Brachtel EF, Rusby JE, Michaelson JS, Smith BL, Koerner FC (2009) Occult nipple involvement in breast cancer: Clinicopathologic findings in 316 consecutive mastectomy specimens. J Clin Oncol 27:4948–4954

44. Wijayanayagam A, Kumar AS, Foster RD, Esserman LJ (2008) Optimizing the total skin-sparing mastectomy. Arch Surg 143:38–45

45. Bresser PJ, Seynaeve C, Van Gool AR et al (2006) Satisfaction with prophylactic surgery and breast reconstruction in genetically predisposed women. Plast Reconstr Surg 118:1496–1497

46. Black DS, Specht MC, Lee JM et al (2007) Detecting occult malignancy in prophylactic mastectomy: preoperative MRI vs. sentinel lymph node biopsy. Ann Surg Oncol 14:2477–2484

47. McLaughlin SA, Stempal M, Morris EA, Liberman L, King TA (2007) Can magnetic resonance imaging be used to select patients for sentinel lymph node biopsy in prophylactic mastectomy? Cancer 112:1214–1221

48. Pierce LJ, Strawderman M, Narod SA et al (2000) Effect of radiotherapy after breast-conserving treatment in women with breast cancer and germline BRCA1/2 mutations. J Clin Oncol 19:3360–3369

49. Pierce LJ, Levin AM, Rebbeck TR et al (2006) Ten-year multi-institutional results of breast conserving surgery and radiotherapy in BRCA ½-associated Stage I or II breast cancer. J Clin Oncol 24:2437–2443

50. De Bock GH, Tollenaar RA, Papelard H et al (2001) Clinical and pathological features of BRCA 1 associated carcinomas in a hospital-based sample of Dutch breast cancer patients. Br J Cancer 85: 347–350

51. Lakhani SR, van De Vijver MJ, Jacquemier J et al (2002) The pathology of familial breast cancer: predictive value of immunohistochemical markers estrogen receptor, progesterone receptor, HER2, and p53 in patients with mutations in BRCA 1 and BRCA2. J Clin Oncol 20:2310–2318

52. Veronesi A, de Giacomi C, Magri MD et al (2005) Familial breast cancer: characteristics and outcome of BRCA1-2 positive and negative cases. BMC Cancer 5:70–75

53. Robson M, Svahn T, McCormick B et al (2005) Appropriateness of breast-conserving treatment of breast carcinoma in women with germline mutations in BRCA1 or BRCA2: a clinic-based series. Cancer 103:44–51

54. Metcalfe K, Lynch HT, Ghadirian P et al (2004) Contralateral breast cancer in BRCA1 and BRCA2 mutation carriers. J Clin Oncol 22:2328–2335

55. Disa JJ, McCarthy CM, Mehrara BJ, Pusic AL, Cordeiro PG (2008) Immediate latissimus dorsi/prosthetic breast reconstruction following salvage mastectomy after failed lumpectomy/irradiation. Plastic Reconstr Surg 121:159–164

56. ACS (2009) Cancer facts and figures 2009, American Cancer Society, Atlanta, GA

57. Garber JE, Offit K (2005) Hereditary cancer predisposition syndromes. J Clin Oncol 23:276–292

58. Struewing JP, Hartge P, Wacholder S et al (1997) The risk of cancer associated with specific mutations of BRCA1 and BRCA2 among Ashkenazi Jews. N Engl J Med 336:1401–1408

59. Frank TS (2001) Hereditary cancer syndromes. Arch Pathol Lab Med 125:85–90

60. Chen S, Parmigiani G (2007) Meta-analysis of BRCA1 and BRCA2 penetrance. J Clin Oncol 25:1329–1333

61. Ford D, Easton DF, Bishop DT et al (1994) Risk of cancer in BRCA1 mutation carriers. Lancet 343:692–695

62. Levine DA, Argenta PA, Yee CJ et al (2005) Fallopian tube and primary peritoneal carcinomas associated with BRCA mutations. J Clin Oncol 21:4222–4227

63. Struewing JP, Watson P, Eaton DF et al (1995) Prophylactic oophorectomy in inherited breast/ovarian cancer families. J Natl Cancer Inst Monogr 17:33–35

64. Weber BL, Punzalan C, Eisen A et al (2000) Ovarian cancer risk reduction after bilateral prophylactic oophorectomy in BRCA1 and BRCA2 mitation carriers. Am Soc Hum Genet 67(Suppl 2):59 (abstract 251)

65. Piver MS, Jishi MF, Tsukada Y, Nava G (1993) Primary peritoneal carcinoma after prophylactic oophorectomy in women with a family history of ovarian cancer. A report of the Gilda Radner Familial Ovarian Cancer Registry. Cancer 71:2751–2755

66. Kauff ND, Satagopan JM, Robson ME et al (2002) Risk-reducing salpingo-oophorectomy in women with a BRCA 1 or BRCA 2 mutation. N Engl J Med 346:1609–1615

67. Schrag D, Kuntz KM, Garber JE, Weeks JC (1997) Decision analysis-effects of prophylactic mastectomy and oophorectomy on life expectancy among women with BRCA1 or BRCA2 mutations. N Engl J Med 336:1465–1471

68. Kauff ND, Domchek SM, Friebel TM et al (2008) Risk-reducing salpingo-oophrectomy for the prevention of BRCA 1 and BRCA 2 associated breast and gynecologic cancer: A multicenter, prospective study. J Clin Oncol 26:1331–1337

69. Rosen B, Kwon K, Fung K, Fung M et al (2004) Systematic review of management options of women with a hereditary predisposition to ovarian cancer. Gynecol Oncol 93:280–286

70. Finch A, Beiner M, Lubinski J et al (2006) Salpingo-oophrectomy in women with a BRCA 1 or BRCA2 mutation. JAMA 296:185–192

71. Domchek SM, Friebel TM, Neuhausen SL et al (2006) Mortality after bilateral salpingo-oophorectomy for the prevention of BRCA1 and BRCA2 mutation carriers: a prospective cohort study. Lancet Oncol 7:223–229

72. Brose MS, Rebbeck TR, Calzone KA et al (2002) Cancer risk estimates for BRCA1 mutation carriers indentified in a risk evaluation program. J Natl Cancer Inst 94:1365–1372

73. Finch A, Shaw P, Rosen B et al (2006) Clinical and pathologic findings of prophylactic salpingo-oophorectomies in 159 BRCA1 and BRCA2 mutation carriers. Gynecol Oncol 100:58–64

74. Zhou J, Iwasa Y, Konishi I et al (1995) Papillary serous carcinoma of the peritoneum in women. A clinicopathologic and immunohistochemical study. Cancer 76:429–436

75. Eisen A, Rebbeck TR, Wood WC, Webber BL (2000) Prophylactic surgery in women with a hereditary predisposition to breast and ovarian cancer. J Clin Oncol 18:1980–1995

76. Dowdy SC, Stefanek M, Hartmann LC (2004) Surgical risk reduction: prophylactic salpingo-oophorectomy and prophylactic mastectomy. Am J Obstet Gynecol 191:1113–1123

77. Powell CB, Kenley E, Chen LM et al (2005) Risk-reducing salpingo-oophorectomy in BRCA mutation carriers: role of serial sectioning in the detection of occult malignancy. J Clin Oncol 23:127–132

78. Powell CB (2006) Occult ovarian cancer at the time of risk-reducing salpingo-oophorectomy. Gynecol Oncol 100:1

79. Guillem JG, Wood WC, Moley JF et al (2006) ASCO/SSO review of current role of risk-reducing surgery in common hereditary cancer syndromes. J Clin Oncol 24:4642–4660

80. Lu KH, Garber JE, Cramer DW et al (2000) Occult ovarian tumors in women with BRCA1 or BRCA2 mutations undergoing prophylactic oophorectomy. J Clin Oncol 18:2728–2732

81. Kauff ND, Barakat RR (2004) Surgical risk-reduction in carriers of BRCA mutations: where do we go from here? Gynecol Oncol 93:277–279

82. (2005) Society of Gynecologic Oncologists Clinical Practice Committee Statement on Prophylactic Salpingo-oophorectomy. Gynecol Oncol 98:179–181

83. Watson P, Lynch HT (1993) Extracolonic cancer in hereditary non-polyposis colorectal cancer. Cancer 71:677–685

84. Lavie O, Hornreich G, Ben Arie A et al (2000) BRCA1 germline mutations in women with uterine serous papillary carcinoma. Obstet Gynecol 96:28–32

85. Hornreich G, Beller U, Lavie O et al (1999) Is uterine serous papillary carcinoma a BRACA1-related disease? Case report and review of the literature. Gynecol Oncol 75:300–304

86. Lavie O, Hornreich G, Ben Arie A et al (2004) BRCA germline mutations in Jewish women with uterine serous papillary carcinoma. Gynecol Oncol 92:521–524

87. Goshen R, Chu W, Elit L et al (2000) Is uterine papillary serous adenocarcinoma a manifestation of the hereditary breast-ovarian cancer syndrome? Gynecol Oncol 79:477–481

88. Rubinstein WS (2005) Surgical management of BRCA1 and BRCA2 carriers: bitter choices slightly sweetened. J Clin Oncol 23:7772–7774

89. Villella JA, Parmar M, Donohue K et al (2006) Role of prophylactic hysterectomy in patients at high risk for hereditary cancers. Gynecol Oncol 102:475–479

Chapter 5
Hereditary Colon Cancer: Colonic Polyposis Syndromes

Andrew T. Chan and Daniel C. Chung

Keywords Familial Adenomatous Polyposis • MYH-Associated Polyposis • Juvenile Polyposis • Peutz-Jeghers Syndrome • PTEN-Hamartoma Syndrome • Hyperplastic Polyposis • APC • MYH • LKB1 • MADH4 • BMPR1A • PTEN

Introduction

In the U.S., the lifetime risk of colorectal cancer among both men and women is approximately 6% [1]. Although as many as 25% of colorectal cancers are associated with a family history of the disease, approximately 3–5% of cases arise in the setting of well-described familial genetic syndromes [2]. The most prevalent familial colorectal cancer syndrome is Lynch syndrome or hereditary nonpolyposis colorectal cancer (HNPCC). Patients with Lynch do not present clinically with an unusually heavy burden of adenomatous polyps, the precursor to the vast majority of colorectal cancers. On the other hand, the remaining 1–2% of hereditary colorectal cancer syndromes are characterized by significant polyposis. These syndromes can be broadly classified as adenomatous polyposis syndromes, hamartomatous polyposis syndromes, and the hyperplastic polyposis syndrome (Table 5.1). In this chapter, we review the salient clinical and genetic features of each of these polyposis syndromes.

Adenomatous Polyposis Syndromes

The adenomatous polyp syndromes include familial adenomatous polyposis (FAP), attenuated familial adenomatous polyposis (AFAP), and MUTYH-associated polyposis

(MAP). Collectively, they have provided tremendous insights into the molecular and pathological changes in the adenoma to carcinoma sequence that characterizes the development of the vast majority of sporadic colorectal cancers. However, the substantially greater burden of polyps that present at an earlier age among patients with these syndromes results in an almost certain risk of colorectal cancer when compared to patients with sporadic adenomas.

FAP/Attenuated FAP

Clinical Features/Distinguishing Characteristics

FAP is the most common polyposis syndrome, with an estimated prevalence of one in 5,000–7,500 individuals [3]. FAP is transmitted in an autosomal-dominant manner, with 100% penetrance. As perhaps the most dramatic of the colorectal cancer syndromes, the key distinguishing feature of classic FAP is the development of hundreds to thousands of adenomatous polyps throughout the colon, often beginning as early as the second decade of life (Fig. 5.1). Colorectal adenocarcinomas inevitably develop, typically by age 40, or approximately 10–15 years after the initial appearance of polyposis. In contrast, the vast majority of sporadic colorectal cancers are diagnosed after age 50, with a median age of 71 [4].

Individuals with AFAP may be more difficult to distinguish from those who develop sporadic adenomas or cancers. Although some AFAP patients can develop polyp numbers that are similar to classic FAP patients, they typically present with an oligopolyposis phenotype with fewer than 100 adenomas. The cumulative lifetime risk of colorectal cancer is not as high as in classic FAP but is still estimated to be at least 69%. The older age of diagnosis (age 50–60) can overlap with the ages more typically seen in sporadic cancer, making clinical recognition of the syndrome more challenging. In addition, polyps and cancer in AFAP tend to arise in the right colon and may have a "flat" morphology [5]. Although some AFAP patients may have a polyposis phenotype that is not dissimilar to classic FAP,

A.T. Chan (✉) and D.C. Chung (✉)
GI Cancer Genetics Program, Gastrointestinal Unit and Cancer Center, MA, USA;
Harvard Medical School, Boston, MA, USA
e-mail: achan@partners.org; dchung@partners.org

Table 5.1 Inherited colonic polyposis syndromes

Syndrome	Genes	Inheritance pattern	Risk of colorectal cancer (CRC)	Average age of diagnosis of CRC (years)	Number of polyps	Polyp histology	Predominant location of polyps/cancer in colon	Extracolonic features
High risk								
Classic familial adenomatous polyposis (FAP)	APC	Autosomal dominant	100%	39	Hundreds to thousands	Adenomatous	Entire colon	Fundic gland polyps, duodenal/ampullary adenomas, desmoid tumors, thyroid tumors, brain tumors, osteomas, CHRPE
Attenuated FAP (AFAP)	APC	Autosomal dominant	69%	56	<100	Adenomatous	Proximal colon	Fundic gland polyps, duodenal/ampullary adenomas
MYH associated polyposis (MAP)	MYH	Autosomal recessive	80%	50 [52]	<100, but highly variable	Adenomatous	Entire colon	Undetermined
Lynch/hereditary non-polyposis colorectal cancer (HNPCC)	MLH1, MSH2, MSH6, PMS2	Autosomal dominant	60–80%	45	Few	Adenomatous	Proximal colon	Tumors of the uterus, ovary, stomach, urinary tract, biliary tree, small intestine, and skin
Moderate risk								
Peutz-Jegher's syndrome (PJS)	LKB1	Autosomal dominant	39% [71]	45 [71]	Few	Hamartomatous	Entire colon	Mucocutaneous pigmentation, tumors of the uterus, breast, lungs, reproductive organs, pancreas, and gallbladder
Juvenile polyposis syndrome (JPS)	MADH4, BMPR1A, ENG	Autosomal dominant	10–38% [106–108]	34 [109]	Few	Hamartomatous	Entire colon	Tumors of the stomach and duodenum, HHT
Hyperplastic polyposis syndrome (HPS)	Unknown	Unknown	25–35% [110, 111]	66 [112]	Many	Hyperplastic/serrated	Entire colon	None described
Low risk								
Bloom's syndrome	BLM	Autosomal recessive	8% [113]	33 [113]	Few	Adenomatous	Entire colon	Leukemia, lymphoma, carcinomas of the head and neck, respiratory tract, female reproductive organs, breast, and upper gastrointestinal tract
I1307K APC polymorphism	APC	Autosomal dominant	8–11% [114]	64–70 [115]	Few	Adenomatous	Entire colon	None described
Cowden's syndrome	PTEN	Autosomal dominant	Low		Multiple	Hamartomatous, juvenile, inflammatory, ganglioneuromas	Entire colon	Facial trichilemmoma, breast cancer, follicular thyroid cancer, endometrial cancer

CHRPE = congenital hypertrophy of the retinal pigmented epithelium, HHT = hereditary hemorrhagic telangiectasia

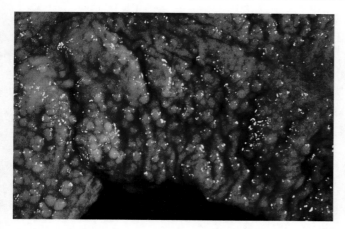

Fig. 5.1 Surgical specimen from a total colectomy for FAP. The entire mucosal surface is carpeted with small adenomatous polyps. (Photo courtesy of Fiona Graeme-Cook, MD, Massachusetts General Hospital Department of Pathology)

some patients display polyp numbers at the lower end of the spectrum that can be difficult to differentiate from Lynch syndrome [6].

Associated Extracolonic Manifestations

Individuals with FAP are at substantially higher risk of developing other gastrointestinal cancers. Duodenal, periampullary, or ampullary adenomas occur in over 90% of FAP patients, with approximately 10% of patients developing duodenal adenocarcinoma by age 60. The lifetime risk of periampullary and duodenal cancer is 3–5%, with many cancers often discovered incidentally during surgery for duodenal polyps [7]. Distal small bowel adenomas are common, but small bowel cancer is rare [8]. Gastric polyps, particularly fundic gland polyps, are also commonly observed. Although low-grade dysplasia is frequently found on the surface of these fundic gland polyps, the lifetime risk of gastric cancer is less than 1% [9]. Gastric adenomas and adenocarcinomas may be more prevalent among FAP kindreds from Japan and Korea [10]. In AFAP, the risk of upper gastrointestinal tract lesions appears to be comparable to the risk associated with classic FAP [6]. Interestingly, some studies have noted that patients with duodenal cancers have fewer colonic polyps than patients with ampullary cancers [7].

FAP is also associated with extraintestinal malignancies. Follicular and papillary thyroid cancers have been described in as many as 12% of FAP patients [11]. The cribiform morula variant of papillary thyroid cancer is particularly associated with FAP and can be the initial presentation of the syndrome. Turcot's syndrome describes families with hereditary colon cancer and central nervous system (CNS) tumors. Among FAP individuals, these are most commonly medulloblastomas and

more rarely gliomas. The lifetime risk of a CNS tumor in FAP is 1.5%. Hepatoblastomas are also associated with FAP in young children [12]. Finally, there has been a suggestion of an increased risk of pancreatic cancer in FAP [13].

Nonmalignant growths, such as osteomas, supernumerary teeth, epidermoid cysts, desmoid tumors, congenital hypertrophy of the retinal epithelium (CHRPE), adrenal adenomas, and nasal fibromas are also observed in FAP patients. The presence of any of these manifestations in the setting of colonic polyposis has been described as Gardner's syndrome. Osteomas, observed in approximately 20% of FAP patients, are bony growths that widely vary in size and number, often located in the jaw or mandible [14]. Dental anomalies such as supernumerary teeth are also common [15]. Although epidermoid cysts are frequently seen in the general population, they can present at a very early age and can precede the onset of polyposis [3]. Approximately 10% of FAP patients will develop desmoid tumors at an average age of 28–31 years [16]. Desmoid tumors are benign connective tissue tumors that most typically occur intraabdominally or in the tissues of the abdominal wall. Desmoids commonly develop after abdominal surgery, such as colectomy, but can also precede the onset of polyposis.

Despite their lack of metastatic potential, these tumors can be locally aggressive by encasing intraabdominal organs and recur despite treatment [17]. Thus, they can be a considerable source of morbidity and mortality. The estimated 10-year survival rate of FAP patients with desmoid tumors is 63%, ranking second as a cause of mortality in FAP behind metastatic colon or duodenal carcinoma [18]. CHRPE are common pigmented ocular fundus lesions that develop bilaterally. Although these are clinically inconsequential, detection of CHRPE lesions can serve as a useful diagnostic clue. Finally, associations with adrenal adenomas as well as nasal angiofibromas have been described in FAP [19, 20].

Genetics

In 1991, three groups identified mutations in the Adenomatous Polyposis Coli (APC) gene as the genetic alteration underlying FAP and AFAP [21–23]. Located on chromosome 5q21, the wild-type APC gene functions as a tumor suppressor that inhibits the oncogenic Wnt signaling pathway. A Wnt signal directs the translocation of β-catenin from the cell membrane into the nucleus, where it interacts with the transcription factor T-cell factor 4 (TCF4) to activate transcription of key growth-regulatory genes, including cyclinD1, c-Myc, PPAR-δ, and VEGF. Wild-type APC forms a complex with axin, β-catenin, and GSK-3β. GSK-3β subsequently phosphorylates β-catenin, which targets it for degradation as opposed to nuclear translocation. Mutations in the APC gene disrupt its binding to β-catenin, thereby inhibiting β-catenin phosphorylation. Excess β-catenin is translocated into the nucleus, resulting in constitutive activation of the Wnt pathway [24].

The APC gene contains 15 exons and 2,843 codons, encoding a large protein of 311.8 kD. Although mutations have been identified throughout each exon, most are found in the largest coding region, exon 15. More than 90% of the mutations in the APC gene are nonsense mutations that result in a truncated protein product [25]. More recently, deletions of all or part of the APC gene have been recognized as an alternative mechanism of gene inactivation in 12% of patients with classic polyposis but without an identifiable APC gene mutation [26].

Genotype/Phenotype Correlations

Specific germline mutations in the APC gene appear to correlate with phenotypic severity. Classic FAP is associated with mutations between codons 169 and 1393, and a particularly severe phenotype with very early onset of thousands of polyps is observed with mutations between codons 1,250 and 1,464, the so-called "mutation cluster region." APC gene deletions are also associated with a classic APC phenotype [26]. In contrast, mutations in the extreme 5′ (proximal to codon 157) and 3′ ends of the APC gene (distal to codon 1596), or in exon 9 correlate with AFAP [27]. One proposed mechanism for the attenuated phenotype is an alternate internal translation start site in attenuated APC alleles [28]. The I1307K allele in the APC gene found in 6% of Ashkenazi Jews appears to be associated with a particularly low disease penetrance, few adenomas, and an older age of onset, typically in the seventh decade of life (Fig. 5.2).

The location of mutations in the APC gene also correlates with specific extracolonic manifestions. For example, mutations distal to exon 9 and between codons 463 and 1,444 are associated with CHRPE while mutations between codons 1,310 and 2,011 are associated with desmoid tumors [29, 30]. Mutations between codons 976 and 1,067 appear to be related to a higher risk of duodenal adenomas. Medulloblastomas appear to be preferentially associated with mutations between codons 457 and 1,309 [31].

Genetic Testing

Genetic assays for mutations in the APC gene were one of the first commercially developed tests for cancer predisposition. These assays include DNA sequencing, conformation strand gel electrophoresis, protein truncation test, and linkage analysis. The current standard is full gene sequencing of all exons, exon–intron boundaries, and gene deletion analysis by Multiplex Ligation-Dependent Probe Amplification.

Evaluation of at-risk families should begin with individuals exhibiting polyposis to determine if a detectable mutation is present. If a mutation is identified in the affected individual (proband), then all at-risk family members can be tested for this specific family's mutation. The presence of the mutation in an at-risk family member is a true positive test result for the disease whereas the presence of a negative result in an at-risk family member is a true negative test result. Family members with a true negative test result do not require further evaluation for polyposis or more intensive cancer screening. However, if no mutation is detected in the proband, then further testing of family members will not be informative. A specific mutation can be identified in approximately 80% of patients who have clinical features of FAP [32]. Some of those without a detectable APC mutation may have MUTYH-associated polyposis (MAP). About 20% of tests that detect

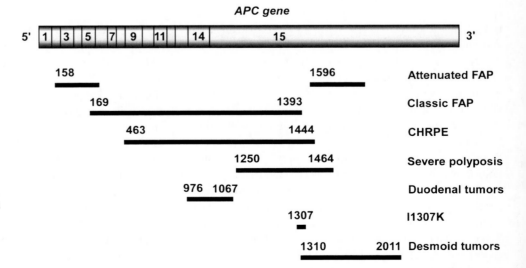

Fig. 5.2 Genotype–phenotype correlations in FAP. A schematic view of the APC gene exons is illustrated at the top. Specific phenotypic features associated with mutations in APC at the indicated amino acid positions are outlined. CHRPE: congenital hypertrophy of retinal pigmented epithelium

an APC mutation occur in individuals without a family history of polyposis in either parent, indicating a de novo, or spontaneously acquired, germline mutation [33]. In addition, mosaicism in a parent may potentially explain some of these de novo cases [34].

Management Implications

In classic FAP, annual sigmoidoscopy beginning at age 10–12 years is recommended. In AFAP, colonoscopies should be initiated beginning at age 25 given the predilection for right-sided adenomas and the relatively delayed onset of disease compared to classic FAP. Screening for extracolonic manifestations of AFAP and FAP should be undertaken as well. Because symptomatic duodenal cancer is almost uniformly lethal, surveillance for ampullary or duodenal cancer with an upper endoscopy using both forward- and side-viewing instruments should be started at the time of colectomy or by age 30 and then repeated at 1–3 year intervals [7]. Screening for hepatoblastoma with measurement of blood alpha-fetoprotein levels and liver ultrasound can be considered annually in children through age 10. Beginning at age 12, annual thyroid ultrasound has been advocated by some authorities.

Strategies for Prevention of Cancer

In classic FAP, a prophylactic colectomy is the only definitive treatment and the only option once the colon is carpeted with adenomatous polyps. The preferred approach is a total proctocolectomy with ileostomy or ileoanal anastomosis with J pouch. After a total proctocolectomy, the residual pouch should be surveyed every 6–12 months because polyps and cancer can arise within the residual cuff tissue, even in the absence of polyposis [35]. Adenomas can also develop within the ileal pouch itself, and a recent study of patients who underwent an ileal pouch–anal anastomosis (IPAA) suggested that the 10-year cumulative risk of developing a pouch adenoma was 45% and a pouch carcinoma was 1% [36].

In rare cases of classic FAP and most cases of AFAP in which there is a relatively low burden of polyps in the rectum, a subtotal colectomy with ileorectal anastamosis rather than IPAA may also be considered. However, because cancer in the resected colon or a mutation between codons 1,250 and 1,464 are strongly associated with the development of cancer in the rectal remnant, an IPAA may still be preferable in patients with these risk factors despite a small number of polyps [37]. For all patients with a retained rectum, close follow-up with sigmoidoscopy every 6–12 months is mandatory. Chemoprevention with agents targeting the cyclooxygenase-2 (COX-2) pathway, such as sulindac and celecoxib, may play an adjunctive role in reducing the number and size

Table 5.2 The Spiegelman Classification System for Duodenal Polyps

Factor	Score		
	1 Point	2 Points	3 Points
No. of polyps	1–4	5–20	>20
Polyp size, mm	1–4	5–10	>10
Histology	Tubular adenoma	Tubulovillous adenoma	Villous adenoma
Dysplasia	Low grade	–	High grade

Final classification
Stage 0, 0 polyps; stage I, 1–4 total points; stage II, 5–10 total points; stage III, 7–8 total points; stage IV, 9–12 total points
Adapted from JCO, Saurin et al. [41]

of adenomas in the residual rectum [38, 39]. However, there does not appear to be a primary role for these drugs to prevent disease expression among young patients with APC gene mutations that have not yet developed polyposis [40].

Duodenal adenomas are more difficult to manage and typically require definitive treatment if they are large (≥2 cm in diameter) or exhibit villous architecture or high grade dysplasia [41]. Adenomas can be resected or ablated with an argon plasma coagulation (APC) laser endoscopically; however, surgical resection, including pancreaticoduodenectomy (Whipple procedure) may be necessary depending on the location, extent, and severity of the dysplastic lesion. The Spigelman classification system is used to classify risk of adenocarcinoma based on the number of duodenal polyps, polyp size, histology, and degree of dysplasia (Table 5.2). Patients with Spigelman Stage IV disease should be considered for a Whipple [42].

Management of desmoid tumors is particularly challenging since desmoids are often quite bulky and their growth may be stimulated by surgery. For extraabdominal and abdominal wall tumors, surgery can successfully treat the disease. However, intraabdominal desmoids are very difficult to manage surgically. Other options for therapy include sulindac, antiestrogens such as tamoxifen, chemotherapy typically used for soft tissue sarcomas, or radiation therapy [43–45].

MUTYH-Associated Polyposis Syndrome

Clinical Features/Distinguishing Characteristics

MUTYH-associated polyposis (MAP) is the first inherited colon cancer syndrome described with an autosomal recessive pattern of inheritance [46]; biallelic mutations in the MutY homolog (MUTYH or MYH) gene are associated with the early development of multiple adenomatous polyps. Although large population-based studies are lacking, it is estimated that about 1 in 2,500–10,000 individuals have biallelic MUTYH mutations, and their lifetime risk of colorectal

Fig. 5.3 Distinguishing adenomatous polyposis syndromes by polyp counts. Although there can be overlap among the syndromes, they can be divided into the categories of "nonpolyposis," "oligopolyposis," and "polyposis" syndromes. The MUTYH-associated polyposis syndrome most often exhibits an oligopolyposis phenotype, but there is considerable variability at both ends of the spectrum

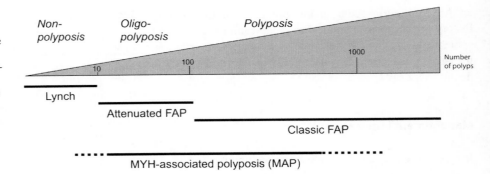

cancer is estimated to be 80% [47]. In European cohorts, 22–29% of individuals with more than 10 adenomas and no APC mutation were found to possess biallelic MUTYH mutations [48–51].

Polyp number in MAP is highly variable, ranging from a few polyps to greater than 100 (Fig. 5.3). However, the vast majority of MAP individuals exhibit an oligopolyposis phenotype and are diagnosed with 10–100 adenomas, similar to patients with AFAP [49, 52]. Nonetheless, 7.5% of individuals who exhibit diffuse polyposis akin to classic FAP have been found to carry biallelic MUTYH mutations. Some series also identified a group of MAP patients with relatively few adenomas (<15) and early onset colon cancer (<50 years) [53]. Also, like individuals with AFAP, those with MAP are usually diagnosed between 45 and 55 years of age [52]. Heterozygosity for MUTYH mutations does not appear to be strongly related to an increased risk of colorectal cancer; however, a modest association cannot be definitively ruled out since studies thus far are limited to small populations [54, 55].

Colorectal cancers that develop among MAP patients are histologically indistinguishable from cancer due to sporadic disease or FAP. However, the G:C to T:A somatic transversions associated with MUTYH mutations (see Genetics) result in cancers with a high frequency of acquired mutations in APC and K-Ras. MUTYH cancers generally develop through chromosomal instability, yielding microsatellite stable tumors. However, unlike FAP and most chromosomally unstable sporadic cancers, MAP-related tumors tend to be diploid rather than aneuploid [56]. Interestingly, recent data suggest an association between MUTYH mutations and not just adenomatous polyps but also hyperplastic polyps and sessile serrated adenomas [57].

Extracolonic features typically seen in FAP/AFAP have also been described in MAP, including CHRPE, osteomas, dental anomalies, and gastric cancer. About 5% of MAP patients develop duodenal adenomas or adenocarcinomas [49, 50, 52, 58].

Genetics

In 2002, MAP was first described in a Welsh family with three of seven siblings that presented with multiple adenomas or adenocarcinomas despite negative germline APC testing. Subsequent analysis of the somatic changes in the tumors revealed excess somatic transversions of guanine-cytosine pairs to a thymine-adenine pairs (G:C → T:A) in the APC gene. This finding was suggestive of defective base-excision repair, which eventually led to the identification of biallelic mutations in MUTYH in the three affected individuals. In contrast, unaffected siblings were either heterozygous for MUTYH mutations or wild-type, supporting an autosomal recessive mode of transmission [46].

Reactive oxygen species generated by cellular metabolism as well as environmental insults such as ionizing radiation can result in DNA damage, including production of 8-oxo guanine, which mispairs with adenine residues. MUTYH is a DNA glycosylase that identifies and removes adenine residues that have been incorrectly paired with 8-oxo guanine [59]. Mutations in MUTYH result in an inability to repair these mismatches, leading to a high frequency of G:C to T:A transversions; curiously, the APC gene is a preferred somatic target [46, 48, 60–62].

Genetic Testing

Although there have been more than 80 MUTYH variants reported, there is considerable variation in their functional significance [63]. The most common point mutations are found in exons 7 and 13, Y165C and G382D, which result in missense mutations. Thus, genetic testing is focused on these two mutations, which account for 87% of all MUTYH mutations reported in Caucasian populations. Other mutations are more common in non-Caucasian (e.g., Indian or Pakistani) populations [49]. If initial testing is negative for these mutations, further sequencing to identify frameshift mutations or functional single nucleotide polymorphisms can be undertaken [63]. Similar to FAP/AFAP, initial testing should be focused on individuals with polyposis before additional at-risk family members are offered testing.

Genotype/Phenotype Correlation

Patients homozygous for G382D mutations or patients with compound heterozygous G382D/Y165C mutations are typically diagnosed with colorectal cancer at an older age (mean age, 58 years) than patients with homozygous Y165C mutations (mean age, 46 years) [64]. These data seem to correlate with in vitro studies which suggest greater impairment of DNA hydroxylase activity with Y165C mutations [63]. Unlike FAP, there do not yet appear to be clear correlations between MUTYH genotype and extraintestinal manifestions of MAP.

Genetic Testing

Testing for MUTYH should be considered for any patient with more than 15 adenomas, particularly if the pattern of inheritance is autosomal recessive. Testing should be offered to anyone exhibiting an AFAP phenotype who has tested negative for APC mutations [65]. About 1/3 of patients with more than 15 adenomas who test negative for APC mutations will have biallelic MUTYH mutations [49]. In addition, the clinical features of MAP can occasionally overlap with those of Lynch syndrome; in one series, 22% of cases with biallelic MUTYH mutations did not have significant polyposis (<15 polyps). Among these cases, the majority did have strong family histories that were actually more consistent with Lynch syndrome. Thus, cases of suspected Lynch syndrome that do not display the typical molecular features associated with Lynch syndrome should also be considered for MUTYH mutation testing [53].

Management Implications

Because MAP is transmitted in an autosomal recessive manner, cancer risk is limited primarily to siblings of an affected individual rather than children or parents. Thus, the approach to genetic counseling for MAP families will differ compared to FAP or Lynch syndrome.

Heightened screening for colon cancer is necessary, but there are no consensus screening or surveillance guidelines. Among patients with biallelic MUTYH mutations, some authorities recommend colonoscopic screening beginning at age 18 [58]; the National Comprehensive Cancer Network has recommended initiating colonoscopies between ages 25

and 30 years, and then repeating every 3–5 years if normal. For older patients, more frequent colonoscopies may be reasonable. Beginning at ages 30–35 years, upper endoscopy with a side viewing duodenoscope to visualize the ampulla should be considered and repeated every 3–5 years if normal. Because monoallelic carriers may have a slightly increased risk of colorectal cancer, screening beginning prior to age 50 has also been suggested by some authorities. In the absence of adenomatous polyps on the baseline exam, a screening interval of 3–5 years would be reasonable [66].

Strategies for Prevention of Cancer

Treatment recommendations for MAP vary depending upon the number and distribution of polyps. Subtotal colectomy with ileorectal anastomosis can be considered for patients with relative rectal sparing of polyps. Otherwise, total proctocolectomy with ileoanal pouch formation would be definitive treatment. For patients with an intact rectum, surveillance with flexible sigmoidoscopy should be considered in the same manner as patients with AFAP. The role for chemoprevention has not been examined [4].

Hamartomatous Polyposis Syndromes

The three major hamartomatous polyposis syndromes associated with an increased colorectal cancer risk are Peutz–Jeghers syndrome (PJS), Juvenile Polyposis Syndrome (JPS), and PTEN hamartoma syndrome (PTHS). Overall, hamartomatous polyposis syndromes are extremely rare and account for less than 1% of the colon cancers in the U.S. These syndromes may represent a model of a "hamartoma to carcinoma" sequence that is analogous to FAP as a model for the adenoma–carcinoma sequence that characterizes most sporadic cancers [67]. JPS result from alterations in genes in the transforming growth factor-β (TGF-β) signaling pathway. In PTHS, profuse polyposis is not the defining feature although hamartomatous polyps are observed. Most cases of PTHS are due to mutations of the phosphatase and tensin homolog (PTEN) gene on chromosome ten [68].

Peutz–Jeghers Syndrome

Clinical Features/Distinguishing Characteristics

PJS is an extremely rare (1 in 150,000 persons) autosomal-dominant condition uniquely characterized by pigmented (dark blue to dark brown) macules on mucocutaneous areas, such as the vermillion border of the lips, perioral area, and buccal mucosa, as well as the hands and feet. Perinasal, perigenital, perianal, and periorbital lesions can be seen, but often fade after puberty. Individuals with PJS develop histologically characteristic hamartomatous polyps consisting of glandular epithelium and a central core of arborizing smooth muscle bands contiguous with the muscularis mucosae. Diagnostic criteria for a clinical diagnosis of PJS include (1) two or more PJS polyps in the gastrointestinal tract; (2) one or more PJS polyps in conjunction with the characteristic mucocutaneous pigmented lesions; or (3) one or more PJS polyps in conjunction with a family history of PJS [69]. PJS polyps arise throughout the gastrointestinal tract but have an especially strong predilection for the small intestine. PJS polyps can grow to be quite large, causing intestinal obstruction, bleeding, and intussusception [70].

PJS is associated with an extremely high risk of cancer, with a 93% cumulative lifetime risk of any malignancy and a 39% risk of colon cancer [71]. Adenocarcinomas can arise in the esophagus, stomach, duodenum, jejunum, ileum, and colon and are believed to originate from adenomatous tissue that develops within PJS polyps [72]. Extraintestinal cancers associated with PJS include melanoma, sex cord, ovarian, uterine, breast, lung, pancreatic, gallbladder, and biliary tumors [73–78] PJS is also specifically associated with cervical adenoma malignum, a rare and extremely aggressive adenocarcinoma of the cervix [79]. The average age of diagnosis of PJS is 23–26 years, and the mean age of any cancer diagnosis is approximately 40–50 years [72, 80]. The mean age of diagnosis of colorectal cancer is 45.8 years [71].

Genetics

PJS has been linked to germline mutations or deletions of STK11 (also known as LKB1), a serine-threonine kinase on chromosome 19p. STK11 regulates p53-mediated apoptosis and also inhibits adenosine monophosphate (AMP)-activated protein kinase, which in turn inhibits the mTOR pathway [81].

Genetic Testing

Mutation testing for STK11 is available, but STK11 mutations are identified in only 50–60% of cases of suspected PJS with classic clinical features. Thus, defining a mutation in an affected individual is a mandatory first step before further testing of at-risk family members. Because the clinical and histopathological features of PJS are so distinct, identification of an STK11 mutation may not always be necessary to establish the diagnosis [69].

Genotype/Phenotype Correlation

Patients with STK11 mutations that result in a premature truncation have a significantly earlier age of onset of polyposis (median age 18 years) than those with missense STK11 mutations (median age 28 years). Interestingly, those without any identifiable STK11 mutations also have an early age of onset of polyposis (median age 14 years). Patients with missense mutations may also be less likely to develop intussusception [82].

Management

Given the high risk of multiple cancers, the following screening guidelines have been suggested: (1) colonoscopy every 3 years starting at age 18; (2) upper endoscopy every 3 years starting at age 25; (3) small bowel series or small bowel capsule endoscopy every 2 years starting at age 25; (4) endoscopic or abdominal ultrasound every 1–2 years starting at age 30; (5) annual breast examination with mammogram every 2–3 years starting at age 25 for women; (6) annual pelvic examination, PAP smear, pelvic ultrasound starting at age 20; (7) annual testicular exam starting at age 10. Other authorities have also advocated endoscopic ultrasound and/or CT scan of the pancreas with CA19-9 levels every 1–2 years, breast MRI starting at age 25, and biannual testicular ultrasound for boys less than age 12. Chemoprevention with drugs active against COX-2 have been examined in patients with PJS with promising results [83]. In a mouse model of PJS, inhibition of the mTOR pathway significantly reduced the polyp and tumor burden [84].

Juvenile Polyposis Syndrome

Clinical Features/Distinguishing Characteristics

Although they are the most common polyp seen in the pediatric population, juvenile polyps can occur at any age. Sporadic juvenile polyps are relatively common, with as many as 2% of children under 10 presenting with an isolated juvenile polyp. In contrast, the juvenile polyposis syndrome (JPS) is characterized by multiple juvenile polyps, sometimes numbering in the hundreds. JPS polyps can grow quite large (up to 4 cm in diameter) and patients often present clinically with rectal bleeding, abdominal pain, prolapse of polyps from the rectum, or intussusception. Diagnostic criteria for a clinical diagnosis of JPS include (1) greater than 3–10 juvenile polyps in the colon; (2) any juvenile polyp in the gastrointestinal tract outside of the colon; or (3) any juvenile polyp with a family history of JPS. JPS usually becomes clinically evident in childhood, with the average age of symptom development at 9.5 years. In contrast to PJS, JPS polyps are most commonly seen in the colon and rectum and are less frequently in the stomach or small intestine. Histologically, juvenile polyps are hamartomatous with a prominent lamina propria and dilated cystic glands, often with an inflammatory infiltrate. Unlike PJS polyps, however, there is no proliferation of smooth muscle within the polyp. Nonetheless, the histological features of JPS polyps can be similar to those seen in other hamartomatous polyp syndromes. Thus, patients suspected of having JPS should also be scrutinized for other clinical features suggestive of PJS or PTHS [69].

Sporadic juvenile polyps do not appear to have neoplastic potential. However, patients with JPS have a 10–38% lifetime risk of colon cancer with an average age of diagnosis of 34 years. In addition, JPS patients have a 15–21% lifetime risk of gastric and duodenal cancers. Like PJS, cancer is believed to originate from adenomatous tissue that develops within the juvenile polyps of patients with JPS. In contrast with sporadic juvenile polyps, polyps in patients with JPS appear to have molecular changes associated with progression to carcinoma, including overexpression of COX-2 [85]. JPS is also associated with cancer of the stomach, duodenum, pancreas, and biliary tree, as well as congenital abnormalities of the heart, gastrointestinal tract, genitourinary system, and central nervous system.

Genetics

JPS has been linked to mutations in three genes related to the TGF-β/SMAD signaling pathway: MADH4, BMPR1A, and ENG. The MADH4 gene on chromosome 18q encodes the Smad4 protein that regulates the intracellular signal of TGF-β. The BMPR1A gene on chromosome 10q encodes a receptor for bone morphogenic protein, a member of the TGF-β superfamily. Finally, the endoglin (ENG) gene, previously associated with only hereditary hemorrhagic telangiectasia (HHT), is an accessory component of the TGF-β receptor complex. The TGF-β signaling pathway regulates multiple cellular processes, including proliferation, differentiation, adhesion, and apoptosis [68, 86].

Genetic Testing

Direct sequencing for mutations in MADH4, BMPR1A, and ENG forms the basis for JPS testing. Most mutations occur in the MADH4 or BMPR1A gene. However, mutations in one of these genes are responsible for only 40–50% of all JPS cases [68].

Genotype/Phenotype Correlation

Patients with MADH4 mutations tend to have more gastric polyps than patients with BMPR1A mutations. Although ENG mutations are classically associated with HHT, they have also been associated with early onset JPS [68]. A subset of patients MADH4 mutations also exhibit classic features of HHT [87].

Management

Because of the early age of onset of polyposis, patients with JPS should have their initial colonoscopy at age 15–18 years, and this should be repeated every 1–2 years. To evaluate for gastric and duodenal cancers, patients should have an upper endoscopy beginning in the teens and then repeated every 1–3 years. Juvenile polyps in JPS do appear to share a pattern of COX-2 overexpression with polyps in FAP [85]. Thus, agents with COX-2 activity, such as sulindac and celecoxib, which are chemopreventive in FAP may ultimately have a role in JPS [88]. Some authorities recommend that patients with JPS and MADH4 mutations should be screened for HHT-related vascular lesions, such as arteriovenous malformations, which may spontaneously rupture [87].

PTEN Hamartoma Syndrome

Clinical Features/Distinguishing Characteristics

Phosphatase and tensin homolog (PTEN) hamartoma syndrome (PHTS) includes Cowden syndrome (CS), Bannayan–Riley–Ruvalcaba (BRRS), and Proteus syndrome. CS is an autosomal dominantly inherited syndrome with an estimated incidence of 1 per 200,000 in European and North American populations [69]. A pathognomonic clinical feature of CS are facial trichilemmomas. CS patients also frequently have macrocephaly and benign breast (e.g., fibrocystic disease), thyroid (e.g., goiters), and endometrial (e.g., fibroids) lesions. CS patients have a 50% lifetime risk of breast cancer, 10% lifetime risk of follicular thyroid cancer, and a 5–10% lifetime risk of endometrial cancer. The risk of colorectal cancer, though elevated, is not well characterized and is likely to be modest. However, CS patients typically develop polyps that can be found throughout the gastrointestinal tract, particularly in the stomach, esophagus, and colon. Most polyps in CS are characterized histologically as hamartomatous or juvenile polyps, although other types, including adenomatous polyps, are often seen. Rarely, lipomas, inflammatory polyps, and ganglioneuromas are observed. In the esophagus, a common feature of CS are elevated gray-white plaques in the distal esophagus that are characterized histologically as glycogen acanthoses [89]. When dysplastic gangliocytoma of the cerebellum occurs in the setting of other features of CS, the syndrome has been termed Lhermitte–Duclos disease [90].

There are several other rare syndromes associated with PTEN mutations, including both BRRS and Proteus syndrome, but the increase in risk of any cancer, including colorectal cancer, is not well defined [89]. BRRS syndrome, like CS, is characterized by the presence of multiple intestinal hamartomatous polyps and macrocephaly. In contrast with CS, BRRS syndrome also appears to be associated with multiple lipomas, hemangiomas, development delay, and in males, pigmented lesions on the penis [91]. Finally, Proteus syndrome includes hamartomatous growths as well as several congenital malformations, hemihypertrophy, epidermal nevi, and hyperostosis [92, 93].

Genetics

CS results from mutations in the PTEN gene, a tumor suppressor on chromosome 10q. Approximately 80% of CS and 60% of BRRS patients diagnosed by clinical criteria have an associated PTEN mutation. PTEN is a ubiquitously expressed protein with phosphatase activity that negatively regulates the AKT and mTOR pathway. Thus, PTEN serves as a key tumor suppressor, controlling cell growth, proliferation, and angiogenesis [94]. Recently, germline mutations in the succinate dehydrogenase subunits SDHB-D have been identified among a subset of CS or patients with CS-like features who are negative for PTEN mutations [95].

Genetic Testing

Testing includes an analysis of the coding regions of the PTEN gene, as well as an analysis of the promoter region [89]. In addition, genomic approaches may be required to identify deletions of PTEN, which have been observed in BRRS [90].

Genotype/Phenotype Correlation

There have been reports of patients with mutations in both PTEN and BMPR1A, the latter being associated with JPS. These patients developed generalized polyposis within the first 2 years of life, often with early mortality secondary to intussusception, rectal bleeding, and a profound protein-losing enteropathy [68, 96]. Although there is significant overlap in the spectrum of PTEN mutations associated with Cowden's and BRRS, there appears to be a clustering of Cowden's-associated mutations in the first 5 exons of PTEN whereas most BRRS-associated mutations are seen in the most 3' four exons [97].

Management

All patients with PTEN mutations should be managed according to guidelines recommended for CS patients. Because the exact magnitude of colon cancer risk in CS is not known, but not likely to be significantly elevated, recommendations for gastrointestinal cancer screening have not been established. However, colonoscopies every 3 years after polyps are found have been recommended. Because of the significantly increased risk of thyroid cancer, annual thyroid examination and ultrasound beginning in the teens has been recommended. For women, the extremely high risk of breast cancer necessitates annual breast examination and mammograms beginning at age 25–30 years [69].

Hyperplastic Polyposis Syndrome

In addition to adenomatous and hamartomatous polyposis syndromes, there appears to be a third, distinct histological form of polyposis characterized by numerous hyperplastic polyps. This syndrome represents a model for the recently described serrated pathway to colorectal cancer development.

Clinical Features/Distinguishing Characteristics

Sporadic hyperplastic polyps are generally small (<5 mm in greatest diameter) and commonly observed in the distal sigmoid and rectum. Numerous studies have suggested that these polyps have no malignant potential and do not predict future neoplasia. However, there appears to be a familial hyperplastic polyposis syndrome (HPS) characterized by numerous hyperplastic polyps throughout the colon, some of which may be as large as 1 cm in greatest diameter. Although the genetic basis of HPS is not known, it is estimated that HPS arises in approximately 1 in 2,000 individuals. Because it appears to be transmitted as a recessive or codominant allele, it has been suggested that as many as 1 in 25 individuals may carry the HPS allele [98].

Typically, individuals with HPS have more than 20 hyperplastic polyps throughout the colon, with the largest lesions often in the right colon. The mean age of diagnosis is 66 years. Diagnostic criteria for HPS include (1) greater than 5 hyperplastic polyps proximal to the sigmoid colon, two of which measure more than 10 mm in diameter; (2) any number of hyperplastic polyps proximal to the sigmoid colon in an individual with a first degree relative with HPS; or (3) greater than 20 hyperplastic polyps of any size distributed throughout the colon [99]. In contrast with patients with sporadic hyperplastic polyps, patients with HPS appear to have an elevated risk of colorectal cancer. The magnitude of the risk is not well-defined and appears to be primarily seen among those with large hyperplastic polyps. Cancer typically presents in the fifth to seventh decades of life [98]. Some studies suggest that up to 50% of individuals with HPS have at least one colorectal cancer at the time of initial presentation [98].

Genetics

The inheritance pattern of HPS is unclear. Although patients clinically diagnosed with HPS often have a first-degree relative with HPS or colorectal cancer, this is not a consistent finding. Thus, it has been suggested that HPS may be transmitted in a recessive or codominant fashion. However, to date, the genetic basis for HPS is unknown. Thus, no genetic testing is available [98].

The mechanism that underlies the potential cancer risk associated with hyperplastic polyposis is poorly understood. However, it appears that in contrast to sporadic hyperplastic polyps, the polyps in hyperplastic polyposis progress to cancer through an admixed hyperplastic-adenomatous polyp or a sessile serrated adenoma. These polyps have high rates of the CpG island methylator phenotype (CIMP), BRAF somatic mutations, and MLH1 promoter methylation [98, 100, 101]. Thus, it has been hypothesized that the hyperplastic polyp/sessile serrated adenoma is the precursor lesion to CIMP positive cancers. The CIMP pathway is proposed as an alternative mechanism of colonic carcinogenesis to the classic pathway of chromosomal instability observed in most sporadic cancers and FAP. The CIMP pathway also appears distinct from the pathway of microsatellite instability associated with germline mutations in DNA mismatch repair genes (Lynch syndrome). CIMP cancers appear to arise through inactivation of DNA repair genes by promoter methylation. Clinical features associated with CIMP cancers include female predominance, proximal tumor location, mucinous or poorly differentiated histology, and acquired mutations in BRAF [102]. Recent studies also suggest a potential overlap between HPS and MAP. In a small series of 17 MAP patients, 47% had hyperplastic polyps or serrated adenomas, with 18% meeting criteria for HPS [57].

Management

There are no precise screening and surveillance guidelines for HPS. However, it has been reported that the rate of malignant transformation of sessile serrated adenomas may be accelerated compared to sporadic adenomas, and may account for a large proportion of interval cancers often seen in the proximal colon [103–105]. Thus, all patients with HPS as well as family members should have regular colonoscopy at 1–3 year intervals. An effort should be made to remove, or at least biopsy, as many of polyps as possible. If the entire colorectum cannot be completely cleared of visible polyps due to size or number, then more frequent surveillance or even prophylactic colectomy is warranted.

Summary

Colonic polyposis syndromes are fascinating conditions that have provided invaluable insights into the diverse genetic pathways that underlie colorectal cancer development. The polyposis syndromes are categorized by the underlying histology of the polyp types (adenomatous, hamartomatous, and hyperplastic). Most are associated with a dramatically increased lifetime risk of colon cancer, and there are effective surveillance as well as risk-reducing surgical approaches. The unique spectrum of extracolonic cancers associated with each of these syndromes dictates the need for a multidisciplinary approach to clinical management. Genetic testing is an invaluable component of the management in these families, and the variable and overlapping phenotypes combined with the large number of genes involved can make the genetic evaluation complex.

References

1. Jemal A, Thun MJ, Ries LA, Howe HL, Weir HK et al (2008) Annual Report to the Nation on the Status of Cancer, 1975–2005, Featuring Trends in Lung Cancer, Tobacco Use, and Tobacco Control. J Natl Cancer Inst 100(23):1672–1694
2. Johns LE, Houlston RS (2001) A systematic review and meta-analysis of familial colorectal cancer risk. Am J Gastroenterol 96:2992–3003
3. Bussey HJ, Veale AM, Morson BC (1978) Genetics of gastrointestinal polyposis. Gastroenterology 74:1325–1330
4. Jo WS, Chung DC (2005) Genetics of hereditary colorectal cancer. Semin Oncol 32:11–23
5. Burt RW, Leppert MF, Slattery ML, Samowitz WS, Spirio LN et al (2004) Genetic testing and phenotype in a large kindred with attenuated familial adenomatous polyposis. Gastroenterology 127:444–451
6. Lynch HT, Smyrk T, McGinn T, Lanspa S, Cavalieri J et al (1995) Attenuated familial adenomatous polyposis (AFAP). A phenotypically and genotypically distinctive variant of FAP. Cancer 76:2427–2433
7. Latchford AR, Neale KF, Spigelman AD, Phillips RK, Clark SK (2009) Features of duodenal cancer in patients with familial adenomatous polyposis. Clin Gastroenterol Hepatol 7(6):659–663
8. Wong RF, Tuteja AK, Haslem DS, Pappas L, Szabo A et al (2006) Video capsule endoscopy compared with standard endoscopy for the evaluation of small-bowel polyps in persons with familial adenomatous polyposis (with video). Gastrointest Endosc 64:530–537
9. Bianchi LK, Burke CA, Bennett AE, Lopez R, Hasson H et al (2008) Fundic gland polyp dysplasia is common in familial adenomatous polyposis. Clin Gastroenterol Hepatol 6:180–185
10. Park YJ, Shin KH, Park JG (2000) Risk of gastric cancer in hereditary nonpolyposis colorectal cancer in Korea. Clin Cancer Res 6:2994–2998

11. Herraiz M, Barbesino G, Faquin W, Chan-Smutko G, Patel D et al (2007) Prevalence of thyroid cancer in familial adenomatous polyposis syndrome and the role of screening ultrasound examinations. Clin Gastroenterol Hepatol 5:367–373

12. Hamilton SR, Liu B, Parsons RE, Papadopoulos N, Jen J et al (1995) The molecular basis of Turcot's syndrome. N Engl J Med 332:839–847

13. Giardiello FM, Offerhaus GJ, Lee DH, Krush AJ, Tersmette AC et al (1993) Increased risk of thyroid and pancreatic carcinoma in familial adenomatous polyposis. Gut 34:1394–1396

14. Gardner EJ, Plenk HP (1952) Hereditary pattern for multiple osteomas in a family group. Am J Hum Genet 4:31–36

15. Gardner EJ (1962) Follow-up study of a family group exhibiting dominant inheritance for a syndrome including intestinal polyps, osteomas, fibromas and epidermal cysts. Am J Hum Genet 14:376–390

16. Speake D, Evans DG, Lalloo F, Scott NA, Hill J (2007) Desmoid tumours in patients with familial adenomatous polyposis and desmoid region adenomatous polyposis coli mutations. Br J Surg 94:1009–1013

17. Nieuwenhuis MH, De Vos Tot Nederveen Cappel W, Botma A, Nagengast FM, Kleibeuker JH et al (2008) Desmoid tumors in a dutch cohort of patients with familial adenomatous polyposis. Clin Gastroenterol Hepatol 6:215–219

18. Gurbuz AK, Giardiello FM, Petersen GM, Krush AJ, Offerhaus GJ et al (1994) Desmoid tumours in familial adenomatous polyposis. Gut 35:377–381

19. Smith TG, Clark SK, Katz DE, Reznek RH, Phillips RK (2000) Adrenal masses are associated with familial adenomatous polyposis. Dis Colon Rectum 43:1739–1742

20. Giardiello FM, Hamilton SR, Krush AJ, Offerhaus JA, Booker SV et al (1993) Nasopharyngeal angiofibroma in patients with familial adenomatous polyposis. Gastroenterology 105:1550–1552

21. Kinzler KW, Nilbert MC, Su LK, Vogelstein B, Bryan TM et al (1991) Identification of FAP locus genes from chromosome 5q21. Science 253:661–665

22. Nishisho I, Nakamura Y, Miyoshi Y, Miki Y, Ando H et al (1991) Mutations of chromosome 5q21 genes in FAP and colorectal cancer patients. Science 253:665–669

23. Groden J, Thliveris A, Samowitz W, Carlson M, Gelbert L et al (1991) Identification and characterization of the familial adenomatous polyposis coli gene. Cell 66:589–600

24. Chung DC (2000) The genetic basis of colorectal cancer: insights into critical pathways of tumorigenesis. Gastroenterology 119:854–865

25. Miyoshi Y, Ando H, Nagase H, Nishisho I, Horii A et al (1992) Germ-line mutations of the APC gene in 53 familial adenomatous polyposis patients. Proc Natl Acad Sci USA 89:4452–4456

26. Sieber OM, Lamlum H, Crabtree MD, Rowan AJ, Barclay E et al (2002) Whole-gene APC deletions cause classical familial adenomatous polyposis, but not attenuated polyposis or "multiple" colorectal adenomas. Proc Natl Acad Sci USA 99:2954–2958

27. Sieber OM, Segditsas S, Knudsen AL, Zhang J, Luz J et al (2006) Disease severity and genetic pathways in attenuated familial adenomatous polyposis vary greatly but depend on the site of the germline mutation. Gut 55:1440–1448

28. Heppner Goss K, Trzepacz C, Tuohy TM, Groden J (2002) Attenuated APC alleles produce functional protein from internal translation initiation. Proc Natl Acad Sci USA 99:8161–8166

29. Caspari R, Olschwang S, Friedl W, Mandl M, Boisson C et al (1995) Familial adenomatous polyposis: desmoid tumours and lack of ophthalmic lesions (CHRPE) associated with APC mutations beyond codon 1444. Hum Mol Genet 4:337–340

30. Bertario L, Russo A, Sala P, Varesco L, Giarola M et al (2003) Multiple approach to the exploration of genotype-phenotype correlations in familial adenomatous polyposis. J Clin Oncol 21:1698–1707

31. Wallis YL, Morton DG, McKeown CM, Macdonald F (1999) Molecular analysis of the APC gene in 205 families: extended genotype-phenotype correlations in FAP and evidence for the role of APC amino acid changes in colorectal cancer predisposition. J Med Genet 36:14–20

32. Burt R, Neklason DW (2005) Genetic testing for inherited colon cancer. Gastroenterology 128:1696–1716

33. Grady WM (2003) Genetic testing for high-risk colon cancer patients. Gastroenterology 124:1574–1594

34. Aretz S, Stienen D, Friedrichs N, Stemmler S, Uhlhaas S et al (2007) Somatic APC mosaicism: a frequent cause of familial adenomatous polyposis (FAP). Hum Mutat 28:985–992

35. Zimmer V, Lammert F, Raedle J (2010) Gardner variant of familial adenomatous polyposis: from extensive skull osteomatosis to metastatic rectal remnant cancer. Clin Gastroenterol Hepatol 8(1):A34

36. Friederich P, de Jong AE, Mathus-Vliegen LM, Dekker E, Krieken HH et al (2008) Risk of developing adenomas and carcinomas in the ileal pouch in patients with familial adenomatous polyposis. Clin Gastroenterol Hepatol 6:1237–1242

37. Bertario L, Russo A, Radice P, Varesco L, Eboli M et al (2000) Genotype and phenotype factors as determinants for rectal stump cancer in patients with familial adenomatous polyposis. Hereditary Colorectal Tumors Registry. Ann Surg 231:538–543

38. Giardiello FM, Hamilton SR, Krush AJ, Piantadosi S, Hylind LM et al (1993) Treatment of colonic and rectal adenomas with sulindac in familial adenomatous polyposis. N Engl J Med 328:1313–1316

39. Steinbach G, Lynch PM, Phillips RK, Wallace MH, Hawk E et al (2000) The effect of celecoxib, a cyclooxygenase-2 inhibitor, in familial adenomatous polyposis. N Engl J Med 342:1946–1952

40. Giardiello FM, Yang VW, Hylind LM, Krush AJ, Petersen GM et al (2002) Primary chemoprevention of familial adenomatous polyposis with sulindac. N Engl J Med 346:1054–1059

41. Saurin JC, Gutknecht C, Napoleon B, Chavaillon A, Ecochard R et al (2004) Surveillance of duodenal adenomas in familial adenomatous polyposis reveals high cumulative risk of advanced disease. J Clin Oncol 22:493–498

42. Gallagher MC, Phillips RK, Bulow S (2006) Surveillance and management of upper gastrointestinal disease in familial adenomatous polyposis. Fam Cancer 5:263–273

43. Ray ME, Lawrence TS (2006) Radiation therapy for aggressive fibromatosis (desmoid tumor). J Clin Oncol 24:3714–3715; author reply 3715

44. Gega M, Yanagi H, Yoshikawa R, Noda M, Ikeuchi H et al (2006) Successful chemotherapeutic modality of doxorubicin plus dacarbazine for the treatment of desmoid tumors in association with familial adenomatous polyposis. J Clin Oncol 24:102–105

45. Lev D, Kotilingam D, Wei C, Ballo MT, Zagars GK et al (2007) Optimizing treatment of desmoid tumors. J Clin Oncol 25:1785–1791

46. Al-Tassan N, Chmiel NH, Maynard J, Fleming N, Livingston AL et al (2002) Inherited variants of MYH associated with somatic $G:C \rightarrow T:A$ mutations in colorectal tumors. Nat Genet 30:227–232

47. Jenkins MA, Croitoru ME, Monga N, Cleary SP, Cotterchio M et al (2006) Risk of colorectal cancer in monoallelic and biallelic carriers of MYH mutations: a population-based case-family study. Cancer Epidemiol Biomarkers Prev 15:312–314

48. Jones S, Emmerson P, Maynard J, Best JM, Jordan S et al (2002) Biallelic germline mutations in MYH predispose to multiple colorectal adenoma and somatic $G:C \rightarrow T:A$ mutations. Hum Mol Genet 11:2961–2967

49. Sieber OM, Lipton L, Crabtree M, Heinimann K, Fidalgo P et al (2003) Multiple colorectal adenomas, classic adenomatous polyposis, and germ-line mutations in MYH. N Engl J Med 348:791–799

50. Enholm S, Hienonen T, Suomalainen A, Lipton L, Tomlinson I et al (2003) Proportion and phenotype of MYH-associated colorectal neoplasia in a population-based series of Finnish colorectal cancer patients. Am J Pathol 163:827–832

51. Halford SE, Rowan AJ, Lipton L, Sieber OM, Pack K et al (2003) Germline mutations but not somatic changes at the MYH locus contribute to the pathogenesis of unselected colorectal cancers. Am J Pathol 162:1545–1548

52. Sampson JR, Dolwani S, Jones S, Eccles D, Ellis A et al (2003) Autosomal recessive colorectal adenomatous polyposis due to inherited mutations of MYH. Lancet 362:39–41

53. Jo WS, Bandipalliam P, Shannon KM, Niendorf KB, Chan-Smutko G et al (2005) Correlation of polyp number and family history of colon cancer with germline MYH mutations. Clin Gastroenterol Hepatol 3:1022–1028

54. Tenesa A, Campbell H, Barnetson R, Porteous M, Dunlop M et al (2006) Association of MUTYH and colorectal cancer. Br J Cancer 95:239–242

55. Webb EL, Rudd MF, Houlston RS (2006) Colorectal cancer risk in monoallelic carriers of MYH variants. Am J Hum Genet 79:768–771; author reply 771–762

56. Lipton L, Halford SE, Johnson V, Novelli MR, Jones A et al (2003) Carcinogenesis in MYH-associated polyposis follows a distinct genetic pathway. Cancer Res 63:7595–7599

57. Boparai KS, Dekker E, Van Eeden S, Polak MM, Bartelsman JF et al (2008) Hyperplastic polyps and sessile serrated adenomas as a phenotypic expression of MYH-associated polyposis. Gastroenterology 135:2014–2018

58. Aretz S, Uhlhaas S, Goergens H, Siberg K, Vogel M et al (2006) MUTYH-associated polyposis: 70 of 71 patients with biallelic mutations present with an attenuated or atypical phenotype. Int J Cancer 119:807–814

59. Slupska MM, Baikalov C, Luther WM, Chiang JH, Wei YF et al (1996) Cloning and sequencing a human homolog (hMYH) of the Escherichia coli mutY gene whose function is required for the repair of oxidative DNA damage. J Bacteriol 178:3885–3892

60. Nghiem Y, Cabrera M, Cupples CG, Miller JH (1988) The mutY gene: a mutator locus in Escherichia coli that generates G.C–T.A transversions. Proc Natl Acad Sci USA 85:2709–2713

61. Michaels ML, Miller JH (1992) The GO system protects organisms from the mutagenic effect of the spontaneous lesion 8-hydroxyguanine (7, 8-dihydro-8-oxoguanine). J Bacteriol 174:6321–6325

62. Moriya M, Grollman AP (1993) Mutations in the mutY gene of Escherichia coli enhance the frequency of targeted G:C → T: a transversions induced by a single 8-oxoguanine residue in single-stranded DNA. Mol Gen Genet 239:72–76

63. Ali M, Kim H, Cleary S, Cupples C, Gallinger S et al (2008) Characterization of mutant MUTYH proteins associated with familial colorectal cancer. Gastroenterology 135:499–507

64. Nielsen M, Joerink-van de Beld MC, Jones N, Vogt S, Tops CM et al (2009) Analysis of MUTYH genotypes and colorectal phenotypes in patients with MUTYH-associated polyposis. Gastroenterology 136:471–476

65. Balaguer F, Castellvi-Bel S, Castells A, Andreu M, Munoz J et al (2007) Identification of MYH mutation carriers in colorectal cancer: a multicenter, case-control, population-based study. Clin Gastroenterol Hepatol 5:379–387

66. Wang L, Baudhuin LM, Boardman LA, Steenblock KJ, Petersen GM et al (2004) MYH mutations in patients with attenuated and classic polyposis and with young-onset colorectal cancer without polyps. Gastroenterology 127:9–16

67. Wang ZJ, Ellis I, Zauber P, Iwama T, Marchese C et al (1999) Allelic imbalance at the LKB1 (STK11) locus in tumours from patients with Peutz-Jeghers' syndrome provides evidence for a hamartoma-(adenoma)-carcinoma sequence. J Pathol 188:9–13

68. Sweet K, Willis J, Zhou XP, Gallione C, Sawada T et al (2005) Molecular classification of patients with unexplained hamartomatous and hyperplastic polyposis. JAMA 294:2465–2473

69. Zbuk KM, Eng C (2007) Hamartomatous polyposis syndromes. Nat Clin Pract Gastroenterol Hepatol 4:492–502

70. McGarrity TJ, Amos C (2006) Peutz-Jeghers syndrome: clinicopathology and molecular alterations. Cell Mol Life Sci 63:2135–2144

71. Giardiello FM, Brensinger JD, Tersmette AC, Goodman SN, Petersen GM et al (2000) Very high risk of cancer in familial Peutz-Jeghers syndrome. Gastroenterology 119:1447–1453

72. Burdick D, Prior JT (1982) Peutz-Jeghers syndrome. A clinicopathologic study of a large family with a 27-year follow-up. Cancer 50:2139–2146

73. Rowan A, Bataille V, MacKie R, Healy E, Bicknell D et al (1999) Somatic mutations in the Peutz-Jeghers (LKB1/STKII) gene in sporadic malignant melanomas. J Invest Dermatol 112:509–511

74. Su GH, Hruban RH, Bansal RK, Bova GS, Tang DJ et al (1999) Germline and somatic mutations of the STK11/LKB1 Peutz-Jeghers gene in pancreatic and biliary cancers. Am J Pathol 154:1835–1840

75. Wang ZJ, Churchman M, Campbell IG, Xu WH, Yan ZY et al (1999) Allele loss and mutation screen at the Peutz-Jeghers (LKB1) locus (19p13.3) in sporadic ovarian tumours. Br J Cancer 80:70–72

76. Wilson DM, Pitts WC, Hintz RL, Rosenfeld RG (1986) Testicular tumors with Peutz-Jeghers syndrome. Cancer 57:2238–2240

77. Cantu JM, Rivera H, Ocampo-Campos R, Bedolla N, Cortes-Gallegos V et al (1980) Peutz-Jeghers syndrome with feminizing sertoli cell tumor. Cancer 46:223–228

78. Trau H, Schewach-Millet M, Fisher BK, Tsur H (1982) Peutz-Jeghers syndrome and bilateral breast carcinoma. Cancer 50:788–792

79. Srivatsa PJ, Keeney GL, Podratz KC (1994) Disseminated cervical adenoma malignum and bilateral ovarian sex cord tumors with annular tubules associated with Peutz-Jeghers syndrome. Gynecol Oncol 53:256–264

80. Foley TR, McGarrity TJ, Abt AB (1988) Peutz-Jeghers syndrome: a clinicopathologic survey of the "Harrisburg family" with a 49-year follow-up. Gastroenterology 95:1535–1540

81. Aretz S, Stienen D, Uhlhaas S, Loff S, Back W et al (2005) High proportion of large genomic STK11 deletions in Peutz-Jeghers syndrome. Hum Mutat 26:513–519

82. Amos CI, Keitheri-Cheteri MB, Sabripour M, Wei C, McGarrity TJ et al (2004) Genotype-phenotype correlations in Peutz-Jeghers syndrome. J Med Genet 41:327–333

83. Udd L, Katajisto P, Rossi DJ, Lepisto A, Lahesmaa AM et al (2004) Suppression of Peutz-Jeghers polyposis by inhibition of cyclooxygenase-2. Gastroenterology 127:1030–1037

84. Wei C, Amos CI, Zhang N, Wang X, Rashid A et al (2008) Suppression of Peutz-Jeghers polyposis by targeting mammalian target of rapamycin signaling. Clin Cancer Res 14:1167–1171

85. van Hattem WA, Brosens LA, Marks SY, Milne AN, van Eeden S et al (2009) Increased cyclooxygenase-2 expression in juvenile polyposis syndrome. Clin Gastroenterol Hepatol 7:93–97

86. Waite KA, Eng C (2003) From developmental disorder to heritable cancer: it's all in the BMP/TGF-beta family. Nat Rev Genet 4:763–773

87. Gallione CJ, Repetto GM, Legius E, Rustgi AK, Schelley SL et al (2004) A combined syndrome of juvenile polyposis and hereditary haemorrhagic telangiectasia associated with mutations in MADH4 (SMAD4). Lancet 363:852–859

88. Brazowski E, Rozen P, Misonzhnick-Bedny F, Gitstein G (2005) Characteristics of familial juvenile polyps expressing cyclooxygenase-2. Am J Gastroenterol 100:130–138

89. Gustafson S, Zbuk KM, Scacheri C, Eng C (2007) Cowden syndrome. Semin Oncol 34:428–434

90. Zhou XP, Marsh DJ, Morrison CD, Chaudhury AR, Maxwell M et al (2003) Germline inactivation of PTEN and dysregulation of the phosphoinositol-3-kinase/Akt pathway cause human Lhermitte-Duclos disease in adults. Am J Hum Genet 73:1191–1198

91. Gorlin RJ, Cohen MM Jr, Condon LM, Burke BA (1992) Bannayan-Riley-Ruvalcaba syndrome. Am J Med Genet 44:307–314

92. Zhou X, Hampel H, Thiele H, Gorlin RJ, Hennekam RC et al (2001) Association of germline mutation in the PTEN tumour suppressor gene and Proteus and Proteus-like syndromes. Lancet 358:210–211

93. Wiedemann HR, Burgio GR, Aldenhoff P, Kunze J, Kaufmann HJ et al (1983) The proteus syndrome. Partial gigantism of the hands and/or feet, nevi, hemihypertrophy, subcutaneous tumors, macrocephaly or other skull anomalies and possible accelerated growth and visceral affections. Eur J Pediatr 140:5–12

94. Waite KA, Eng C (2002) Protean PTEN: form and function. Am J Hum Genet 70:829–844

95. Ni Y, Zbuk KM, Sadler T, Patocs A, Lobo G et al (2008) Germline mutations and variants in the succinate dehydrogenase genes in Cowden and Cowden-like syndromes. Am J Hum Genet 83:261–268

96. Delnatte C, Sanlaville D, Mougenot JF, Vermeesch JR, Houdayer C et al (2006) Contiguous gene deletion within chromosome arm 10q is associated with juvenile polyposis of infancy, reflecting cooperation between the BMPR1A and PTEN tumor-suppressor genes. Am J Hum Genet 78:1066–1074

97. Eng C (2003) PTEN: one gene, many syndromes. Hum Mutat 22:183–198

98. Young J, Jenkins M, Parry S, Young B, Nancarrow D et al (2007) Serrated pathway colorectal cancer in the population: genetic consideration. Gut 56:1453–1459

99. Burt R, Jass J (2000) Hyperplastic polyposis. World Health Organization classification of tumours Pathology and genetics of tumours of the digestive system. IARC Press, Lyon

100. Rashid A, Houlihan PS, Booker S, Petersen GM, Giardiello FM et al (2000) Phenotypic and molecular characteristics of hyperplastic polyposis. Gastroenterology 119:323–332

101. Jass JR, Whitehall VL, Young J, Leggett BA (2002) Emerging concepts in colorectal neoplasia. Gastroenterology 123:862–876

102. Hawkins N, Norrie M, Cheong K, Mokany E, Ku SL et al (2002) CpG island methylation in sporadic colorectal cancers and its relationship to microsatellite instability. Gastroenterology 122:1376–1387

103. Hyman NH, Anderson P, Blasyk H (2004) Hyperplastic polyposis and the risk of colorectal cancer. Dis Colon Rectum 47:2101–2104

104. Azimuddin K, Stasik JJ, Khubchandani IT, Rosen L, Riether RD et al (2000) Hyperplastic polyps: "more than meets the eye"? Report of sixteen cases. Dis Colon Rectum 43:1309–1313

105. Lazarus R, Junttila OE, Karttunen TJ, Makinen MJ (2005) The risk of metachronous neoplasia in patients with serrated adenoma. Am J Clin Pathol 123:349–359

106. Desai DC, Murday V, Phillips RK, Neale KF, Milla P et al (1998) A survey of phenotypic features in juvenile polyposis. J Med Genet 35:476–481

107. Howe JR, Mitros FA, Summers RW (1998) The risk of gastrointestinal carcinoma in familial juvenile polyposis. Ann Surg Oncol 5:751–756

108. Scott-Conner CE, Hausmann M, Hall TJ, Skelton DS, Anglin BL et al (1995) Familial juvenile polyposis: patterns of recurrence and implications for surgical management. J Am Coll Surg 181:407–413

109. Jass JR, Williams CB, Bussey HJ, Morson BC (1988) Juvenile polyposis – a precancerous condition. Histopathology 13:619–630

110. Hawkins NJ, Gorman P, Tomlinson IP, Bullpitt P, Ward RL (2000) Colorectal carcinomas arising in the hyperplastic polyposis syndrome progress through the chromosomal instability pathway. Am J Pathol 157:385–392

111. Renaut AJ, Douglas PR, Newstead GL (2002) Hyperplastic polyposis of the colon and rectum. Colorectal Dis 4:213–215

112. Place RJ, Simmang CL (1999) Hyperplastic-adenomatous polyposis syndrome. J Am Coll Surg 188:503–507

113. Lowy AM, Kordich JJ, Gismondi V, Varesco L, Blough RI et al (2001) Numerous colonic adenomas in an individual with Bloom's syndrome. Gastroenterology 121:435–439

114. Laken SJ, Petersen GM, Gruber SB, Oddoux C, Ostrer H et al (1997) Familial colorectal cancer in Ashkenazim due to a hypermutable tract in APC. Nat Genet 17:79–83

115. Gryfe R, Di Nicola N, Lal G, Gallinger S, Redston M (1999) Inherited colorectal polyposis and cancer risk of the APC I1307K polymorphism. Am J Hum Genet 64:378–384

Chapter 6
Hereditary Colon Cancer: Lynch Syndrome

Eunice L. Kwak and Daniel C. Chung

Keywords Lynch syndrome • Hereditary nonpolyposis colon cancer syndrome • DNA mismatch repair • Microsatellite instability • MSH2 gene • MLH1 gene • MSH6 gene • PMS2 gene • Endometrial cancer • Immunohistochemistry • Amsterdam criteria • Bethesda guidelines • Muir–Torre syndrome

Introduction

Colorectal cancer is the second leading cause of cancer-related deaths in the United States, with approximately 140,000 cases diagnosed and 50,000 deaths annually [1]. The majority of these cases are sporadic, occurring in individuals without any known familial predisposition. Approximately 10–30% of all colorectal cancer cases occur in the context of a family history [2], but most of the predisposing genetic factors have not yet been identified. Highly penetrant inherited colorectal cancer syndromes such as familial adenomatous polyposis (FAP), MYH-associated polyposis (MAP), and Lynch syndrome/hereditary nonpolyposis colon cancer (HNPCC) are less common but account for as many as 5% of colorectal cancer cases [3]. However, it is likely that this is an underestimate. With appropriate screening, an estimated 12,000 individuals could be diagnosed with Lynch syndrome on a yearly basis in the United States [4]. The ability to dramatically alter the clinical course of families with these syndromes mandates that clinicians understand the key features in the diagnosis and management of these hereditary colorectal cancer syndromes. Because of the absence of an overt polyposis phenotype, Lynch syndrome can be the most challenging hereditary colorectal syndrome to recognize.

E.L. Kwak (✉)
Department of Hematology and Oncology, Massachusetts General Hospital Cancer Center,
Boston, MA, USA
e-mail: ekwak@partners.org

D.C. Chung (✉)
GI Cancer Genetics Program, Gastrointestinal Unit and Cancer Center Massachusetts General Hospital, Boston, MA, USA
and
Harvard Medical School, Boston, MA, USA.
e-mail: dchung@partners.org

Clinical Features of Lynch Syndrome

In 1913, the pathologist Alfred Warthin described an unusual clustering of endometrial and gastric cancers in "family G" [5]. The subsequent analysis of this family as well as others over the next several decades led to the recognition of a "cancer family syndrome" by Henry Lynch [6]. It is now recognized that Lynch syndrome is transmitted in an autosomal-dominant fashion, and affected individuals are at high risk for the development of early-onset colorectal cancers, which are typically located in the right colon (cecum, ascending, or transverse colon). Lynch syndrome is the most common of the known causes of inherited predisposition to colorectal cancer, accounting for 1–4% of all colorectal cancers and up to 10% of colorectal cancers in patients younger than 50 years of age [7]. In contrast to polyposis syndromes, relatively few adenomas are seen in Lynch Syndrome. When they occur, adenomas present at younger ages, are more commonly located in the right colon, and are associated with a rapid progression to dysplasia and cancer (1–3 years) compared to adenomas occurring in the general population [8]. While initial studies of selected Lynch families estimated a 70–80% lifetime risk of colon cancer with a mean age at diagnosis in the mid-forties [9, 10], more recent studies have suggested a somewhat lower lifetime colorectal cancer risk (52.2% in women and 68.7% in men) and a higher median age at diagnosis of 61.2 years [11].

Importantly, Lynch syndrome is also associated with an increased risk of extracolonic cancers. While Lynch syndrome is associated with increased risks for malignancies of the gastrointestinal tract (stomach, small bowel, biliary tract) and urinary collecting system (renal pelvis, ureter), the increased risk of female reproductive system cancers (uterus, ovaries) is particularly striking (Table 6.1). Women with Lynch syndrome have an approximate 12% lifetime risk of developing ovarian cancer, and a 40–60% lifetime risk of endometrial cancer, making it the second most common cancer seen in Lynch syndrome [12]. Unique variants of the syndrome characterized by the presence of skin tumors (keratoacanthomas, sebaceous neoplasms) or brain tumors

Table 6.1 Gene-specific lifetime cancer risks in Lynch

	MSH2 (%)	MLH1 (%)	MSH6[a] (%)	PMS2[a] (%)
Colorectal	52–69	52–69	20–44	15–20
Endometrial	50–60	50–60	44–71	15
Ovarian	12	6		
Gastric	5	6		
Urinary tract				
Men	28	4		
Women	12	1		
Small bowel	6	4		

[a]Cancers typically diagnosed at older ages

(glioblastoma) are termed Muir–Torre and Turcot syndromes, respectively [12]. It is important to recognize that these extracolonic tumors may precede a diagnosis of colorectal cancer in many Lynch syndrome families.

Clinical Criteria for Lynch Syndrome

The clinical diagnosis of Lynch syndrome has been traditionally defined by the Amsterdam Criteria: (1) colorectal cancer in three family members, (2) two of whom are first-degree relatives, in two or more successive generations, and (3) at least one colorectal cancer diagnosed before age 50 without a diagnosis of familial adenomatous polyposis. These criteria (Amsterdam I) were established in 1991 as a means of standardizing patients recruited for Lynch syndrome studies prior to the discovery of the causative genes [13, 14]. The Amsterdam Criteria I have an estimated sensitivity of 60% and specificity of 70% [15–17]. Over time, it became increasingly recognized that Amsterdam I did not fully account for the presenting features of Lynch patients, and the Amsterdam Criteria II were introduced in 1999 to include the extracolonic tumors seen in the syndrome (uterine, gastric, ovarian, renal pelvis). Although initial reports indicated a sensitivity for Amsterdam II of 78% and specificity of greater than 60% [15, 18], recent population-based studies report a disappointing sensitivity of only 39% [19].

Because the Amsterdam Criteria are too restrictive in identifying patients at risk, a broader set of guidelines was proposed. The Bethesda Guidelines in 1996 (revised in 2004; see Table 6.2) were primarily established to identify which colorectal tumors should be considered for microsatellite instability testing (MSI; [20]) and/or mismatch repair protein immunohistochemistry (IHC), both of which can serve as screening tests for Lynch syndrome (see next section below). Germline sequencing of the genes of interest could then be pursued in those patients with a positive MSI or IHC test. The Bethesda Guidelines not only incorporate broader age and family history criteria but also include the unique

Table 6.2 The revised Bethesda Guidelines for testing colorectal tumors for microsatellite instability (MSI)

Tumors from individuals should be tested for MSI in the following situations:

1. Colorectal cancer diagnosed in a patient who is less than 50 years of age
2. Presence of synchronous, metachronous colorectal, or other Lynch-associated tumors,[a] regardless of age
3. Colorectal cancer with the MSI-H histology (characterized by the presence of tumor infiltrating lymphocytes, Crohn's-like lymphocytic reaction, mucinous/signet-ring differentiation, or medullary growth pattern) diagnosed in a patient who is less than 60 years of age
4. Colorectal cancer diagnosed in one or more first-degree relatives with a Lynch-related tumor, with one of the cancers being diagnosed under age 50 years
5. Colorectal cancer diagnosed in two or more first- or second-degree relatives with Lynch-related tumors, regardless of age

[a]Lynch-associated tumors include colorectal, endometrial, stomach, ovarian, pancreas, ureter and renal pelvis, biliary tract, and small bowel. Brain tumors (usually glioblastoma as seen in Turcot syndrome) or sebaceous gland adenomas and keratoacanthomas as seen in Muir–Torre syndrome are less common [26]

histopathologic features associated with MSI tumors, including tumor-infiltrating lymphocytes and signet ring cell/poorly differentiated histology (Fig. 6.1). When used alone, the revised Bethesda Guidelines are associated with an increased sensitivity of ~94% in identifying an individual with Lynch syndrome but a lower specificity of 25% [15].

Genetics of Lynch Syndrome and DNA Microsatellite Instability

The genes underlying Lynch syndrome were identified in 1993 when it was recognized that tumors from patients with Lynch syndrome exhibited a unique molecular phenotype designated microsatellite instability. Lynch syndrome can be caused by a germline mutation in one of several genes involved in DNA mismatch repair (MMR). The four most commonly mutated genes, MSH2, MLH1, MSH6, or PMS2, encode proteins that maintain the integrity of short tracts of nucleotide repeats (DNA microsatellite sequences) during replication. To date, most germline mutations have been identified in the MSH2 or MLH1 genes. Pathogenic mutations in any one of these genes can lead to aberrant stretches of mono- or dinucleotide sequences, leading to microsatellite instability and the creation of a "mutator phenotype" within the cell (Fig. 6.2). Most DNA microsatellite sequences are located within intronic sequences, but selected genes have DNA microsatellite sequences within their coding sequences. Cells with mismatch repair deficiency can rapidly accumulate mutations in these genes that contribute to tumorigenesis

Fig. 6.1 Photomicrograph of histologic features associated with colon cancers with microsatellite instability. (**a**) Medullary adenocarcinoma, (**b**) mucinous adenocarcinoma, (**c**) peritumoral Crohn's like reaction, (**d**) tumor-infiltrating lymphocytes. Courtesy of Mari Mino-Kenudson, Massachusetts General Hospital Department of Pathology

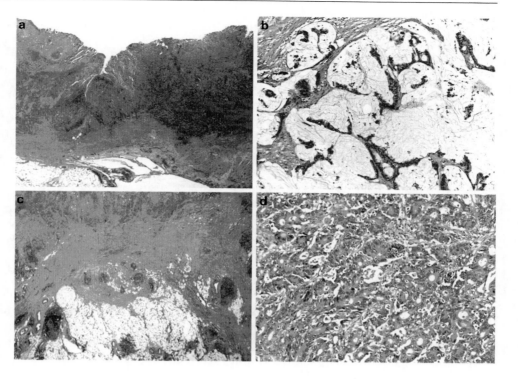

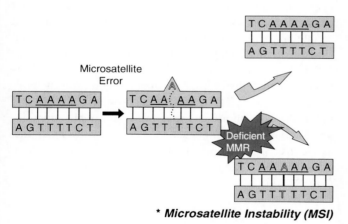

Fig. 6.2 Schematic view of the DNA mismatch repair process and MSI. The DNA mismatch repair system normally corrects base-pair mismatches that can occur during DNA replication. Microsatellite DNA sequences are particularly prone to error, and these errors result in the addition or deletion of one or more microsatellite sequences. Mutations in one of the DNA mismatch repair genes render this process ineffective, and the failure to correct the errors in DNA microsatellites results in "microsatellite instability"

[12]. These target genes include receptors for growth factors (transforming growth factor-β receptor, insulin-like growth factor II receptor, activin receptor type 2), cell cycle regulators (E2F4), regulators of apoptosis (BAX), and some of the MMR genes themselves (MSH3 and MSH6). Thus, defective mismatch repair does not directly result in cellular transformation, but rather establishes a milieu in which mutations develop in key growth-regulatory genes. This has been designated the "MSI pathway" of tumorigenesis, which contrasts with the "chromosomal instability" pathway that is characterized by aneuploidy, frequent loss of heterozygosity, and mutations in the APC, K-Ras, and p53 genes.

The integrity of mismatch repair is routinely analyzed by extracting DNA from an individual's paraffin-embedded tumor sample as well as control normal tissue, and subjecting that DNA to polymerase chain reaction (PCR) amplification of five genetic loci (BAT25, BAT26, D2S123, D5S346, D17S250; [13]). These PCR products can be separated electrophoretically. Differences in fragment size of tumor-derived DNA vs. DNA from normal tissue are scored, leading to an assessment of instability, with instability at ≥2/5 loci, or >30%, being defined as MSI-high (MSI-H). Recently, there has been recognition that an alternative panel of mononucleotide microsatellites may be more effective in detecting MSI and identifying Lynch syndrome [21].

Defects in the MMR genes may also be assessed indirectly in tumor tissue through immunohistochemistry. Absence of MSH2, MLH1, MSH6, or PMS2 protein staining in the nuclei of tumor cells is indicative of a functional mutation that results in protein loss. Adjacent normal colonic

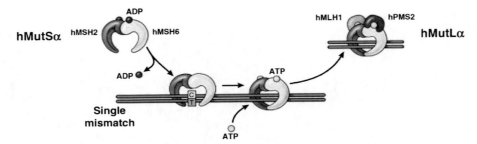

From Grady WM, Carethers JM. Gastroenterology 2008 Oct;135(4):1083

Fig. 6.3 Schematic view of DNA mismatch repair protein function. The heterodimer of MSH2 and MSH6 (also known as hMutSα) recognizes single nucleotide mispairs and binds to DNA as a sliding clamp. The heterodimer of MLH1 and PMS2 (also known as hMutLα) then binds to hMutSα to guide an exonuclease to remove several bases from the newly synthesized DNA strand, with subsequent resynthesis of

DNA with the correct base pairing. When the MutS complexes bind DNA, they exchange ADP for ATP. For the MMR proteins to be released from DNA, ATP is hydrolyzed to ADP. (Reprinted from Gastroenterology, vol. 135, WM Grady and JM Carethers, Genomic and epigenetic instability in colorectal cancer pathogenesis, 136, p. 1083, copyright 2008, with permission from Elsevier.)

mucosa can serve as a positive control. It is important to recognize that MSH2 and MSH6 function as heterodimers, as do MLH1 and PMS2 (Fig. 6.3). A mutation in MLH1 will typically result in immunohistochemical loss of both MLH1 and PMS2, and a mutation in MSH2 will typically result in absence of staining for both MSH2 and MSH6. However, loss of staining of MSH6 or PMS2 alone is typically observed with germline mutations in each of these respective genes. Ultimately, the definitive way to analyze the status of mismatch repair is the direct germline sequencing of MMR genes using DNA isolated from peripheral blood mononuclear cells [13]. An important application of this immunohistochemical approach is that results can direct germline testing to the single gene that displays abnormal staining, rather than the costlier alternative of sequencing all four DNA mismatch repair genes.

There are no consensus "hot-spots" for germline mutations in any of the four DNA mismatch repair genes. Truncating mutations are the most frequent cause of deficient mismatch repair function, but gene rearrangements and epimutations have been increasingly appreciated as potential etiologies of deficient mismatch repair. In a Finnish study, 45 individuals with suspected Lynch syndrome on the basis of abnormal IHC or MSI but without mutations in MLH1, MSH2, or MSH6 were evaluated by multiplex ligation-dependent probe amplification (MLPA) or in some cases, long-range genomic PCR. Twenty-seven percent (12 individuals) were found to have large genomic rearrangements caused by deletions of one or more exons [22]. Genomic rearrangements have also been described in PMS2 [23]. Currently, the standard analysis of DNA mismatch repair genes includes full-gene sequencing of all exons and exon–intron boundaries as well as MLPA to detect large genomic rearrangements or deletions.

Interestingly, two individuals from the Finnish study were found to have germline epimutations in MLH1, as assessed

by methylation-specific multiplex ligation-dependent probe amplification, and confirmed by methylation-specific PCR and sequencing of bisulphite-modified DNA [22]. The phenomenon of germline MLH1 epimutation was first reported by Suter et al. in two individuals meeting clinical criteria for Lynch syndrome but lacking mismatch repair gene mutations. In these individuals, methylation was detected in one of the MLH1 alleles and this was observed in normal tissues. One individual had MLH1 epimutations in a fraction of spermatozoa, suggesting that epimutations may be transmitted among generations [24]. While Gylling et al. did not find epimutations in other mismatch repair genes, Dutch and Chinese families with heritable germline epimutations in MSH2 have been reported [25, 26]. Interestingly, this germline methylation of MSH2 resulted from deletions in the 3′ exons of the TACSTD1 gene that lies upstream of the MSH2 promoter. This observation has important implications for technical approaches to genetic testing in Lynch syndrome, as the loss of MSH2 protein may result from a mutation in either the MSH2 gene itself or an adjacent regulatory gene (TACSTD1).

Screening Tests for Lynch Syndrome

Both IHC and MSI are important tools in the workup of Lynch syndrome. The relative performances of MSI and IHC were determined by Lindor et al., who compared these two screening tools in 1,144 patients. The correlation between the two techniques was excellent; absence of staining for MLH1 or MSH2 was 92.3% sensitive and 100% specific for detection of microsatellite instability. Furthermore, MLH1 or MSH2 immunohistochemistry as a stand-alone approach to identify mutation carriers was associated with a sensitivity of 81.8% and specificity of 93.9%, as compared to 90.0% sensitivity and 93.9% specificity for MSI as a stand-alone screening test [27]. The use of Bethesda Criteria in conjunction with MSI or loss of IHC has been reported to yield 81.8% sensitivity and 97.8% specificity in identifying carriers of a germline mutations in MSH2 or MLH1 [28]. Though the sensitivity of this approach was lower than using MSI or IHC alone, the advantage of using revised Bethesda Guidelines in conjunction with IHC or MSI was derived from a higher positive predictive value for the presence of a germline mutation, as compared to testing for IHC or MSI alone.

In several reports, a screening strategy using both IHC and MSI analyses offered no significant advantage over IHC evaluation alone, and this has important implications considering the greater availability and lower cost of IHC [4, 29, 30]. Similar results indicating the utility of MSI or IHC for screening in high-risk populations have been reported by Terdiman et al. [31]. It is notable, however, that the presence of MMR proteins on IHC may not completely rule out abnormalities in function [28, 32]. Furthermore, while a screening strategy using MSI alone is sensitive, the absence of MSI can be misleading. This is particularly pertinent to cases involving MSH6 mutation, as tumors with MSH6 mutations frequently lack or have low levels of MSI (<30% of microsatellite markers unstable; [32]). The limitations of screening on the basis of MSI alone were demonstrated by Robinson et al. who tested for mutations in MLH1, MSH2, MSH6, and PMS2 in individuals from families either meeting Amsterdam criteria or known to have a history of MSI tumors. Individuals who had a personal or family history of early-onset colorectal cancer were also tested. From the above groups, a subset of 47 MSI-negative families was tested, and ten germline mutations in mismatch repair genes were found, with mutations in MSH6 predominating [33]. Therefore, our algorithm for testing includes both MSI and IHC, which is the most comprehensive screening approach. For purposes of feasibility, IHC alone may be a reasonable strategy if MSI testing is not available. It should be noted that abnormal MSI and IHC are observed not only in colon cancers but also in extracolonic tumors associated with Lynch syndrome as well as precancerous colonic adenomas. Thus, for cases in which adenomatous polyps are the only tissue available for testing, a combination of MSI and IHC testing is also a sensitive approach to screening for Lynch syndrome [34].

It is important to note that many families may fulfill Amsterdam criteria for Lynch syndrome but fail to demonstrate microsatellite instability on tumor testing. Such families are unlikely to have Lynch syndrome, and this is more likely to represent a new colon cancer syndrome, tentatively designated "familial colorectal cancer type X" [35]. These individuals appear to have a lower risk of extracolonic malignancies.

Hypermethylation and Sporadic Colon Cancers

While 85–92% of Lynch syndrome-associated colorectal cancers demonstrate high levels of MSI (i.e., at least 30% of the markers show instability), up to 15% of sporadic colorectal cancers are also associated with microsatellite instability, and this is usually due to somatic hypermethylation of the MLH1 promoter [12, 13]. Recent studies have demonstrated that tumors with somatic hypermethylation of MLH1 can be distinguished from those arising through a germline mutation of MLH1 by the presence of mutations in the BRAF gene. For instance, Deng et al. found BRAF V599E (also known as V600E) mutations in six of eight primary tumors with hypermethylated MLH1, while no BRAF mutations were found in 20 microsatellite unstable tumors from Lynch patients [36]. The mutually exclusive nature of BRAF mutations and a diagnosis of Lynch syndrome have also been documented in patients who fulfill Amsterdam criteria, or who have germline MSH2, MLH1, or MSH6 mutations [37]. In addition, Weisenberger et al. analyzed 295 primary human colorectal tumors and found that sporadic cases of MLH1 methylation were associated with a CpG island methylator phenotype and BRAF mutations [38]. Therefore, BRAF sequencing and MLH1 promoter hypermethylation assays can define which abnormal MSI and IHC results are due to somatic gene alterations and therefore do not require germline DNA sequencing for mismatch repair gene mutations [39].

Screening for Lynch Syndrome in Unselected Colorectal Cancer Populations

Though a thorough family history is a vital first step to assess the risk of Lynch syndrome, there are cases which would be missed if the diagnosis were made solely on Amsterdam or Bethesda criteria. Therefore, there has been a move toward screening broader populations of individuals at risk for Lynch using molecular techniques. Alone, MSI analysis has a sensitivity of greater than 90% for the detection of pathogenic MMR mutations but also has the disadvantage of not predicting which specific gene carries a mutation. IHC is highly sensitive and specific in predicting germline mutations in either MLH1 or MSH2; however, the studies cited above did not account for the importance of mutations in MSH6 [40], and the contribution of PMS2 mutations is being increasingly appreciated.

A study from Pinol et al. prospectively analyzed 1,222 patients with colon cancer from 20 centers, chosen without regard for age, personal or family history, or tumor characteristics. Of these, 1.8% (22 patients) belonged to families meeting clinical criteria for Lynch syndrome by Amsterdam II, while 23.5% (287 patients) belonged to families meeting at least one of the revised Bethesda guidelines. Eighty-three tumors exhibited MSI, and 81 tumors had loss of MSH2 (21 cases) or MLH1 (60 cases) by IHC. Seventy-three of the MSI tumors had loss of MSH2 or MLH1, and the remaining ten tumors with MSI had intact MSH2 or MLH1 staining. Meanwhile, loss of MSH2 or MLH1 by IHC was seen in eight patients with MSS (stable) tumors. Germline mutations in MSH2 or MLH1 were identified in 11 cases, yielding a detection rate of 0.9% in this unselected population of colorectal cancer patients [28]. It is important to note that this study was performed before routine testing for MSH6 and PMS2.

A study of colorectal patients unselected for family history but selected for age less than 60 years was performed by Schofield et al. One thousand three hundred and ninety-five colorectal cancer patients from Western Australia who were less than 60 years old were screened for Lynch syndrome, irrespective of family history. MSI was tested at a single BAT-26 marker as the initial screen, and MSI was detected in 105 patients. Of these, seven tumors had a BRAF mutation, indicating sporadic loss of MLH1 through promoter hypermethylation. Ninety-eight patients had both MSI and wild-type BRAF, suggesting the possibility of Lynch syndrome. Ninety-five of 97 tested cases were evaluated with IHC: 42 patients had absence of both MLH1 and PMS2, 30 patients had absence of MSH2 and MSH6, seven patients had absence of PMS2 alone, and five patients had absence of MSH6 alone. Germline testing was performed in available cases, and the proportion of mutation carriers among MSI cases, grouped by patient age, was: age <30 years: 8/9 = 89%; age 30–39: 10/12 = 83%; age 40–49: 21/31 = 68%; age 50–59: 9/53 = 17%. This indicates that while MSI testing of young patients is more likely to identify cases of Lynch syndrome, restricting the population for MSI screening to age less than 50 years would fail to detect a sizable percentage of patients with mismatch repair defects. Overall, the frequency of Lynch syndrome was of 3.6% (48 cases out of 1,344 patients), supporting MSI-based screening for Lynch syndrome in colorectal patients regardless of family history, particularly in younger patients [41].

Hampel et al. examined an unselected population of colorectal cancer patients in the U.S., asking whether the prevalence of mismatch repair mutations is high enough to warrant large-scale screening. Five hundred unselected colon cancer cases were tested for MSI and IHC of all four mismatch proteins (MSH2, MLH1, MSH6, and PMS2). All 113 cases exhibiting MSI (high or low) or abnormal IHC underwent genetic analysis. Out of 98 MSI tumors and six MSS tumors with MLH1 loss on IHC, 38 exhibited MLH1 promoter methylation. Overall, 18/500 patients with CRC had deleterious mutations: MSH2 = 10, MLH1 = 4, MSH6 = 3, PMS2 = 1. Furthermore, only 7/18 patients fulfilled Amsterdam II criteria,

and 13/18 patients fulfilled revised Bethesda criteria. Five out of these 18 patients with deleterious mutations did not meet either set of criteria. All 18 patients (3.6%) with deleterious mutations displayed MSI, and 17/18 patients were correctly predicted with IHC. Therefore, MSI and IHC screening of colorectal tumors in an unselected population was highly effective at identifying patients with Lynch syndrome. Furthermore, the use of clinical criteria to guide tumor screening would have missed many of these cases, as only eight (44%) of these 18 patients were diagnosed at age less than 50, only 13 patients (72%) met revised Bethesda criteria, and only 7/18 patients met Amsterdam Criteria, yielding a surprisingly low 39% sensitivity [4].

Hampel et al. had published a previous investigation of 1,066 patients, to which the findings on the more recent 500 patients were added. In this combined larger cohort, the overall prevalence of Lynch syndrome was 2.8% (44/1,566 patients; mutation distribution: MSH2 = 23, MLH1 = 9, MSH6 = 6, and PMS2 = 6). Furthermore, for each affected proband, there were, on average, three additional family members who were identified with mutations. A total of 153 individuals were identified with Lynch syndrome (44 probands together with 109 affected relatives). Surprisingly, out of these 153 individuals, only one had been previously diagnosed with Lynch syndrome, pointing to the low detection rates in the population. Age of colon cancer onset was not a reliable predictor, as equal numbers of patients with Lynch syndrome were identified that were younger than as well as older than 50 years. The 2.8% prevalence rate is likely an underestimate, since mutations of unclear significance were not counted toward the diagnosis of Lynch syndrome in this study. While prescreening with Bethesda guidelines would reduce the number of tests required, it would also decrease the number of carriers detected by 28%, thus supporting a proposal for broader screening of unselected populations with colorectal cancer [19].

In order to more accurately integrate the clinical information used to identify individuals with Lynch Syndrome, multiple mathematical models have been designed. At least four models have been created, and each calculates a risk score that reflects various clinical parameters. For instance, the Leiden model incorporates age at diagnosis of colorectal cancer, family history of endometrial cancer, and Amsterdam I criteria. Meanwhile, MMRpredict utilizes age at diagnosis of colorectal cancer, gender, location of tumor, synchronous or metachronous cancers, and occurrence of colorectal or endometrial cancer in a first-degree relative. For all the models, the resulting risk score represents the probability that a colorectal cancer patient possesses a mismatch repair gene mutation. Several studies have recently compared the performance of these models in the clinic when screening patients for Lynch syndrome [42, 43]. In the largest analysis, Green et al. compared four models – Leiden, MMRpredict,

PREMM 1,2, and MMRpro – to predict the presence of mismatch repair mutations in 725 unselected colorectal cancer patients who were under the age of 75 years. Green et al. found that all the models overestimated the risk of a gene mutation in the studied patient population. Results of the comparison, however, favored the use of MMRpredict to identify those patients appropriate for molecular testing for Lynch syndrome [43].

Genotype/Phenotype Correlations

There are fascinating genotype–phenotype correlations that have begun to emerge in Lynch syndrome. As the number of distinct genes associated with Lynch syndrome increases, it is apparent that the clinical phenotype can differ based upon the specific gene mutated. Kastrinos et al. examined 285 patients with deleterious mutations in MLH1 (112) and MSH2 (173). The mean age for colorectal cancer diagnosis was 42.2 years for MLH1 carriers compared to 44.8 years for MSH2 carriers, with male MLH1 carriers having a significantly younger age at colorectal cancer diagnosis compared with MSH2 carriers (38 years vs. 44 years, $P<0.01$). Endometrial cancer was reported in 41% of female mutation carriers (68/167), with similar prevalence in MLH1 and MSH2 cohorts. With respect to all other Lynch-related cancers, there was a much higher prevalence among MSH2 carriers compared to MLH1 carriers (24% vs. 9%; [44]).

Goecke et al. also studied genotype/phenotype correlations in 988 German patients from 281 families with MLH1 or MSH2 mutations. Colorectal cancers were the most frequent cancers, affecting 78% ($n=600$) of MLH1 carriers and 65% of MSH2 carriers ($n=781$). While the majority of cancers affected the right colon, the rectum was the first site of cancer in ~20% of MLH1 and MSH2 carriers. MLH1 mutations were again associated with an earlier age at diagnosis for CRC (41 years vs. 44 years; $P=0.004$), particularly in males with MLH1 mutations (39 years vs. 42 years; $P<0.001$). Of note, 9% of CRCs occurred in male MLH1 carriers prior to age 25 years. Gastric cancer was the second-most frequent GI cancer, representing 5% of tumors from both groups of mutation carriers with a diagnosis almost universally greater than age 35. Only 26% of Lynch-associated gastric cancer cases had a family history of gastric cancer [45]. While gastric cancer occurred with similar frequency in MLH1 and MSH2 carriers, the incidence of urinary tract cancers has been reported to be significantly higher in male MSH2 carriers (lifetime risk of 28% vs. 4% in male MSH2 carriers) [46]. Skin tumors are also more highly associated with MSH2 defects. Goecke reported that 33/38 skin tumors (86%) (including sebaceous adenomas and carcinomas, squamous cell carcinomas, and epitheliomas) were seen in

MSH2 carriers. The strong association between MSH2 mutations and sebaceous skin neoplasms has also been reported by others [47–49]. However, South et al. defined an overall frequency of Muir–Torre among 152 Lynch family members of 9.2%, and mutations in MSH2 or MLH1 were represented equally among families with germline mutation and a history of sebaceous skin tumors or keratocanthomas [50]. Another Lynch-associated tumor seen in MLH1 and MSH2 mutation carriers is adenocarcinoma of the small bowel. A Dutch study of 1,496 individuals from Lynch families demonstrated a small bowel cancer lifetime risk of 4.4% in MLH1 carriers and a 5.9% risk in MSH2 carriers. No small bowel cancers were observed in families with MSH6 mutations [51].

Interestingly, there appear to be specific mutations that correlate with nontraditional tumor spectra. For instance, the G67E mutation in MLH1 was found in a male individual that developed colon cancer in his thirties, and this was preceded by a diagnosis of breast cancer and leiomyosarcoma. The sarcoma was found to possess microsatellite instability, while testing for p53 and BRCA mutations was negative [52]. Similarly, a Danish registry of Lynch syndrome patients found 14 sarcomas in individuals having an MSH2, MLH1, or MSH6 mutation. Eight of these cases had tissue available for testing, and 6/8 exhibited microsatellite instability and loss of staining by IHC [53].

Mutations in MSH6 and PMS2 account for fewer Lynch syndrome cases; however, they appear to be associated with specific clinical presentations. For example, multiple studies have demonstrated a stronger association between endometrial cancer and mutations in MSH6 when compared to other mismatch repair genes. Matthews et al. [54] retrospectively examined endometrial cancers from 61 patients with onset prior to age 50. Twenty-one tumors (34%) from these patients had IHC and MSI findings indicating mismatch repair defects, and 16 patients had absence of staining for MSH6, as compared to only five patients with PMS2, three patients with MLH1, and one with MSH2. Similarly, Hampel et al. examined 543 unselected endometrial cancer patients and found that ten had a deleterious mutation in a mismatch repair gene, with MLH1 accounting for one case, MSH2 accounting for three cases, and mutations in MSH6 accounting for six cases. MSI and IHC correlated well with presence of germline mutation. Abnormal IHC was detected in 8/10 cases and MSI was detected in 9/10 cases. Of note, the one case that was MSI negative occurred in a MSH6 carrier whose tumor was abnormal by IHC for MSH6 protein. Two of the MSH6 tumors exhibited low levels of MSI. This contrasts with a series of colorectal cancer patients where no mutation carriers were found to have MSI-low tumors, likely due to the higher representation of MSH6 mutations in endometrial cancer patients with Lynch syndrome. In fact, Lynch patients with endometrial cancer had a fivefold higher likelihood of mutations in MSH6 as compared to those with colorectal cancer. It is important to remember that women with Lynch syndrome may present first with endometrial cancer rather than colon cancer. Among 543 unselected endometrial cancer cases, it was found that 1.8% of newly diagnosed endometrial cancer patients had Lynch syndrome [55].

Though less frequently seen, the role of PMS2 mutations in Lynch syndrome has been increasingly appreciated. The presence of multiple highly homologous genes and a nearly identical pseudogene has historically impeded analysis of the PMS2 gene. Recent technologies, however, including PMS2-specific polymerase chain reaction and denaturing gradient gel electrophoresis have facilitated mutation analysis of PMS2. Truncating mutations and large genomic rearrangements have also been reported in patients, many of whom did not meet Amsterdam II criteria [56]. As with the other mismatch repair genes, families with PMS2 gene defects are at highest risk for colorectal cancer, followed in frequency by endometrial cancer. In comparison to MSH2 or MLH1 patients, PMS2 mutations are associated with older age of colorectal cancer onset (mean = 59 years), and carriers have a lower risk of Lynch-associated cancers in general. This suggests that defects in PMS2 may result in an attenuated phenotype compared to MSH2 and MLH1 inactivation [57, 58]. The exception to this is individuals who are homozygous for PMS2 mutations. Biallelic PMS2 mutation carriers exhibit a unique phenotype that includes cancers of the gastrointestinal tract, central nervous system tumors, clinical features of neurofibromatosis, and lymphomas at very young ages [57].

Management of Patients with Lynch Syndrome

For patients who fulfill the Amsterdam Criteria or who have an identified mutation in a mismatch repair gene, aggressive surveillance is recommended for tissues at risk. Colonoscopy every 3 years has been demonstrated to reduce the incidence of colon cancer by 62% and overall mortality by 65% [59], though expert consensus recommends colonoscopy starting in the early twenties and repeating every 1–2 years until age 40, at which point exams should be performed annually [29]. While firm evidence supporting efficacy are lacking, the increased risk of endometrial, ovarian, and urinary collecting system cancers has led to the additional recommendations of annual gynecologic evaluation with endometrial biopsy and transvaginal ultrasound as well as annual urinalysis with cytology [7]. Prophylactic hysterectomy and oophorectomy should be considered in women who have completed childbearing [60]. Other screening tests that have

not been studied rigorously include upper endoscopy and renal ultrasound exams, and some apply these based upon the cancer family history [7].

A diagnosis of Lynch syndrome influences not only cancer surveillance and prevention practices but also the decisions regarding therapy at the time of cancer diagnosis. Because of the 45% rate of metachronous colorectal cancers, patients diagnosed with early-stage colon cancer or more than one advanced adenoma should consider subtotal colectomy with ileorectal anastomosis (IRA). After total colectomy with IRA, regular endoscopic surveillance is required due to the 12% risk of developing cancer in the retained rectum after 10–12 years [61]. A consensus recommendation for surveillance in individuals with Lynch syndrome was provided in 2009 by the National Comprehensive Cancer Network and is summarized in Table 6.3 below [62].

Table 6.3 NCCN practice Guidelines for Lynch syndrome follow-up

Surveillance

Colon cancer

- Colonoscopy at age 20–25 years or 10 years prior to the youngest age at diagnosis in the family, whichever comes first, and repeat every 1–2 years

Extracolonic

- Gastric and duodenal cancer: Consider upper GI endoscopy (including side-viewing examination) at age 25–30 years and repeat every 1–3 years
- Urothelial cancer: Consider annual urinalysis and imaging of the renal collecting system
- Central nervous system cancer: Annual physical examination: no additional screening recommendations have been made
- Pancreatic cancer: No recommendations have been made

For women:

Endometrial and ovarian cancer

- Encourage patient education and prompt response to endometrial cancer symptoms
- Screening for endometrial cancer with transvaginal ultrasound and office endometrial sampling annually and screening for ovarian cancer with concurrent transvaginal ultrasound (preferably day 1–10 of cycle for premenopausal women), plus CA-125 every 6–12 months, starting by age 30–35 years or 5–10 years prior to the earliest age of first diagnosis of these cancers in the family
- Prophylactic hysterectomy and bilateral salpingo-oophorectomy is a risk-reducing option for women who have completed childbearing. Chemoprevention may be considered.

If no pathologic findings: Continue screening. For women, consider prophylactic total abdominal hysterectomy with bilateral salpingo-oophorectomy

If adenomas are found: Endoscopic polypectomy with follow-up colonoscopy every 1–2 years depending on location, character, surgical risk, patient preference

If adenomas found not amenable to endoscopic resection or high-grade dysplasia: Total abdominal colectomy with ileorectal anastomosis. Consider TAH/BSO at time of colon surgery if postmenopausal or family completed. Endoscopic rectal examination of the remaining mucosa every 1–2 years

If adenocarcinoma found: Standard treatment recommendations for colorectal cancer

Based on epidemiologic evidence that nonsteroidal antiinflammatory use is associated with a decreased risk of sporadic colorectal cancer [63–65], a chemoprevention study has been performed to assess reduction of colorectal polyps and cancers in Lynch syndrome. Sulindac is used clinically to slow the development of polyps in patients with familial adenomatous polyposis [66]. In a randomized placebo-controlled trial of 1,071 persons, Burn et al. assessed the role of 600 mg of aspirin daily in reducing adenoma and carcinoma risk in individuals with Lynch syndrome. They also explored the role of resistant starch, based on previous epidemiologic evidence. Aspirin, resistant starch, or both taken for up to 4 years did not reduce the incidence of adenomas or cancer in Lynch syndrome [67].

When colorectal cancer develops, treatment is determined on the basis of disease stage. Though colorectal cancer can arise via a chromosomal instability pathway (responsible for 85% of sporadic colorectal cancers) or a microsatellite instability pathway (responsible for 15% of colorectal cancers), the underlying mechanism of genetic instability has not historically been a consideration in therapy. Only very recently have these characteristics weighed into treatment decisions (Eastern Cooperative Oncology Group, A Randomized Phase III Study Comparing 5-FU, Leucovorin and Oxaliplatin vs. 5-FU, Leucovorin, Oxaliplatin and Bevacizumab in Patients with Stage II Colon Cancer at High Risk for Recurrence to Determine Prospectively the Prognostic Value of Molecular Markers). This is based on the observation that colorectal cancers possessing MSI are associated with a relatively favorable course when compared to cancers with chromosomal instability [68]. The relationship between MSI status and responsiveness to chemotherapy is not straightforward. Ribic et al. performed a retrospective study of microsatellite instability as a predictor of outcome following adjuvant 5-fluorouracil in stage II and stage III colon cancer. Interestingly, patients with MSI-H tumors who did not receive chemotherapy had a higher 5-year overall survival than patients with MSI-L or MSI-stable tumors (88% vs. 68.4%). Furthermore, among patients with MSI-tumors, those who received adjuvant fluorouracil fared worse than those who did not receive adjuvant therapy (5-year overall survival of 70.7% vs. 88%), while patients with MSI-L or MSI-stable tumors benefited from adjuvant therapy (5-year overall survival of 75.5% vs. 68.4%; [69]). Similar findings were recently reported in a prospective study by Jover et al. [70]. Because the majority of these MSI-H tumors were likely to represent sporadic tumors with MLH1 hypermethylation, it is as yet unclear whether these observations hold for patients with Lynch syndrome. Furthermore, it is unknown whether patients with MSI-H tumors would also fail to benefit from current adjuvant chemotherapy regimens containing newer agents such as oxaliplatin.

Genetic Counseling

Incorporating all of these molecular and clinical components into the evaluation of cancer risk is a complex process. Genetic counselors play a pivotal role in this process, as their expertise facilitates multiple facets of patient evaluation and care. One of their essential roles includes the evaluation of family history, which is crucial to the assessment of cancer risk. In addition, their expertise helps crystallize the features of various hereditary syndromes into an algorithm for genetic testing. For example, it has been reported that some families with clinical features consistent with Lynch syndrome did not carry DNA mismatch repair mutations but instead harbored MYH gene mutations [71]. Recognizing that there can be overlap between syndromes is crucial, and this is an important aspect of testing algorithms. While the interpretation of genetic test results is often straightforward, there are inevitably circumstances where results of testing provide limited guidance. For example, mutations of uncertain significance are sometimes identified that do not have any known relationship to disease etiology and risk. Also, the inherent limitations of testing will occasionally result in negative test results that do not reflect true risk within a given family.

Genetic counselors are trained to distill technical jargon and such subtleties of testing into explanations that can be easily understood by the patient, allowing individuals to make informed decisions about the medical, psychological, and social pros and cons of proceeding with genetic testing. As we move forward, continued advances in the understanding of the genetic basis of cancer will present additional challenges for genetic counselors and clinicians. For instance, though not widely used, prenatal testing is already available to determine fetal risk of carrying a mutation in the genes that cause FAP, MAP, and HNPCC. Furthermore, advances in reproductive technology have even made preimplantation genetic diagnosis of these diseases possible [72]. Clearly, the multifaceted issues surrounding genetic testing for colorectal syndromes in adults will be further amplified in these settings, necessitating the expertise of appropriately trained genetic counselors and clinicians.

Summary

It is crucial for clinicians caring for colorectal cancer patients to be fully aware of the inherited predisposition syndromes, particularly Lynch syndrome. High-risk patients should be identified and referred to specially trained teams that include endoscopists, oncologists, surgeons, pathologists, and genetic counselors. There is evidence, however, that the clinical identification of high-risk patients and families is inadequate, and

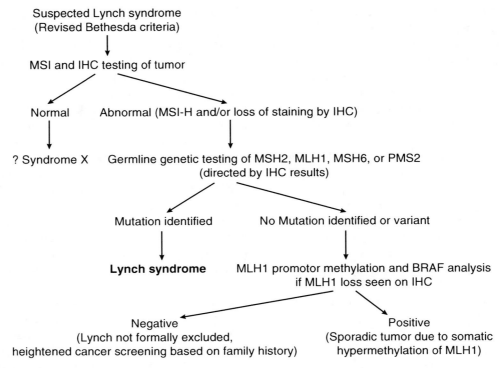

Suspected Lynch syndrome
(Revised Bethesda criteria)

MSI and IHC testing of tumor

Normal   Abnormal (MSI-H and/or loss of staining by IHC)

? Syndrome X   Germline genetic testing of MSH2, MLH1, MSH6, or PMS2
(directed by IHC results)

Mutation identified   No Mutation identified or variant

Lynch syndrome   MLH1 promotor methylation and BRAF analysis
if MLH1 loss seen on IHC

Negative
(Lynch not formally excluded,
heightened cancer screening based on family history)

Positive
(Sporadic tumor due to somatic
hypermethylation of MLH1)

Fig. 6.4 Algorithm of the molecular and genetic workup for suspected Lynch syndrome

therefore, MSI and IHC screening strategies in unselected colon cancer patients may be warranted. Subsequent germline gene testing can then identify pathologic mutations in affected and unaffected family members, and appropriate surveillance and management can be instituted (summarized in Fig. 6.4). Nonetheless, genetic testing is imperfect, and a thorough family history and sound clinical judgment are still essential components in the appropriate workup and management of Lynch syndrome.

References

1. Meyerhardt JA, Mayer RJ (2005) N Engl J Med 352:476–487
2. Lynch HT, de la Chapelle A (2003) Hereditary colorectal cancer. N Engl J Med 348:919–932
3. Smith RA, von Eschenbach AC, Wender R et al (2001) American Cancer Society guidelines for the early detection of cancer: update of early detection guidelines for prostate, colorectal, and endometrial cancers. CA Cancer J Clin 51:38–75
4. Hampel H, Frankel WL, Martin E et al (2008) Feasibility of screening for Lynch syndrome among patients with colorectal cancer. J Clin Oncol 26:5783–5788
5. Warthin AS (1925) The further study of a cancer family. J Cancer Res 9:279–286
6. Lynch HT, Krush AJ (1971) Cancer family G revisited: 1895–1970. Cancer 27:1505–1511
7. Jo WS, Chung DC (2005) Genetics of hereditary colorectal cancer. Sem Oncol 32:11–23
8. Rijcken FE, Hollema H, Kleibeuker JH (2002) Proximal adenomas in hereditary non-polyposis colorectal cancer are prone to rapid malignant transformation. Gut 50:382–386
9. Vasen H, Wijnen J, Menko F et al (1996) Cancer risk in families with hereditary nonpolyposis colorectal cancer diagnosed by mutation analysis. Gastroenterology 110:1020–1028
10. Watson P, Lynch H (2001) Cancer risk in mismatch repair gene mutation carriers. Fam Cancer 1:57–60
11. Hampel H, Stephens JA, Pukkala E et al (2005) Cancer risk in hereditary nonpolyposis colorectal cancer syndrome: later age of onset. Gastroenterology 129:415–421
12. Chung DC, Rustgi AK (2003) The hereditary nonpolyposis colorectal cancer syndrome: genetic and clinical implications. Ann Intern Med 138:560–570
13. Hendriks YMC, de Jong AE, Morreau H et al (2006) Diagnostic approach and management of Lynch syndrome (hereditary nonpolyposis colorectal carcinoma): a guide for clinicians. CA Cancer J Clin 56:213–225
14. Vasen HF, Mecklin JP, Khan PM et al (1991) The international collaborative group on hereditary non-polyposis colorectal cancer (ICG-HNPCC). Dis Colon Rectum 34:424–425
15. Syngal S, Fox EA, Eng C et al (2000) Sensitivity and specificity of clinical criteria for hereditary non-polyposis colorectal cancer associated mutations in MSH2 and MLH1. J Med Genet 37:641–645
16. Liu T, Wahlberg S, Burek E et al (2000) Micro-satellite instability as a predictor of a mutation in a DNA mismatch repair gene in familial colorectal cancer. Genes Chromosomes Cancer 27:17–25
17. Lipton LR, Johnson V, Cummings C et al (2004) Refining the Amsterdam criteria and Bethesda guidelines: testing algorithms for the prediction of mismatch repair mutation status in the familial cancer clinic. J Clin Oncol 22:4934–4943
18. Vasen HF, Watson P, Mecklin JP et al (1999) New clinical criteria for hereditary nonpolyposis colorectal cancer (HNPCC, Lynch

syndrome) proposed by the International Collaborative Group on HNPCC. Gastroenterology 116:1453–1456

19. Hampel H, Frankel WL, Martin E et al (2005) Screening for the Lynch syndrome (hereditary nonpolyposis colorectal cancer). N Engl J Med 352:1851–1860

20. Umar A, Boland CR, Terdiman JP et al (2004) Revised Bethesda guidelines for hereditary nonpolyposis colorectal cancer (Lynch syndrome) and microsatellite instability. J Natl Cancer Inst 96:261–268

21. Laghi L, Bianchi P, Malesci A (2008) Differences and evolution of the methods for the assessment of microsatellite instability. Oncogene 27(49):6313–6321

22. Gylling A, Ridanpaa M, Vierimaa O et al (2009) Large genomic rearrangements and germline epimutations in Lynch syndrome. Int J Cancer 124:2333–2340

23. Van der Klift H, Wijnen J, Wagner A et al (2005) Molecular characterization of the spectrum of genomic deletions in the mismatch repair genes MSH2, MLH1, MSH6, and PMS2 responsible for hereditary nonpolyposis colorectal cancer (HNPCC). Genes Chromosomes Cancer 44:123–138

24. Suter CM, Martin DIK, Ward RL (2004) Germline epimutation of MLH1 in individuals with multiple cancers. Nat Genet 36:497–501

25. Chan TL, Yuen ST, Kong CK et al (2006) Heritable germline epimutation of MSH2 in a family with hereditary nonpolyposis colorectal cancer. Nat Genet 38:1178–1183

26. Ligtenberg MJ, Kuiper RP, Chan TL et al (2009) Heritable somatic methylation and inactivation of MSH2 in families with Lynch syndrome due to deletion of the 3′ exons of TACSTD1. Nat Genet 41:112–117

27. Lindor NM, Burgart LJ, Leontovich O et al (2002) Immunohistochemistry versus microsatellite instability testing in phenotyping colorectal tumors. J Clin Oncol 20:1043–1048

28. Pinol V, Castells A, Andreu M et al (2005) Accuracy of revised Bethesda guidelines, microsatellite instability, and immunohistochemistry for the identification of patients with hereditary nonpolyposis colorectal cancer. JAMA 293:1986–1994

29. Lindor NM, Petersen GM, Hadley DW et al (2006) Recommendations for the care of individuals with an inherited predisposition to Lynch syndrome: a systematic review. JAMA 296:1507–1517

30. Wahlberg SS, Schmeits J, Thomas G et al (2002) Evaluation of microsatellite instability and immunohistochemistry for the prediction of germ-line MSH2 and MLH1 mutations in hereditary nonpolyposis colon cancer families. Cancer Res 62:3485–3492

31. Terdiman JP, Gum JR, Conrad PG et al (2001) Efficient detection of hereditary nonpolyposis colorectal cancer gene carriers by screening for tumor microsatellite instability before germline genetic testing. Gastroenterology 120:21–30

32. Berends MJW, Wu Y, Sijmons RH et al (2002) Molecular and clinical characteristics of MSH6 variants: an analysis of 25 index carriers of a germline variant. Am J Hum Genet 70:26–37

33. Robinson KL, Liu T, Vandrovcova J et al (2007) Lynch syndrome (hereditary nonpolyposis colorectal cancer) diagnostics. J Natl Cancer Inst 99:291–299

34. Pino MS, Mino-Kenudson M, Wildemore BM et al (2009) Deficient DNA mismatch repair is common in Lynch syndrome-associated colorectal adenomas. J Mol Diagn 11:238–247

35. Lindor NM, Rabe K, Petersen GM et al (2005) Lower cancer incidence in Amsterdam-I criteria families without mismatch repair deficiency: familial colorectal cancer type X. JAMA 293(16):1979–1985

36. Deng G, Bell I, Crawley S et al (2004) BRAF mutation is frequently present in sporadic colorectal cancer with methylated hMLH1 but not in hereditary nonpolyposis colorectal cancer. Clin Cancer Res 10:191–195

37. Domingo E, Niessen RC, Oliveira C et al (2005) BRAF-V600E is not involved in the colorectal tumorigenesis of HNPCC in patients with functional MLH1 and MSH2 genes. Oncogene 24:3995–3998

38. Weisenberger DJ, Siegmund KD, Campan M et al (2006) CpG island methylator phenotype underlies sporadic microsatellite instability and is tightly associated with BRAF mutation in colorectal cancer. Nat Genet 38:787–793

39. Bessa X, Ballesté B, Andreu M et al (2008) A prospective, multi-center, population-based study of BRAF mutational analysis for Lynch syndrome screening. Clin Gastroenterol Hepatol 6:206–214

40. Peltomaki P (2005) Lynch syndrome genes. Fam Cancer 4:227–232

41. Schofield L, Watson N, Grieu F et al (2009) Population-based detection of Lynch syndrome in young colorectal cancer patients using microsatellite instability as the initial test. Int J Cancer 124:1097–1102

42. Pouchet CJ, Wong N, Chong G et al (2009) A comparison of models used to predict MLH1, MSH2 and MSH6 mutation carriers. Ann Oncol 20:681–688

43. Green RC, Parfrey PS, Woods MO et al (2009) Prediction of Lynch syndrome in consecutive patients with colorectal cancer. J Natl Cancer Inst 101:331–340

44. Kastrinos F, Stoffel EM, Balmana J et al (2008) Phenotype comparison of MLH1 and MSH2 mutation carriers in a cohort of 1, 914 individuals undergoing clinical genetic testing in the United States. Cancer Epidemiol Biomarkers Prev 17:2044–2051

45. Goecke T, Schulmann K, Engel C et al (2006) Genotype–phenotype comparison of German MLH1 and MSH2 mutation carriers clinically affected with Lynch syndrome: a report by the German HNPCC consortium. J Clin Onc 24:4285–4292

46. Watson P, Vasen HFA, Mecklin J-P et al (2008) The risk of extra-colonic, extra-endometrial cancer in the Lynch syndrome. Int J Cancer 123:444–449

47. Kruse R, Rutten A, Lambert C et al (1998) Muir–Torre phenotype has a frequency of DNA mismatch-repair-gene mutations similar to that in hereditary nonpolyposis colorectal cancer families defined by the Amsterdam criteria. Am J Hum Genet 63:63–70

48. Mangold J, Pagenstecher C, Leister M et al (2004) A genotype–phenotype correlation in HNPCC: strong predominance of MSH2 mutations in 41 patients with Muir–Torre syndrome. J Med Genet 41:567–572

49. Kruse R, Lamberti C, Wang Y et al (1996) Is the mismatch repair deficient type of Muir–Torre syndrome confined to mutations in the hMSH2 gene? Hum Genet 98:747–750

50. South CD, Hampel H, Comeras I et al (2008) The frequency of Muir–Torre syndrome among Lynch syndrome families. J Natl Cancer Inst 100:277–281

51. ten Kate GL, Kleibeuker JH, Nagengast FM et al (2007) Is surveillance of the small bowel indicated for Lynch syndrome families. Gut 56:1198–1201

52. Clyne M, Offman J, Shanley S et al (2009) The G67E mutation in hMLH1 is associated with an unusual presentation of Lynch syndrome. Br J Cancer 100:376–380

53. Nilbert M, Therkildsen C, Nissen A et al (2009). Sarcomas associated with hereditary nonpolyposis colorectal cancer: broad anatomical and morphological spectrum. Fam Cancer 8:209–213

54. Matthews KS, Estes JM, Conner MG et al (2008) Lynch syndrome in women less than 50 years of age with endometrial cancer. Obstet Gynecol 111:1161–1165

55. Hampel H, Frankel W, Panescu J et al (2006) Screening for Lynch syndrome (hereditary nonpolyposis colorectal cancer) among endometrial cancer patients. Cancer Res 66:7810–7817

56. Hendriks YMC, Jagmohan-Changur S, Van Der Klift HM et al (2006) Heterozygous mutations in PMS2 cause hereditary nonpolyposis colorectal carcinoma (Lynch syndrome). Gastroenterology 130:312–322

57. Senter L, Clendenning M, Sotamaa K et al (2008) The clinical phenotype of Lynch syndrome due to germ-line PMS2 mutations. Gastroenterology 135:419–428

58. Niessen RC, Kleibeuker JH, Westers H et al (2009) PMS2 involvement in patients suspected of Lynch syndrome. Genes Chromosomes Cancer 48:322–329

59. Jarvinen HJ, Aarnio M, Mustonen H et al (2000) Controlled 15-year trial on screening for colorectal cancer in families with hereditary nonpolyposis colorectal cancer. Gastroenterology 118:829–834

60. Schmeler KM, Lynch HT, Chen LM et al (2006) Prophylactic surgery to reduce the risk of gynecologic cancers in the Lynch syndrome. N Engl J Med 354:261–269

61. Guillem JG, Wood WC, Moley JF et al (2006) ASCO/SSO review of current role of risk-reducing surgery in common hereditary cancer syndromes. J Clin Oncol 24:4642–4660

62. NCCN Practice Guidelines in Oncology – v.1.2009. Colorectal cancer screening, Hereditary predisposition, Lynch syndrome. CSCR-10

63. Dube C, Rostom A, Lewin G et al (2007) The use of aspirin for primary prevention of colorectal cancer: a systematic review prepared for the U.S. Preventive Services Task Force. Ann Intern Med 146:365

64. Rostom A, Dube C, Lewin G et al (2007) Nonsteroidal anti-inflammatory drugs and cyclooxygenase-2 inhibitors for primary prevention of colorectal cancer: a systematic review prepared for the U.S. Preventive Services Task Force. Ann Intern Med 146:376

65. Flossmann E, Rothwell PM (2007) Effect of aspirin on long-term risk of colorectal cancer: consistent evidence from randomised and observational studies. Lancet 369:1603

66. Cruz-Correa M, Hylind LM, Romans KE et al (2002) Long-term treatment with Sulindac in familial adenomatous polyposis: a prospective cohort study. Gastroenterology 122:641

67. Burn J, Bishop T, Mecklin J-P et al (2008) Effect of aspirin or resistant starch on colorectal neoplasia in the Lynch syndrome. N Engl J Med 359:2567–2578

68. Gryfe R, Kim H, Hsieh ETK et al (2000) Tumor microsatellite instability and clinical outcome in young patients with colorectal cancer. N Engl J Med 342:69–77

69. Ribic CM, Sargent DJ, Moore MJ et al (2003) Tumor microsatellite-instability status as a predictor of benefit from fluorouracil-based adjuvant chemotherapy for colon cancer. N Engl J Med 349:247–257

70. Jover R, Zapater P, Castells A et al (2006) Mismatch repair status in the prediction of benefit from adjuvant fluorouracil chemotherapy in colorectal cancer. Gut 55:848–855

71. Jo WS, Bandipalliam P, Shannon KM, Niendorf KB, Chan-Smutko G, Hur C, Syngal S, Chung DC (2005) Correlation of polyp number and family history of colon cancer with germline MYH mutations. Clin Gastroenterol Hepatol 3:1022–1028

72. Offit K, Kohut K, Clagett B et al (2006) Cancer genetic testing and assisted reproduction. J Clin Oncol 24:4775–4782

Chapter 7
Hereditary Pancreatic Cancer

Janivette Alsina and Sarah P. Thayer

Keywords Pancreatic cancer • PANIN • BRCA2 • p16 gene • Endoscopic ultrasound • MRI • ERCP • Hereditary pancreatitis • Pancreatic endocrine tumor

Introduction

Neoplastic processes of the pancreas can be divided into two broad categories based on the histopathologic properties of the tumor. Tumors of exocrine differentiation include those resembling pancreatic ducts or acinar cells. This category includes pancreatic adenocarcinoma, intraductal mucinous tumors, solid pseudopapillary tumors, and acinar cell carcinoma. Tumors of endocrine differentiation exhibit characteristics of the various islet cell populations and include, among others, insulinomas, glucagonomas, and gastrinomas.

The majority of cases of pancreatic cancer are sporadic in nature. Approximately 90–95% of all pancreatic cancers are of the exocrine type; most of these are ductal adenocarcinomas (PDAC). Pancreatic malignancies are now the fourth leading cause of cancer-related deaths in the US in both men and women, with an estimated 37,680 new pancreatic cancer cases and 34,290 deaths in 2008 [1, 2]. The recognition that pancreatic cancer aggregates in some families, in a manner similar to familial colon cancer, is providing new insights into the molecular pathogenesis of this disease that will likely be applied to cases of sporadic cancer, which express some of the same mutations found in hereditary cases.

Early studies suggested a hereditary component in the pathogenesis of pancreatic cancer; in some families multiple family members across generations are affected.

In a case-control study published in 1991, approximately 8% of patients with pancreatic cancer reported at least one family member with the disease, whereas less than 1% of unaffected controls reported an affected family member [3].

An estimated 5–10% of pancreatic cancer cases are believed to arise as part of a familial cancer syndrome. These familial clusterings of pancreatic cancer are divided into one of three broad categories: (1) families who develop pancreatic cancer in the setting of a known familial cancer syndrome in which pancreatic cancer is not the predominant phenotype (Peutz–Jeghers, Lynch/HNPCC, BRCA2) [4–7], (2) families with hereditary pancreatitis, and (3) families where multiple members develop pancreatic cancer with no association with known tumor syndromes.

The term "familial pancreatic cancer" is generally used to denote kindred which include at least two first-degree relatives (FDR) with pancreatic adenocarcinoma but exhibit no clustering of other cancers [8]. The variability of phenotypes in affected kindred carrying known mutations has been attributed to the types of mutations involved, environmental exposures, and expression of potentially modifying genes [9, 10]. Identifying the causative genes and the actual risk of developing pancreatic cancer in these families is difficult, given the low incidence of pancreatic cancer in the general population, the relatively small number of affected families, and the fact that kindred affected can be quite small. Despite these limitations, a number of inherited genetic alterations that increase the risk of pancreatic cancer have been discovered. These include germline mutations in DNA repair genes (BRCA1, BRCA 2, hMLH1), cell cycle regulators (p16), pancreatic enzymes (PRSS1), and their regulators, among others [11–13]. Some of these mutations are also found as somatic alterations in sporadic cases of pancreatic cancer, which highlights the potential for developing diagnostic and therapeutic interventions based on studies of this high-risk population.

A smaller proportion of pancreatic cancers are well-differentiated endocrine neoplasms, often referred to as islet cell tumors or neuroendocrine tumors. Endocrine tumors of the pancreas differ from exocrine tumors in their growth characteristics, ability to produce hormones that lead to

S.P. Thayer (✉)
Department of Surgery, Harvard Medical School, Boston, MA, USA;
Director, Pancreatic Biology Laboratory, Massachusetts General Hospital, Boston, MA, USA
e-mail: sthayer@partners.org

characteristic clinical symptoms, and overall better prognosis compared with PDAC. In general, endocrine tumors of the pancreas are categorized by the hormones they produce. They tend to grow at slower rates, show less propensity to become metastatic, and in most cases are amenable to less radical surgical resections, such as local enucleation. Their rates of recurrence are also more favorable than those of exocrine tumors, and overall 5-year survival rates are better than those of PDAC. In cases of advanced, non-resectable or metastatic disease, palliation can sometimes be achieved using anti-hormonal agents in combination with chemotherapy.

Hereditary Pancreatic Endocrine Tumors

Pancreatic endocrine neoplasms can occur sporadically or in association with genetic syndromes (see Chap. 11). Because of their low incidence, estimated at one to five cases per million annually, little is known about the underlying genetics of sporadic endocrine tumors. The association with inherited disorders is better understood. These tumors can be associated with multiple endocrine neoplasia type 1 syndrome (MEN-1), neurofibromatosis, tuberous sclerosis, and von-Hippel Lindau (vHL). Of these, the highest risk for the development of these tumors is seen in the MEN-1 (multiple endocrine neoplasia) syndrome [14].

The MEN-1 syndrome is a rare, autosomal-dominant condition with the potential for multiple tumor formation, primarily in the parathyroid, pituitary, and pancreatic islets in affected individuals. Germline mutations of the *MEN1* gene were linked to this syndrome in 1997 [15]. The *MEN1* gene product, menin, is believed to act as a tumor suppressor via its interactions with transcription factors, proteins involved in cell-cycle progression, and cell division regulators. Most recently, it has been shown to regulate gene expression through histone methylation [16]. The age-dependent penetrance of pancreatic endocrine tumors in MEN-1 carriers has been estimated at 45% at 30 years, 82% at 50 years, and 96% at 70 years, highlighting the importance of early detection and treatment [17]. Current genetic tests can identify mutations in approximately 50% of suspected MEN-1 patients; clinical guidelines for testing and screening of the pancreatic tumors in this population are discussed in Chap. 11.

Exocrine Neoplasms of the Pancreas

Given the poor prognosis of pancreatic adenocarcinoma, its association with hereditary syndromes presents an opportunity not only to better characterize the origin and progression of this disease, but also to test early screening strategies to identify those likely to be affected. In a prospective registry-based study to estimate the risk of pancreatic cancer in individuals with a known family history of pancreatic cancer, 22 of the 25 individuals who developed pancreatic cancer during the study presented with advanced, metastatic disease [5]. Given that the only curative treatment at this time is early eradication of the tumor using surgical strategies, early detection and intervention are key in the treatment of this disease.

Hereditary Tumor Syndromes Associated with Exocrine Pancreatic Neoplasms

Several hereditary tumor syndromes that are well-recognized for their risks of non-pancreatic tumors are also associated with an increased risk of pancreatic ductal adenocarcinoma (PDAC). To date, four genetic syndromes have been described that carry an increased risk for the development of pancreatic cancer: Peutz–Jeghers syndrome (PJS), hereditary non-polyposis colon cancer syndrome (HNPCC), familial atypical mole melanoma syndrome (FAMM), and hereditary breast/ovarian cancer (HBOC).

Peutz–Jeghers

Peutz–Jeghers is an autosomal-dominant condition first described in 1921 by Jan Peutz, who described a relationship between mucocutaneous lesions and intestinal polyps in a Dutch family [18] (Chap. 5). Approximately 50% of Peutz–Jeghers cases have been associated with mutations in a serine-threonine kinase, LKB1/STK11, which is involved in the regulation of cell polarity, proliferation, and the mTOR pathway. The product of this gene is believed to act as a tumor suppressor.

The phenotypic presentation in affected individuals includes the finding of characteristic mucocutaneous pigmentation and gastrointestinal hamartomatous polyps. Relative to the general population, these individuals are estimated to have a 132-fold greater risk of developing PDAC, or a 36% cumulative risk of developing pancreatic cancer by age 64 [19], a risk significantly above that for the general population. Peutz–Jeghers syndrome has also been associated with intrapapillary mucinous neoplasms (IPMN). These lesions are cystic neoplasms of the pancreas with malignant potential. It has been estimated that approximately 32% of IPMN demonstrate a loss of heterozygosity at the LKB1/STK11 locus. However, the percentage of patients presenting with PDAC who have this in the setting of an IPMN is unknown.

Hereditary Non-polyposis Colon Cancer: Lynch Syndrome

Also known as Lynch Syndrome, HNPCC is an inherited autosomal-dominant condition with a high predisposition for the development of malignant colorectal tumors (see Chap. 6). The mutations responsible for this syndrome have been mapped to several DNA repair genes, including hMLH1, hMSH2, hMSH6, and hPMS2. These mutations lead to the accumulation of DNA replication errors that ultimately result in microsatellite instability. Affected individuals have a lifetime risk of up to 80% for developing colorectal cancer; the tumors tend to cluster proximal to the splenic flexure. Based on clinical presentation, those affected are traditionally classified into two categories: those presenting with colorectal tumors only are classified as Lynch I, whereas a separate group, designated Lynch II, present with colon cancers and extracolonic tumors, including uterine, ovarian, gastric, pancreatic, biliary and urinary tract cancers. Although there appear to be trends for a slightly increased risk of pancreatic cancer in Lynch syndrome, the exact risk for the development of pancreatic cancer is unknown.

Familial Atypical Mole Melanoma Syndrome

This syndrome is characterized by the presence of dysplastic nevi and melanoma in association with other malignancies that include pancreatic cancer (see Chap. 10). FAMM is caused by a germline mutation in the p16/CDKN2A gene, which is located on chromosome 9p. It is inherited in an autosomal-dominant fashion, with an estimated 80–100% penetrance. Somatic mutations in p16 are also identified in more than 90% of sporadic pancreatic cancer cases. In the FAMM syndrome, melanoma is the most frequent malignancy, followed by pancreatic cancer. The relative risk for the development of pancreatic cancer is estimated to be between 12- and 38-fold. The cumulative risk has been estimated to be 17% by age 75 [11, 20]. Only a subset of FAMM kindred with p16 mutations will develop pancreatic cancer, and which factors increase this risk is unknown. Family history is an important diagnostic tool, as most patients with pancreatic cancer associated with germline mutations of CDKN2A also have a family or personal history of melanoma.

Hereditary Breast/Ovarian Cancer Syndrome

The association between germline mutations in the breast cancer genes BRCA1 and BRCA2 and an increased risk of breast and ovarian cancers is well established (see Chap. 3). These mutations exhibit an autosomal-dominant pattern of inheritance, with incomplete penetrance. Their gene products act as tumor suppressors via their roles in transcriptional regulation and DNA damage repair. It is estimated that 5–10% of all breast and ovarian tumors are associated with BRCA1/2 mutations, and that the incidence of carrying a mutated gene in the general population of the U.S. is approximately 1/345–1/1,000. Pancreatic cancer has been associated with BRCA2 mutations since the discovery of the gene.

A link between BRCA2 genes and pancreatic cancer was established during the mapping and cloning of a region of chromosome 13q from pancreatic carcinoma samples that later mapped to the BRCA2 gene, already known for its role in breast cancer development. Pancreatic cancer is the third most common tumor detected in mutation carriers. BRCA2 mutations have been shown to account for approximately 6–17% of familial pancreatic cancers [21, 22], making it the most common genetic alteration underlying familial pancreatic cancer. Interestingly, several of the families known to have BRCA2-associated familial pancreatic cancer did not manifest a history of breast cancer. A germline mutation thus cannot be excluded solely on the basis of lack of history of breast cancer. BRCA2 is also found to be inactivated somatically in ~10% of sporadic pancreatic cancer cases, with mutations detected in the advanced precursor lesions of PDAC. Overall, BRCA2 mutation carriers are estimated to have an up to tenfold higher risk of developing PDAC; the average age at presentation (66 years) is unchanged compared to controls [23, 24].

The product of BRCA2 interacts with other proteins that also function in the repair of double-stranded DNA breaks. These proteins include several of the Fanconi anemia genes, FANCC and FANCG [25]. More recently, the PALB2 protein (partner and localizer of BRCA2), a BRCA2 interacting protein that acts to stabilize BRCA2 complexes during genome recombination and repair, has been identified as a pancreatic cancer susceptibility gene in patients with familial pancreatic cancer. In 96 cases of familial cancer samples tested in this study, 3% harbored a mutation in PALB2 [26].

Hereditary Pancreatitis and Pancreatic Neoplasms

Hereditary Pancreatitis

Hereditary pancreatitis has been implicated in the development of PDAC by various groups. Mutations that lead to the development of early-onset and recurrent pancreatitis include mutations in pancreatic enzymes and their regulators (PRSS1, SPINK1) and genes whose function is not limited to the pancreas (CFTR) [27–30]. In these patients, onset of pancreatitis with sometimes subclinical episodes of acute pancreatitis usually occurs by age 20.

PRSS1 encodes the cationic trypsinogen enzyme, a serine protease normally produced and then excreted from the pancreas in an inactive form which is converted to its active product, trypsin, in the small intestine. Germline mutations of the PRSS1 gene lead to an autosomal-dominant form of the disease. Mutations at R122H and N29I are the most commonly encountered in hereditary pancreatitis cases; these are believed to lead to the activation of trypsinogen within the pancreas, which in turn leads to autodigestion with recurrent acute pancreatitis and then to chronic pancreatitis [31]. These mutations are associated with a predisposition for the development of PDAC, not through direct effects of the mutations, but rather through the effects of chronic pancreatitis and inflammation after autoactivation of pancreatic enzymes, which causes repeated cycles of injury and epithelial growth [13].

The lifetime risk of developing pancreatic cancer in cases of hereditary pancreatitis has been estimated to be as high as 40–70% by age 70 for those carrying the PRSS1 mutation [32].

Recently, mutations in the most abundant trypsin inhibitor Kasal type 1, also known as SPINK1 or pancreatic secretory trypsin inhibitor, PSTI, have been linked to hereditary pancreatitis [33]. It is unclear whether this trait is inherited through an autosomal-recessive pattern of inheritance with variable penetrance, or whether it is a disease modifier leading to enhanced susceptibility to environmental or other genetic mutations. Most individuals with SPINK1 mutations do not exhibit a family history of pancreatitis. Although the mechanism of disease remains to be conclusively determined, it is believed that mutations in SPINK1 could affect the balance between proteases and protease inhibitors within the pancreas and result in premature pancreatic activation of trypsin. The clinical manifestations result in recurrent episodes of pancreatitis, starting in childhood or young adulthood and resulting in pancreatic exocrine and endocrine insufficiency. The cumulative risk of pancreatic cancer with these chronic forms of pancreatitis is high, but the specific risk of pancreatic cancer in this group remains to be defined.

Mutations in cystic fibrosis transmembrane receptor (CFTR) are also associated with idiopathic and familial forms of pancreatitis [34]. These mutations are present in 5% of the population, but are found in 50% of patients with idiopathic pancreatitis [35]. Cystic fibrosis is inherited as an autosomal-recessive disorder, but most patients affected by recurrent pancreatitis are heterozygous for a CFTR mutation. These patients are also affected by exocrine and endocrine deficiencies that require close monitoring and management.

The major contributor to chronic pancreatitis remains heavy alcohol consumption; this accounts for approximately 80% of cases. It is estimated that only 5% of patients with "sporadic" forms of pancreatitis will develop cancer, while patients with these genetic forms have been found to have increased risk, as high as 40%, by age 65 [36]. It appears to be clear that environmental factors can increase this risk. Current recommendations for those affected by hereditary pancreatitis include the reduction of risk factors associated with the development and progression of pancreatic cancer (smoking) and pancreatitis (alcohol, hypertriglyceridemia, hypercalcemia). In particular, smoking has been implicated in the development and acceleration of pancreatic cancer in multiple studies, where it can double the risk of pancreatic cancer in high-risk individuals [37].

Familial Pancreatic Cancer

Familial clustering of pancreatic cancer is estimated to occur in approximately 10% of cases [20]. Patients who have no association with a known hereditary cancer syndrome and who have at least two first-degree relatives diagnosed with pancreatic cancer are defined as "familial pancreatic cancer" (FPC). Prospective analyses of data collected by pancreatic cancer registries have estimated the risk of developing PDAC to be as high as 18-fold in affected families where two first-degree relatives are diagnosed with pancreatic cancer. Those kindred with more than three affected members have a risk as high as 57-fold [5] (Table 7.1).

Attempts at identifying the genes involved in cases of familial pancreatic cancer have yielded mixed results. A susceptibility locus for familial pancreatic cancer was identified in 2002 from a pancreatic cancer-prone family of western European descent (Family X) [38]. The mutation in this family was inherited in an autosomal-dominant fashion with high penetrance. The actin-binding protein palladin was later identified as the gene responsible for pancreatic cancer susceptibility in kindred [39]. Sequencing of the target gene from this family revealed a P239S mutation that affects its predicted actin-binding site, suggesting a link between its role in cell motility/cytoskeletal organization and the development of pancreatic cancer. Further analysis showed that palladin is overexpressed in early pancreatic lesions, in cancers of Family X members, and also in samples from sporadic cancers. However, the degree of overexpression is small (<1.2-fold increase), and several more recent publications have failed to support the role of palladin mutations in other pancreatic cancer specimens from both sporadic and familial cases [40]. At this time, the genetic basis of most cases of familial pancreatic cancer remains unknown.

Table 7.1 Estimated risk of developing pancreatic cancer in familial pancreatic cancer kindred

Number of affected first-degree relatives	Increased risk
1	4.5-fold
2	18-fold
>3	32- to 57-fold

Screening and Surveillance Strategies in High-Risk Patients

The ultimate goal of screening and surveillance is early diagnosis of pancreatic cancer before the development of invasion, when a tumor becomes unresectable. Precursor lesions include PanINs (pancreatic intra-epithelial neoplasia) and mucinous cystic tumors (IPMN, MCN). IPMN and MCN are macroscopic lesions that are easily identifiable by present-day imaging modalities. How to treat and follow these lesions is still debated; however, some guidelines and consensus statements have been published for non-familial patients [41]. Most PDACs, however, do not arise in the setting of a mucinous lesion; rather, they are the result of progressive precursor lesions, PanINs 1–3. PanIN-3 represents carcinoma in situ. At present, there is no imaging modality or tumor marker that can reliably detect PanIN-3 lesions. Thus, the realistic goal of screening and surveillance is to identify small, surgically resectable lesions. There are data to support claims that these early lesions have a better prognosis. Presently, however, there is no reliable, highly sensitive and specific screening test for pancreatic cancer. Furthermore, unlike breast cancer, there are no data supporting the concept that high-risk screening will be able to find early cancers, or for that matter, that early diagnosis of invasive pancreatic cancer will improve survival. Many questions essentially remain to be determined such as: who, when, and how.

Who Should Undergo Screening and Surveillance for Pancreatic Cancer?

Currently, screening and early detection protocols are limited to high-risk patients only. The reason is that the diagnostic value of screening and surveillance tests is dependent on the pretest probability of disease. Some studies have suggested that for screening and surveillance to be cost-effective, the probability of finding disease needs to be greater than or equal to 16% [42]. Most recent screening and surveillance strategies have focused on a small handful of high-risk groups.

Who then is at high risk? This is still a matter of some debate. At-risk patients are categorized according to their estimated degree of risk for developing pancreatic cancer. Patients estimated to have a greater than tenfold increased risk of developing the disease are considered at high risk. Patients who do not meet the above criteria are considered to be at either low risk (<5-fold increase) or moderate risk (5- to 10-fold increase).

Low-risk patients (<5-fold risk) include those with only one first-degree relative with pancreatic cancer, patients with HNPCC or FAP, or BRCA1 mutation carriers. Patients at

Table 7.2 Categories of at-risk patients

Low risk (<5-fold)	Moderate risk (5- to 10-fold)	High risk (>10-fold)
One first-degree relative with PDAC	BRCA2 mutation carriers	Two or more relatives with PDAC
HNPCC patients	Cystic fibrosis patients	Hereditary pancreatitis
FAP patients	History of chronic pancreatitis	PJS patients
BRCA1 mutation carriers		FAMM patients

Table 7.3 Genetic syndromes associated with development of pancreatic cancer

Syndrome	Mutations	Relative risk
Peutz–Jeghers	STK11/LKB1	36-fold
HNPCC	MLH1, MSH2	Increased, <5-fold
FAMM	CDKN2A	16-fold
FOBC	BRCA2	10-fold, with + FH
Hereditary pancreatitis	PRSS1, SPINK1	50-fold
Familial pancreatic cancer	Unknown	18- to 57-fold

moderate (5- to 10-fold) risk of developing pancreatic cancer include BRCA-2 mutation carriers, cystic fibrosis patients, and those with a history of chronic pancreatitis [6] (Table 7.2).

It is currently recommended that patients with a greater than tenfold increase of risk be screened (Table 7.3). This includes patients having two or more first-degree family members afflicted with pancreatic cancer, or patients who are known mutation carriers of syndromes strongly associated with the disease, such as FAMM, PJS, or HP. BRCA2 mutations have a relative risk that falls below this theoretical level; however, BRCA2 mutation families appear to have several distinct phenotypes, including those with primarily breast and ovarian cancers and those with primarily pancreatic cancer. The latter group is believed to be at much higher risk. Thus, screening should be offered to BRCA2 mutation carriers who have at least one family member afflicted with PDAC.

When Should Screening and Surveillance Begin and How Frequently Should They Be Performed?

Unlike hereditary breast or colon cancer, the literature on hereditary pancreatic cancer has very little data to assist with decision-making. Initially, recommendations were suggested based on extrapolations of colon cancer screening and surveillance guidelines. Screening and surveillance were recommended to start at 50 years of age or 10 years before the youngest age of diagnosis in the family. However, recently published studies indicate that successive generations of pancreatic cancer families are affected at progressively earlier ages (genetic anticipation) [43], suggesting that screening should actually begin earlier. Earlier screening should also be advocated in cancer-prone patients engaged in high-risk activities such as smoking. In terms of frequency, current recommendations vary between 1 and 3 years; however, most studies use a yearly interval.

How to Screen for Pancreatic Cancer

One of the most pressing questions is how to screen and survey these patients. Currently, there is no consensus opinion as to the best screening method. What is known comes from published data on a small number of high-risk families [44–46]. One approach from the University of Washington used a combination of EUS and ERCP. EUS was the initial modality. If abnormalities were identified, then ERCP was used to further investigate these findings. Patients found to have an abnormal EUS and ERCP were then offered distal pancreatectomy. If patients were found to have diffuse changes, they were offered total pancreatectomy. By this method, 43 patients were identified to have abnormal EUS/ERCP findings. Twelve of the 43 were found by pancreatic biopsy to have diffuse PanIN-2,-3 changes; all underwent total pancreatectomy. No invasive cancer was identified in these samples

or in the remaining 31 patients who were returned to annual surveillance [47]. A similar EUS-based prospective screening strategy has also been used at Johns Hopkins. This study used EUS and CT followed by ERCP. Of 78 high-risk patients screened, eight (four identified initially and four within the first year) underwent subtotal pancreatectomy. These patients were found to have precursor lesions; one IPMN was a pre-invasive cancer. The yield of screening was thus estimated at 10%; the authors interpreted this yield to be high enough to support screening, as many of these asymptomatic high-risk individuals harbored neoplastic lesions [47].

It is clear that there are families at high risk for pancreatic cancer. Much uncertainty remains, however, as to how best to manage these patients. At present, no data are available as to any survival benefit from aggressive surveillance or from prophylactic surgeries driven by abnormal findings at the time of screening. Thus, we recommend that all patients in a surveillance program be enrolled in a clinical study.

MGH Screening Program for Pancreatic Cancer

Based on some of these early studies, the MGH has developed a program of screening and surveillance to follow these patients (Fig. 7.1). This program is based on MRI/MRCP and EUS-based screens to limit the risks of radiation from

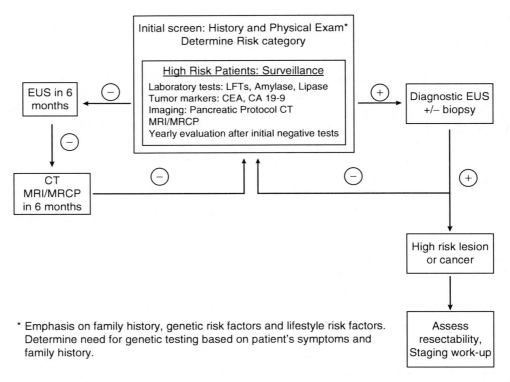

Fig. 7.1 MGH screening program for pancreatic cancer

CT and pancreatitis from ERCP. Patients or physicians who are concerned and seek risk evaluation should be referred for initial consultation (see below).

During this evaluation, a comprehensive history will be taken regarding genetic and lifestyle risk factors. Appropriate patients will be screened and referred to the genetic risk assessment clinic for possible genetic testing, looking for the aforementioned known syndromes. All patients, regardless of risk, will be counseled regarding risk reduction strategies, such as smoking cessation. Patients determined to be at high risk will be offered surveillance starting at age 40 years, or 10 years younger than the earliest diagnosis of pancreatic cancer in the family. If they are interested, initial investigation will entail laboratory tests which include tumor markers (CEA, CA19-9), LFTs, amylase, and lipase. The initial radiologic evaluation will consist of a pancreatic protocol CT and an MRI/MRCP. Patients with normal CT and MRI/MRCP will be placed on surveillance. Surveillance will include a yearly EUS and/or MRI/MRCP. If any mass or cyst is identified during initial CT or MRI, a diagnostic EUS with or without biopsy will be performed shortly after identification of the lesion in question. If this is a cancer or a high-risk cystic lesion, then patients will be subject to the standard-of-care workup and will be evaluated for resectional therapy. At present, we do not advocate prophylactic surgeries or total pancreatectomies unless there is histopathologic proof of high-grade lesions that cannot be extirpated by segmental resection.

References

1. American Cancer Society (2009). Cancer Facts & Figures 2009
2. Horner MJ, Ries LAG, Krapcho M, Neyman N, Aminou R, Howlader N, Altekruse SF, Feuer EJ, Huang L, Mariotto A, Miller BA, Lewis DR, Eisner MP, Stinchcomb DG, Edwards BK (eds) (2009) SEER Cancer Statistics Review, 1975–2006, National Cancer Institute. Bethesda, MD, http://seer.cancer.gov/csr/1975_2006/, based on November 2008 SEER data submission, posted to the SEER web site
3. Ghadirian P, Boyle P, Simard A et al (1991) Reported family aggregation of pancreatic cancer within a population-based case-control study in the Francophone community in Montreal, Canada. Int J Pancreatol 10(3–4):183–196
4. Hemminki K, Li X (2003) Familial and second primary pancreatic cancers: a nationwide epidemiologic study from Sweden. Int J Cancer 103:525–530
5. Klein AP, Brune KA, Petersen GM et al (2004) Prospective risk of pancreatic cancer in familial pancreatic cancer kindreds. Cancer Res 64:2634–2638
6. Brand RE, Lynch HT (2006) Genotype/phenotype of familial pancreatic cancer. Endocrinol Metab Clin North Am 35(2):405–415, xi
7. Shi C, Hruban RH, Klein AP (2009) Familial pancreatic cancer. Arch Pathol Lab Med 133:365–374
8. Habbe N, Langer P, Sina-Frey M, et al (2006) Familial pancreatic cancer syndromes. Endocrinol Metab Clin North Am 35:417–430, xi
9. Lynch HT, Fitzsimmons ML, Smyrk TC et al (1990) Familial pancreatic cancer: clinicopathologic study of 18 nuclear families. Am J Gastroenterol 85:54–60
10. Vitone L, Greenhalf W, McFaul C et al (2006) The inherited genetics of pancreatic cancer and prospects for secondary screening. Best Pract Res Clin Gastroenterol 20:253–283
11. Goldstein AM, Fraser MC, Strewing JP et al (1995) Increased risk of pancreatic cancer in melanoma-prone kindreds with p16INK4 mutations. N Engl J Med 333:970–974
12. Ghimenti C, Tannergard P, Wahlberg S et al (1999) Microsatellite instability and mismatch repair gene inactivation in sporadic pancreatic and colon tumours. Br J Cancer 80:11–16
13. Rebours V, Boutron-Ruault MC, Schnee M et al (2009) The natural history of hereditary pancreatitis: a national series. Gut 58: 97–103
14. Jensen RT, Berna MJ, Bingham DB et al (2008) Inherited pancreatic endocrine tumor syndromes: advances in molecular pathogenesis, diagnosis, management, and controversies. Cancer 113(7 Suppl): 1807–1843
15. Chandrasekharappa SC, Guru SC, Manickam P et al (1997) Positional cloning of the gene for multiple endocrine neoplasia-type 1. Science 276:404–407
16. Karnik SK, Hughes CM, Gu X et al (2005) Menin regulates pancreatic islet growth by promoting histone methylation and expression of genes encoding p27Kip1 and p18INK4c. Proc Natl Acad Sci U S A 102:14659–14664
17. Nagy R, Sweet K, Eng C (2004) Highly penetrant hereditary cancer syndromes. Oncogene 23:6445–6470
18. Peutz JLA (1921) [Very remarkable case of familial polyposis of mucous membrane of intestinal tract and nasopharynx accompanied by peculiar pigmentation of skin and mucous membranes.] Nederlandsch Maandschrift voor Geneeskunde 10:134–136
19. Giardiello FM, Brensinger J, Tersmette A et al (2000) Very high risk of cancer in familial Peutz–Jeghers syndrome. Gastroenterology 199:1447–1453
20. Hruban RH, Petersen GM, Goggins M et al (1999) Familial pancreatic cancer. Ann Oncol 10:569–573
21. White K, Held KR, Weber BHF (2001) A BRCA2 germ-line mutation in familial pancreatic carcinoma. Int J Cancer 91:742–744
22. Couch FJ, Johnson MR, Rabe KG et al (2007) The prevalence of BRCA2 mutations in familial pancreatic cancer. Cancer Epidemiol Biomarkers Prev 16:342–346
23. Brentnall TA (2000) Cancer surveillance of patients from familial pancreatic cancer kindreds. Med Clin N Am 84:707–718
24. Greer JB, Whitcomb DC (2007) Role of BRCA1 and BRCA2 mutations in pancreatic cancer. Gut 56:601–605
25. Goggins M, Schutte M, Lu J et al (1996) Germline BRCA2 gene mutations in patients with apparently sporadic pancreatic carcinomas. Cancer Res 56:5360–5364
26. Jones S, Hruban RH, Kamiyama M et al (2009) Exomic sequencing identifies PALB2 as a pancreatic cancer susceptibility gene. Science 324(5924):217
27. Whitcomb DC, Preston RA, Aston CE et al (1996) A gene for hereditary pancreatitis maps to chromosome 7q35. Gastroenterology 110:1975–1980
28. Lowenfels AB, Maisonneuve P, DiMagno EP et al (1997) Hereditary pancreatitis and the risk of pancreatic cancer. International Hereditary Pancreatitis Study Group. J Natl Cancer Inst 89: 442–446
29. Creighton JE, Lyall R, Wilson DI et al (2000) Mutations of the cationic trypsinogen gene in patients with hereditary pancreatitis. Br J Surg 87:170–175
30. Witt H, Luck W, Hennies HC et al (2000) Mutations in the gene encoding the serine protease inhibitor, Kazal type 1 are associated with chronic pancreatitis. Nat Genet 25:213–216
31. Simon P, Weiss FU, Sahin-Toth M et al (2002) Hereditary pancreatitis caused by a novel PRSS1 mutation (Arg-122 → Cys) that alters autoactivation and autodegradation of cationic trypsinogen. J Biol Chem 277:5404–5410

32. Rebours V, Boutron-Ruault M-C, Schnee M et al (2008) Risk of pancreatic adenocarcinoma in patients with hereditary pancreatitis: a national exhaustive series. Am J Gastroenterol 103:111–119

33. Drenth JP, te Morsche R, Jansen JB (2002) Mutations in serine protease inhibitor Kazal type 1 are strongly associated with chronic pancreatitis. Gut 50:590–591

34. Teich N, Mössner J (2008) Hereditary chronic pancreatitis. Best Pract Res Clin Gastroenterol 22:115–130

35. Behrman SW, Fowler ES (2007) Pathophysiology of chronic pancreatitis. Surg Clin North Am 87:1309–1324

36. Lowenfels AB, Maisonneuve P, Cavallini G et al (1993) Pancreatitis and the risk of pancreatic cancer. N Engl J Med 328:1433–1437

37. Yeo TP, Hruban RH, Brody J et al (2009) Assessment of "gene–environment" interaction in cases of familial and sporadic pancreatic cancer. J Gastrointest Surg 13:1487–1494

38. Evans JP, Burke W, Chen R et al (1995) Familial pancreatic adenocarcinoma: association with diabetes and early molecular diagnosis. J Med Genet 32:330–335

39. Pogue-Geile K, Chen R, Bronner MP et al (2006) *Palladin* mutation causes familial pancreatic cancer and suggests a new cancer mechanism. PLoS Med 3:e516

40. Slater E, Amrillaeva V, Fendrich V, Bartsch D, Earl J et al (2007) Palladin mutation causes familial pancreatic cancer: absence in European families. PLoS Med 4:e164. doi:10.1371/journalpmed. 0040164

41. Tanaka M, Chari S, Adsay V et al (2006) International consensus guidelines for management of intraductal papillary mucinous neoplasms and mucinous cystic neoplasms of the pancreas. Pancreatology 6:17–32

42. Rulyak SJ, Kimmey M, Veenstra D et al (2003) Cost-effectiveness of pancreatic cancer screening in familial pancreatic cancer kindreds. Gastrointest Endosc 57:23–29

43. McFaul CD, Greenhalf W, Earl J et al (2006) Anticipation in familial pancreatic cancer. Gut 55:252–258

44. Rulyak SJ, Brentnall TA (2001) Inherited pancreatic cancer: surveillance and treatment strategies for affected families. Pancreatology 1:477–485

45. Canto MI, Goggins M, Yeo CJ et al (2004) Screening for pancreatic neoplasia in high-risk individuals: an EUS-based approach. Clin Gastroenterol Hepatol 2:606–621

46. Canto MI, Goggins M, Hruban RH, et al (2006) Screening for early pancreatic neoplasia in high-risk individuals: a prospective controlled study. Clin Gastroenterol Hepatol 4:766–781; quiz 665

47. Kimmey MB, Bronner MP, Bird D et al (2002) Screening and surveillance for hereditary pancreatic cancer. Gastrointest Endosc 56:S82–S86

Chapter 8
Hereditary Diffuse Gastric Cancer

Prakash K. Pandalai and Sam S. Yoon

Keywords Diffuse gastric cancer • CDH1 gene • E-cadherin • Gastrectomy • Lobular breast cancer • Signet ring cells • Endoscopy

Introduction

Gastric cancer is one of the leading worldwide causes of cancer death with about 866,000 deaths each year. The incidence varies tremendously throughout the world, with the highest incidence occurring in South Korea at 66.5–72.5 per 100,000 males and 19.5–30.4 per 100,000 females [1]. In contrast, incidence in the United States is about one-tenth that of South Korea, and the estimated number of new gastric cancer cases in the United States in 2008 was 21,500, and the estimated number of deaths was 10,880 [2]. Overall the rates of gastric adenocarcinoma have declined over the past 50 years, but there has been a significant increase in the subset of tumors of the proximal stomach and gastroesophageal junction [3].

In 1965, Lauren described two distinct histological subtypes of gastric adenocarcinomas, intestinal and diffuse [4]. The intestinal type exhibits components of glandular, solid, or intestinal architecture as well as tubular structures. The diffuse type demonstrates single cells or poorly cohesive cells infiltrating the gastric wall, and progressive disease can ultimately lead to linitus plastica. The two Lauren subtypes have distinct clinical profiles [5]. The intestinal type is more common and arises from precancerous areas such as chronic atrophic gastritis or intestinal metaplasia, while the diffuse type does not typically arise from precancerous areas. The intestinal type is more common in men and older patients, and is associated with environmental exposures

such as *Helicobacter pylori* (*H. pylori*) infection. The diffuse type is slightly more common in women and in younger patients, and is more associated with familial occurrence, thus suggesting a genetic contribution. The incidence of the intestinal type has been declining while the incidence of the diffuse type has remained either stable or increased [3].

Etiological factors associated with gastric cancer can be divided into acquired factors, genetic factors, and precursor lesions (Table 8.1) [6]. The vast majority of gastric adenocarcinomas are sporadic and seem to result from the cumulative effects of environmental risk factors such as *H. pylori* infection, smoking, dietary habits, and other exposures [7–9]. There are some genetic factors that can pre-dispose individuals to develop gastric adenocarcinoma, with a mild elevation in risk for those with type A blood [6] to dramatic elevations in risk for those with certain familial syndromes.

Hereditary Diffuse Gastric Cancer

Early onset familial gastric cancer was first described in three families of Maori descent from New Zealand in 1964 [10]. Over the following 30 years, 25 family members died of gastric cancer, the youngest at age 14. Pedigree analysis was consistent with the inheritance of an autosomal-dominant susceptibility gene with incomplete penetrance. In 1998, Guilford and colleagues carried out genetic linkage analysis with microsatellite markers in a large Maori kindred and found significant linkage to markers flanking the gene for E-cadherin, *CDH1* [11–12]. This group ultimately identified germline mutations in the *CDH1* gene in familial gastric cancer. Inactivating *CDH1* germline mutations were subsequently identified in diffuse gastric cancer in families from multiple different countries [13–15].

The first workshop of the International Gastric Cancer Linkage Consortium (IGCLC) was held in June 1999 in Cambridge, United Kingdom. Hereditary diffuse gastric cancer (HDGC) was defined as any family that fits the criteria shown in Table 8.2 [16]. The authors estimated based on limited

S.S. Yoon (✉)
Department of Surgery, Harvard Medical School,
Massachusetts General Hospital, Boston, MA, USA

D.C. Chung and D.A. Haber (eds.), *Principles of Clinical Cancer Genetics: A Handbook from the Massachusetts General Hospital*,
DOI 10.1007/978-0-387-93846-2_8, © Springer Science+Business Media, LLC 2010

Table 8.1 Factors associated with an increased risk of gastric adenocarcinoma

Acquired factors
   Helicobacter pylori infection
   High salt and nitrate consumption
   Low dietary vitamin A and vitamin C
   Smoked, salted, or cured food preparation
   Lack of refrigeration
   Poor drinking water
   Cigarette smoking
   Rubber workers
   Coal workers
   Epstien-Barr virus infection
   Radiation exposure
Prior gastric surgery
Genetic factors
   Hereditary diffuse gastric cancer
   Hereditary nonpolyposis colon cancer
   Li-Fraumeni syndrome
   Peutz-Jehgers syndrome
   Type A blood
Precursor lesions
   Adenomatous gastric polyps
   Chronic atrophic gastritis
   Dysplasia
   Intestinal metaplasia

Table 8.2 Clinical criteria for diagnosis of hereditary diffuse gastric cancer

International gastric cancer linkage consortium (IGCLC) original
   criteria [16]
1. Any family with two or more documented cases of diffuse gastric
   cancer in first- or second-degree relative with one under the age of 50
2. Three documented diffuse gastric cancers in first or second degree
   relative at any age
British Columbia Cancer Agency criteria for HDGC [19]
Modified testing criteria
1. Family with two or more cases of gastric cancer, with at least one
   case of diffuse gastric cancer diagnosed before the age of 50 years
   (38/83 patients; 46%)
2. Family with multiple cases of lobular carcinoma of the breast with
   or without diffuse gastric cancer in first- or second-degree relatives
   (3/13 patients; 23%)
3. Isolated individual diagnosed with diffuse gastric cancer at age less
   than 35 years from a low-incidence population (3/31 patients; 10%)
Potential additional criteria
4. Personal history but no family history of diffuse gastric cancer or
   lobular carcinoma of the breast (risk unknown)
5. Family with three or more cases of gastric cancer diagnosed at any
   age, one or more of which is a documented case of diffuse gastric
   cancer; no other criteria met (1/30 patients, 3%)
6. Family with one or more cases of both diffuse gastric cancer and
   signet-ring colon cancer (1/3 patients, 33%)

data that up to 25% of families that fit the IGCLC criteria would have germline *CDH1* mutations. The International Collaborative Group Hereditary Gastric Cancer (ICG-HGC)

was founded in April 1999 and had an inaugural meeting with 110 participants from six countries in August 1999 in Seoul, South Korea [16]. Because the aims of these two independent groups were concordant, they subsequently merged under the IGCLC designation. *CDH1* germline mutations have been demonstrated in about 30% of patients meeting the IGCLC clinical criteria [17], which represents only about 1% of all gastric cancer cases [18].

The British Columbia Cancer Agency has suggested more relaxed criteria to include a broader group of patients with gastric cancer, lobular breast cancer, age at presentation, and the absence of documentation of diffuse-type histology [18]. These criteria and the rate of identifying germline *CDH1* mutation are shown in Table 8.2. A more recent analysis of 160 families that fulfilled these somewhat looser criteria (three or more diffuse gastric cancers in first degree relatives diagnosed at any age, or two or more gastric cancers in first degree relatives with at least one diffuse gastric cancer diagnosed before age 50) revealed a *CDH1* mutation detection rate of 46% [19].

CDH1 Gene

The *CDH1* gene maps to chromosome 16q22.1 and consists of 16 exons occupying about 100 kb of genomic DNA. The *CDH1* gene is transcribed into a 4.5-kb mRNA that encodes the 120-kDa protein E-cadherin [20]. E-cadherin is a transmembrane glycoprotein expressed on epithelial tissue and is responsible for calcium-dependent cell-to-cell adhesion. It is important for establishing cellular polarity and maintaining normal tissue morphology and cellular differentiation. It has five tandemly repeated extracellular domains and a cytoplasmic domain that connects to the actin cytoskeleton through a complex with alpha, beta, and gamma catenins [21]. The cadherin–catenin complexes are involved in intracellular signaling and promote tumor growth via the Wnt signaling pathway [22].

CDH1 mutations or inactivation have been described in numerous malignancies including colon, prostate, and thyroid cancers [28]. *CDH1* was first implicated in gastric carcinogenesis by Becker et al. [23] in 1994. They identified somatic *CDH1* mutations in 50% of primary diffuse gastric cancer specimens. Subsequently, somatic mutations in *CDH1* have been identified in 40–83% of sporadic diffuse type gastric cancer but not in sporadic intestinal type gastric cancer [24]. Somatic loss of *CDH1* has also been described as an important feature of lobular breast cancer, explaining why women who harbor the germline mutation also have an increased lifetime risk of lobular carcinoma of the breast [25, 26].

CDH1 acts as a classic tumor suppressor gene, with mutation leading to the loss of cell adhesion, proliferation, invasion, and metastasis [27] [23, 28–30]. For patients with germline *CDH1* mutation, a second hit must occur that inactivates the wild-type *CDH1* allele. The mechanisms leading to the inactivation of the wild-type CDH1 allele include somatic mutations, loss of heterozygosity (LOH), and promoter hypermethylation [24, 31]. Oliveira and colleagues examined 28 primary tumors and metastases from 17 patients with germline *CDH1* mutations and demonstrated somatic *CDH1* epigenetic or genetic alterations in 75% of lesions. Specifically, promoter hypermethylation was seen in 32%, LOH in 25%, both promoter hypermethylation and LOH in 18%, and neither promoter hypermethylation or LOH in 25% of specimens analyzed [31]. In both diffuse as well as intestinal gastric cancer, LOH is reported within a broad range of 3–60% [23, 32]. Hypermethylation of the *CDH1* gene promoter is also common in sporadic gastric cancer [24, 32–34]. Tamura and colleagues demonstrated *CDH1* promoter hypermethylation in 56% of diffuse gastric cancers and 29% of intestinal gastric cancers [34]. The importance of promoter hypermethylation was demonstrated by investigating the relationship between *CDH1* mutations and outcome in 73 patients with resected diffuse gastric cancer [35]. Graziano et al. identified *CDH1* promoter hypermethylation in 54% of patients (40) and demonstrated a significant adverse association between the neoplasms with hypermethylation and the distribution of disease relapse and disease-free survival in these patients [35]. Some investigators have postulated that promoter hypermethylation may be reversible, thus making it an attractive target for novel anticancer therapies [24, 36].

Genotype and Phenotype

There are now well over 50 different pathogenic germline mutations in *CDH1* that have been described [14]. As with other autosomal dominant cancer-predisposing genes, most genetic changes lead to truncation of the protein and subsequent loss of function. About three-quarters of the mutations are truncating mutations while the remaining quarter includes splice site and missense mutations [14, 17]. Recently, germline deletions of *CDH1* have also been reported in 4% of diffuse gastric cancer families [19].

Although the pathogenic role of *CDH1* truncating mutations in the development of diffuse gastric cancer has been clearly demonstrated, certain missense mutations may confer a lower risk of developing diffuse gastric cancer [5, 11]. Missense mutations do not display any preferential hot spots. The identification of missense mutations represents a challenge to both genetic counseling and the management of patients who are *CDH1* mutation carriers. Suriano and colleagues developed an *in vitro* functional assay to help infer the possible nature of these germline missense variants [37, 38]. They were able to characterize 13 missense mutations and demonstrated that 11 of these limited the ability of E-cadherin to mediate cell-to-cell adhesion and to suppress invasion.

CDH1 mutations in HDGC families can arise from independent mutational events as well as common ancestry. Kaurah and colleagues performed mutational analysis on 38 families with clinically diagnosed HDGC in order to estimate the frequency and penetrance of mutations in the *CDH1* gene [14]. Germline mutations were found in 15 of 38 families, representing a 40% detection rate. Utilizing haplotype analysis, they demonstrated that two families in their study along with two families found in other studies shared a common mutation (2398delC), and all four families originated from the southeast coast of Newfoundland. This mutation was the first report of a founder mutation in the CDH1 gene with respect to HDGC.

As noted earlier, about 30–46% of families that meet clinical criteria for HDGC will be found to have a germline mutation in the *CDH1* gene [14, 19]. Thus, as many as two-thirds of suspected HDGC families do not harbor *CDH1* mutations. Beta-catenin and gamma catenin compete for the same binding site on the E-cadherin cytoplasmic tail and link this adhesion complex to the cytoskeleton via alpha catenin. Beta-catenin mutations have recently been described in intestinal-type gastric cancers [39]. Oliveira et al. examined 32 families with a history of gastric cancer and 23 patients with early onset gastric cancer for beta-catenin exon 3 germline mutations, but failed to identify any abnormalities [40]. Similarly, Huntsman and colleagues examined 29 HDGC families who were negative for CDH1 mutation for beta-catenin and gamma catenin germline mutations but all were negative [5]. This same group of families was also negative for *TP53* germline mutations.

Penetrance of HDGC in patients who carry a *CDH1* mutation is estimated overall at 40–67% for men and 63–83% for women [14, 41]. Women with CDH1 mutations carry an additional 20–40% risk of lobular breast cancer [25, 42]. Pharoah and colleagues estimated the risk of gastric and breast cancer in CDH1 mutation carriers using 11 families with germline CDH1 mutations which included 476 individuals [42]. They estimated the cumulative risk of diffuse gastric cancer by age 80 at 67% in men (95% CI, 39–99%) and 83% in women (95% CI, 58–99%). They also estimated a low risk of gastric cancer in children, less than 1% at age 20 and increasing to 4% by the age of 30, but by the age of 50 this risk increases to 21% for men and 46% for women. For women, the risk of breast cancer was 39% (95% CI, 12–84%), and the combined risk of gastric and breast cancer was 90% by the age of 80 years. A more recent analysis of 15 families carrying CDH1 mutations demonstrated a cumulative risk of clinically detected diffuse gastric cancer was

40% (95% CI, 12–91%) for males and 63% (95% CI, 19–99%) for females. The risk of breast cancer in female mutation carriers was 52% (95% CI, 29–94%) [14]. The risk of breast cancer is not associated with any specific *CDH1* mutation.

Other Autosomal Dominant Gastric Cancer Susceptibility Syndromes

For the small minority of patients in whom gastric adenocarcinoma develops due to a genetic predisposition, there are a few syndromes other than HDGC to consider. Hereditary non-polyposis colon cancer (HNPCC) syndrome, also known as Lynch syndrome, is caused by germline mutations in one of several mismatch repair genes. These individuals are predominantly at high risk of colon cancer, but also have an increased risk of extracolonic cancer including gastric cancer. Stomach cancers arise in 11% of HNPCC families and predominate in families with MLH1, MSH2, or MSH6 germline mutations [43, 44]. Vasen and colleagues examined 19 families with HNPCC and found a relative risk of 19.3 for developing gastric cancer [43]. Unlike HDGC, the majority of gastric cancers in HNPCC are of the intestinal type [44]. Li Fraumeni syndrome is caused by germline mutations in *TP53* and results in a marked predisposition to soft-tissue sarcomas and a spectrum of cancers including gastric cancer in some families [40]. These gastric cancers are of both the intestinal and diffuse types. Peutz-Jeghers syndrome is an autosomal dominant, hereditary disease characterized by hamartomatous polyps of the gastrointestinal tract and mucocutaneous melanin deposits. In a large meta-analysis of 210 patients with Peutz-Jeghers syndrome, Giardeillo and colleagues found an increased risk of several malignancies including gastric cancer [45]. The relative risk of gastric cancer in this study was 213, with a 95% confidence limit of 96–368. The cumulative risk of gastric cancer was reported as 29% between age 15 and 64 years. Cancer surveillance programs for patients with HNPCC, Li Fraumeni syndrome and Peutz-Jehgers syndrome all have been impeded by the variability of risk estimates of individual reports. Recommendations for future cancer surveillance may be modeled after guidelines developed for other diseases with similar cancer risk.

Genetic Counseling and Testing

Testing for *CDH1* mutations is currently recommended for families that meet the modified IGCLC criteria [41]. Approximately 30–50% of families meeting these criteria carry a predisposing *CDH1* mutation [41]. Testing for *CDH1* mutation is also recommended for families with multiple cases of lobular breast cancer, with or without diffuse gastric cancer, because germline *CDH1* mutations have also been detected in families with lobular breast cancer alone [46]. HDGC can be diagnosed in patients younger than 20 years of age, with the youngest reported death from HDGC occurring in a 14-year-old child [42]. The average age of onset of HDGC is 38 years, suggesting a long indolent phase of tumor evolution [15]. Because of the morbidity of prophylactic total gastrectomy and its impact on quality of life, counseling with a team that includes a geneticist, genetic counselor, surgical oncologist, gastroenterologist, and nutritionist should take place before surgery. This multidisciplinary team should discuss the possible outcomes of testing, risk incurred for future disease development, management options, and known outcomes. Although there are no clear standards, some authors have advocated reserving genetic testing until the age at which the patient is able to give informed consent [47].

When possible, genetic testing should be performed first on a family member with a known diagnosis of diffuse gastric cancer. Because diffuse gastric cancer is often rapidly fatal, often no living affected individuals are available for testing. In this case, the remaining options include testing an unaffected first-degree relative or testing DNA extracts from archived paraffin blocks if available. Once a *CDH1* mutation is identified in the affected individual, asymptomatic family members should proceed to testing and some recommend performing this in their early 20s [27]. A blood sample from an affected member of the prospective kindred is the best substrate for genetic testing. Primary mutation screening is accomplished by two different approaches. First, denaturing high-performance liquid chromatography is used as an initial screening method [48]. Once abnormal results are obtained, direct sequencing is used to verify and further specify exact mutations [49]. Once a family mutation is identified, a mutation specific assay to assess other family members can be performed [14].

Surveillance for Patients with Germline *CDH1* Mutation

Early stage diffuse gastric cancer identified in patients with HDGC is characterized by the presence of multiple foci of signet-ring cell carcinoma confined to the superficial gastric mucosa [50]. Huntsman and colleagues performed prophylactic gastrectomy in five patients with *CDH1* mutation and demonstrated superficial infiltrates of malignant signet-ring cell carcinoma in all 5 patients [51]. Neoplastic foci tended to be less than 8 mm in diameter, many less than 1 mm, and all lay under apparently normal-appearing gastric surface epithelium. An important observation was that there was no lymphatic or vascular invasion and that all tumor foci were confined to the lamina propria in these patients. All lymph nodes identified in perigastric fat of the specimen were free of metastasis. Some investigators have hypothesized that the natural history of HDGC involves the development of multiple foci of signet-ring cell carcinoma in most mutation carriers by 20–30 years of age. These foci may likely develop following the loss of the second *CDH1* allele. This is then followed by invasion of the lamina propria and submucosa after the acquisition of additional mutations or changes in the microenvironment of the surrounding carcinoma cells [52].

A significant challenge in managing patients with *CDH1* mutations is the inadequacy of current screening techniques. Diffuse gastric adenocarcinoma in HDGC patients is characterized by multiple infiltrates of signet-ring cell carcinoma that underlie normal mucosa. There is usually a wide distribution of small-sized lesions that make them difficult to identify with random endoscopic biopsies [51]. Additionally, conventional white light endoscopy has poor sensitivity to detect these submucosal abnormalities. To reliably detect disease before it spreads, surveillance endoscopy should be able to detect invasive carcinoma at the earliest stage such as invasion into the lamina propria or submucosa. A major concern with surveillance endoscopy is that in HDGC most neoplastic foci lie beneath normal-appearing epithelium.

For those not electing a prophylactic total gastrectomy, it has been recommended that a 30 min endoscopy be performed every 6 months by a team experienced at diagnosing early gastric cancer [52]. Based on experience gained by mass endoscopic screening programs in Japan, chromoendoscopy had been proposed as a superior alternative to traditional white light endoscopy. Clinical experience suggests the use of Congo red-methylene blue method originally described by Tatsuta improves sensitivity and the detection of early gastric cancer in HDGC kindred [53]. Additional studies have demonstrated an increase in the diagnostic accuracy of early gastric cancer using methylene blue-Congo red (89%) compared with traditional endoscopy (28%) [54].

Shaw et al. performed both traditional white-light endoscopy and chromoendoscopy using the congo red-methylene blue technique on 33 members of the original HDGC kindred and demonstrated improved detection of early gastric cancer [55]. All 33 patients underwent a total of 99 surveillance gastroscopies. Traditional endoscopy detected two macroscopically visible lesions in two patients that on pathological analysis demonstrated signet-ring cell cancer. Following chromoendoscopy 56 pale lesions were detected suggesting early gastric cancer. Chromoendosocpy-directed biopsies of these lesions demonstrated signet-ring cell carcinoma in 23 (41%). However, concerns over embryotoxicity and carcinogenic potential have recently resulted in Congo red and methylene blue being withdrawn from clinical use. More recently, Barber et al. suggested that white light endoscopic detection of microscopic foci of signet ring cells is possible when multiple biopsies (>20) are performed [56].

PET scans have been advocated by one group. Van Kouwen and colleagues reported on a single case of an asymptomatic 28-year-old woman with a germline *CDH1* mutation [57]. This patient underwent screening endoscopy and was found to have a well-differentiated signet-ring-cell carcinoma in one of 40 random biopsies. Subsequent [18F] Fluoro-2-deoxy-D-glucose positron emission tomography (FDG-PET) scan revealed increased activity in the proximal stomach and pylorus. She underwent total gastrectomy and pathological analysis confirmed intramucosal carcinoma in the cardia and antrum that matched the result of the FDG-PET. Given many invasive gastric cancers are not FDG avid [58], it does not seem reasonable that FDG-PET could reliably detect non-invasive early lesions. Thus, the routine use of PET scan as surveillance for patients with HDGC requires validation before this can be recommended.

Prophylactic Total Gastrectomy

The first patient who underwent a prophylactic total gastrectomy for HDGC at our institution has been previously reported [59]. Figure 8.1 demonstrates the pedigree of this patient's family. The patient's mother had died of diffuse gastric cancer at the age of 33. The patient's maternal grandfather died of stomach cancer at age 50. The patient's maternal aunt developed invasive ductal breast cancer at age 58 and invasive lobular breast cancer at age 66. This same aunt developed diffuse gastric cancer at age 67 and died less than 1 year later. When this maternal aunt was diagnosed with gastric cancer, she was offered and underwent *CDH1* gene testing and was found to have R732Q mutation. The patient was seen by our genetic counselors, and her testing revealed this same mutation. The patient underwent a total prophylactic gastrectomy 3 months after her positive genetic test and has subsequently undergone bilateral prophylactic mastectomies.

Chun and colleagues published their experience of prophylactic gastrectomy in five patients with germline E-cadherin mutations [60]. Patients ranged in age from 37 to 47 years, and all patients had undergone surveillance endoscopy with random biopsy which did not reveal any malignancy. However, pathological evaluation of the resected stomachs showed multiple microscopic foci of signet-ring-cell carcinoma in all five patients. All lesions were submucosal but did not extend into the lamina propria and all lymph nodes examined were negative for metastasis. The findings of occult carcinoma in an otherwise normal-appearing stomach were further demonstrated by Lewis and colleagues in six members of two different HDGC kindred [61]. The

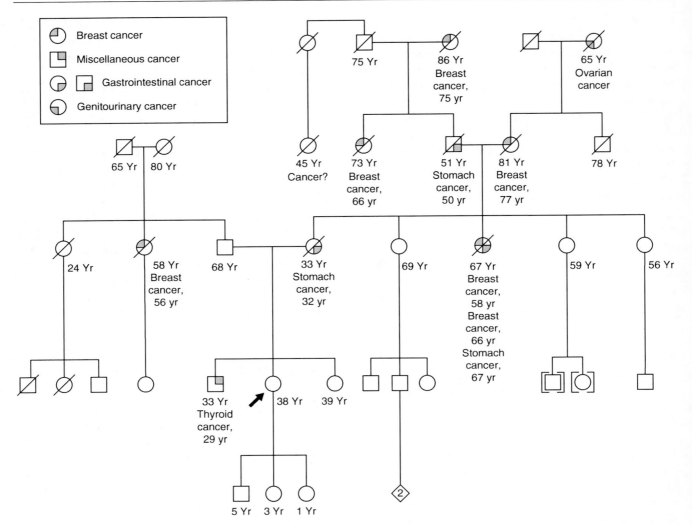

Fig. 8.1 Pedigree of the HDGC patient's family. Circles represent female family members, and squares male family members. Slashes indicate persons who died, and the numbers beneath the circles or squares are age at death (if there is a slash) or, for those living, age at the time the pedigree was created. Yellow represents confirmed cancer. The diamond indicates that sex is unknown; the number inside the diamond indicates the number of persons represented by the diamond. The patient's (*arrow*) maternal aunt had cancer of the right breast at 58 years of age, cancer of the left breast at 66 years of age, and diffuse gastric cancer at 67 years of age, and she died at 67 years of age. The patient's mother had gastric cancer at 32 years of age and died at 33 years of age. The patient's maternal grandmother had breast cancer at 77 years of age, and the maternal great grandmother died of ovarian cancer. The patient's paternal grandfather had gastric cancer at 50 years of age and died at 51 years of age. The patient's brother, 33 years of age, had papillary thyroid cancer at 29 years of age. Her father was of German ancestry, and her mother was of German and English ancestry

gastrectomy specimens appeared normal and underwent "routine" pathological evaluation and were negative for malignancy. However, when the entire specimen was examined microscopically, which in some cases required up to 250 separate blocks, small microscopic foci of diffuse gastric cancer were noted in all six patients.

In total, there have been at least five series with patients with germline E-cadherin mutations who have undergone prophylactic total gastrectomy (Table 8.3) [48, 51, 60–62]. In these five studies, there were a total of 30 patients, and the majority of patients had normal upper endoscopies prior to

their prophylactic total gastrectomies. Twenty-eight patients (94%) had intramucosal or superficially invasive carcinomas identified in the gastrectomy specimen, and 23 patients (76%) had multifocal disease. Our institution has performed prophylactic total gastrectomies on eight patients from five HDGC families (Table 8.3). The eight patients (3 males, 5 females) had a median age of 42 years (range 38–51 years). All patients had a strong family history of diffuse gastric cancer and tested positive for CDH1 gene mutation. Of the five families represented, there were three missense, one frameshift, and one splice site mutation. Median time from

Table 8.3 Surgical series of prophylactic gastrectomy for CDH1 mutations

Author Year	Number of families/pts	Age	Preoperative Endoscopy	Pathology	Complications	LOS
Huntsman DG 2001	2/5	22–40	4/5 Negative within 15 months	5 pts with superficial carcinoma 3 multifocal	NR[a]	NR
Chun YS 2001	1/5	37–47	5 Negative within 3 years	5 pts with intramucosal carcinoma 3 multifocal	None	POD[b] 6–9
Lewis FR 2001	2/6	22–40	NR	5 pts with superficial carcinoma 4 multifocal	1 Septic phlebitis 1 Anastomotic stricture	Averate POD 7
Suriano G 2005	1/6	NR	5 Negative Within 6 months	5 pts with carcinoma (depth NR) 5 multifocal	NR	NR
Newman EA 2006	1/2	28–35	NR	No pt with carcinoma	1 Ileus 1 wound infection	POD 7–15
MGH series 2009	5/8	38–51	8/9 Negative Within 6 months	7 pts with noninvasive carcinoma 2 pts with early invasive carcinoma 1 pt with no carcinoma 8 multifocal	1 pulmonary embolism 2 late SBO	POD 7–8

[a]NR, not reported
[b]POD, postoperative day

genetic testing to surgery was 3 months (range 1–7 months). All patients had an upper endoscopy or chromoendoscopy with random biopsies prior to surgery with only one patient having a focus of diffuse gastric cancer. All patients underwent a total gastrectomy with Roux-en-Y esophagojejunostomy. Median operating time was 201 min (range 187–308 min), and length of stay was 7–8 days. One patient had an early postoperative complication (pulmonary embolism), and two patients had late complications (small bowel obstructions). For the six patients with at least 6 months follow-up, the median weight loss was 19%.

Operative morbidity and mortality is likely to be significantly lower for prophylactic total gastrectomy than for total gastrectomy performed for invasive cancers. The patient population in the former group is generally younger and healthier, and the actual operation does not require any formal lymphadenectomy, which can increase complications [63]. However, even prophylactic operations carry the risk of early complications such as ileus, wound and intra-abdominal infections, and anastomotic leak, and late complications such as anastomotic stricture. Operative mortality following prophylactic total gastrectomy for germline *CDH1* mutation has not been reported to our knowledge. However, there is likely publication bias against such cases and mortality is certainly a possibility. Mortality following gastrectomy for diagnosed gastric cancer ranges from <1% at specialized, high volume centers [64] to 7% in smaller non-tertiary care facilities, so any prophylactic gastrectomy should be performed by an experienced surgeon at a referral center [65]. Discounting complications that are generic to all gastrointestinal operations, the most dreaded complication of a prophylactic total gastrectomy is a leak at the critical esophagojejunostomy anastomosis. Large randomized control trials from both Japan and Europe have demonstrated that the incidence of anastomotic leak, stenosis, morbidity, and length of hospital stay is no different when comparing handsewn versus stapled anastomosis [66, 67]. An anastomotic leak rate of less than 1% has been reported in a large series from Japan with 390 patients [68].

Some technical details of prophylactic total gastrectomy for germline *CDH1* mutation differ from total gastrectomy for known gastric adenocarcinoma. It is critically important to remove all gastric mucosa at risk. There is at least one report of gastric cancer developing 24 years after presumed total prophylactic gastrectomy in the gastric cardia remnant of a patient with a strong family history of gastric cancer [61]. The distal division across the duodenum should be performed at least 1 cm beyond the pylorus, and the proximal division should be performed at least 1 cm above the squamocolumnar junction. Some authors recommend intra-operative endoscopy to ensure accurate identification of the squamocolumnar junction [61]. The gastrectomy specimen should be analyzed grossly by the surgeon to ensure the squamocolumnar junction is included in the specimen, and the specimen should be sent for frozen section analysis of proximal and distal margins to confirm that all gastric mucosa have been removed. Some perigastric lymph nodes, especially those along the lesser and greater curvatures, are more easily removed with the stomach than left *in situ*, but our practice is not to perform a formal D1 or D2 lymph node dissection.

Reconstruction is generally performed with a Roux-en-Y reconstruction with at least a 50 cm Roux limb to prevent bile reflux [69]. Some advocate the formation of a jejunal pouch. At least 15 randomized trials have investigated this issue, and there may be a small benefit of jejunal pouches in terms of early food intake which diminishes with time [70]. In the largest prospective trial to date, Fein and colleagues randomized 138 patients to Roux-en-Y reconstruction with or without a 15 cm pouch and followed patients for a median of 3.6 years [71]. There were no differences in short-term or long-term weight loss. Quality of life was equivalent in the first year but was improved in the pouch group in the third, fourth, and fifth years.

Given we are early in the experience regarding prophylactic total gastrectomy for germline *CDH1* mutation, there remain many unresolved issues. First, the timing of prophylactic surgery is still unclear. The earliest reported case of a germline E-cadherin mutation carrier developing gastric cancer is 14 years old, and the median age in developing clinically apparent gastric cancer is around 38 years old [10]. Second, many elderly patients are currently being identified with germline E-cadherin mutations, and it is unclear at what age the risk of surgery outweighs its potential advantages [72]. Roviello and colleagues reported on a patient with germline CDH1 missense mutation who developed gastric cancer at age 79 and her brother who had no evidence of gastric cancer at age 73. Third, given a total gastrectomy is not an insignificant undertaking, a more accurate ability to estimate risk in relation to specific mutations may improve patient selection for prophylactic surgery and reduce the morbidity associated with radical resection in the individuals who may not ultimately develop gastric cancer. Fourth, there may be selection bias in the current predictions of risk. It is possible that the families with mutations that are more likely to result in the development of diffuse gastric cancer have been identified earlier and risk calculations are based on these families. Subsequent families with lower risk mutations and thus a less pronounced family history may be identified in the future, but such families will be given risk estimates based on the earlier high risk families. Fifth, laparoscopic or laparoscopically assisted total gastrectomies have been described for other benign and malignant gastric diseases by a number of groups with reductions in postoperative ileus and recovery time compared to open surgery [73, 74]. Given no formal lymph node dissection is required, laparoscopic total prophylactic gastrectomy for patients with germline *CDH1* mutations is likely a reasonable option for those highly experienced with this technique.

Pathological analysis of gastrectomy specimens should include a detailed analysis of the gastric mucosa. Pathological mapping of the entire gastric mucosa has been reported for 29 stomachs, 15 of which were from prophylactic total gastrectomy patients from 13 HDGC families [42, 50, 51, 60, 61]. None of the specimens showed *H. pylori* infection, lymphovascular invasion, or lymph node metastasis, highlighting the importance and value of early detection in this high risk population. For pathological analysis in the eight patients treated with total prophylactic gastrectomy at our institution, the entire gastric mucosa was examined microscopically, which required up to 490 sections (Fig. 8.2). Only one patient had unremarkable pathology. The other seven patients had 1–77 foci of noninvasive cancer, and two of these patients had multifocal (4–12) foci of T1 invasive cancer (Fig. 8.3).

There are clear nutritional consequences following total gastrectomy. Nearly all patients lose weight, which nadirs after 3–6 months and averages about 25% of pre-operative weight [75]. Postoperative issues such as early dumping syndrome (secondary to hyperosmotic carbohydrate loads) and diarrhea (secondary to rapid transit or malnutrition) occur in 20–30% of patients, and can be severe immediately following surgery but tend to improve over time (Madura, 2001). Patients can also experience lactose intolerance, and bacterial overgrowth resulting in malabsorption and bloating can

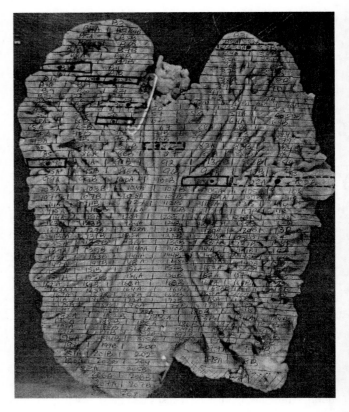

Fig. 8.2 Gross specimen from prophylactic total gastrectomy. The stomach was mapped and entirely submitted for microscopic examination in a total of 340 sections. The sections with solid red outline indicate areas where intramucosal carcinoma was identified, and sections with dotted red outline indicate areas where carcinoma in situ was identified

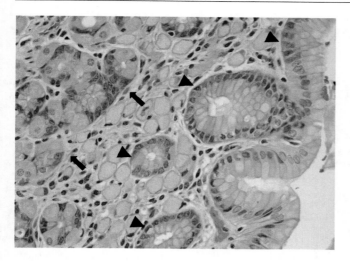

Fig. 8.3 Microscopic view from a section of a prophylactic total gastrectomy with intramucosal carcinoma. Pale, discohesive malignant cells with signet-ring features (*arrows*) infiltrate the lamina propria between normal glands and underneath the gastric mucosa (*arrowheads*)

also occur. Patients in general are initially instructed to eat small amounts continuously over the course of the day, and after several months can reach a point of eating three small to moderate meals per day with snacks in between.

Total gastrectomy results in the loss of intrinsic factor secretion, significantly impairing vitamin B12 absorption, and predisposes to iron malabsorption and deficiency. Additionally, vitamin D and calcium absorption are also diminished. Decreased intestinal transit time is thought to cause some degree of fat malabsorption, contributing to vitamin A, D, E, and K deficiencies. Patients should receive an intramuscular injection of vitamin B12 monthly along with an oral multivitamin with ferrous sulfate daily. There is a minority of patients who have significant difficulty in maintaining an adequate nutritional status following total gastrectomy, and thus regular follow-up visits with the surgeon and nutritionist are essential.

Associated Malignancies: Lobular Breast Cancer

An association between HDGC and breast cancer was first noted in 1999 by Keller and colleagues, who demonstrated a germline *CDH1* mutation in a patient with diffuse gastric cancer and metachronous development of lobular breast cancer [25]. Subsequently, women with *CDH1* germline mutations have been shown to have an increased frequency of breast cancer, predominantly of the lobular type [42]. In an analysis of 11 HDGC families, Pharoah and colleagues

found seven cases of breast cancer and estimated that the risk of breast cancer was 39% (95% CI, 12–84%) by the age of 80 years. These numbers should be cautiously interpreted due to the relatively small number of patients found to have breast cancer in this analysis. Of the 45 HDGC kindreds identified, 18 include a history of at least one case of breast cancer. A total of 32 cases of breast cancer have been identified in these families. Breast cancer histiotype has been confirmed in only nine of these cases, seven of which have been lobular carcinoma. This represents a much higher proportion than would be expected in the normal population, in which less than 10% of sporadic breast cancer are of the lobular type. While the association between HDGC and lobular breast cancer is not concrete, it does suggest that there is a role for increased screening in this population. Unfortunately, patient screening in this setting may be limited by the fact that invasive lobular carcinoma is frequently missed by mammographic surveillance. These lesions are more readily seen with MRI [76]. In *CDH1* afflicted pedigrees, prophylactic bilateral mastectomy, risk reduction strategies using tamoxifen, or surveillance every 6 months with MRI alternating with breast ultrasonography, may be reasonable approaches.

Summary

Hereditary diffuse gastric cancer (HDGC) is a familial cancer syndrome defined in clinical terms by a strong family history of diffuse gastric cancer. About one-third to one-half of these families harbor a germline mutation of the E-cadherin gene (*CDH1*). The cumulative risk for diffuse gastric cancer in patients harboring a germline *CDH1* mutation is roughly 67% in men and 83% in women. Women carrying the mutation also have an increased lifetime risk of lobular breast cancer. Early HDGC in these patients is characterized by multiple microscopic foci of intramucosal signet-ring-cell carcinoma. The time to progression is variable and at this point not predictable. In patients up to 20 years of age, gastric cancer risk is very low, but the median age of patients with germline *CDH1* mutation who develop clinically apparent diffuse gastric cancer is about 38 years old. Improvements in the quality of traditional white light endoscopy with >20 biopsies may improve early detection rates but high variability exists. Definitive management requires prophylactic total gastrectomy. Examination of prophylactic total gastrectomy specimens even after normal endoscopic screening demonstrates that over 90% have microscopic foci of signet-ring-cell cancer, which highlights the importance of prophylactic total gastrectomy as a curative therapy.

References

1. Lee J et al (2007) Cancer incidence among Korean–American immigrants in the United States and native Koreans in South Korea. Cancer Control 14(1):78–85
2. Jemal A et al (2008) Cancer statistics, 2008. CA Cancer J Clin 58(2): 71–96
3. Crew KD, Neugut AI (2006) Epidemiology of gastric cancer. World J Gastroenterol 12(3):354–362
4. Lauren P (1965) The two histological main types of gastric carcinoma: diffuse and so-called intestinal-type carcinoma. An attempt at a histo-clinical classification. Acta Pathol Microbiol Scand 64:31–49
5. Lynch HT et al (2005) Gastric cancer: new genetic developments. J Surg Oncol 90(3):114–133, discussion 133
6. Karpeh MS, Kelsen DP, Tepper JE (2001) Cancer of the stomach. In: DeVita VT, Hellman S, Rosenberg SA (eds) Cancer: principles and practice of oncology, 6th edn. Lippincott Williams & Wilkins, Philadelphia, pp 1092–1126
7. Sasazuki S, Sasaki S, Tsugane S (2002) Cigarette smoking, alcohol consumption and subsequent gastric cancer risk by subsite and histologic type. Int J Cancer 101(6):560–566
8. Kobayashi M et al (2002) Vegetables, fruit and risk of gastric cancer in Japan: a 10-year follow-up of the JPHC Study Cohort I. Int J Cancer 102(1):39–44
9. Serafini M et al (2002) Total antioxidant potential of fruit and vegetables and risk of gastric cancer. Gastroenterology 123(4):985–991
10. Jones EG (1964) Familial gastric cancer. N Z Med J 63:287–296
11. Guilford P et al (1998) E-cadherin germline mutations in familial gastric cancer. Nature 392(6674):402–405
12. Guilford PJ et al (1999) E-cadherin germline mutations define an inherited cancer syndrome dominated by diffuse gastric cancer. Hum Mutat 14(3):249–255
13. Gayther SA et al (1998) Identification of germ-line E-cadherin mutations in gastric cancer families of European origin. Cancer Res 58(18):4086–4089
14. Kaurah P et al (2007) Founder and recurrent CDH1 mutations in families with hereditary diffuse gastric cancer. JAMA 297(21): 2360–2372
15. Richards FM et al (1999) Germline E-cadherin gene (CDH1) mutations predispose to familial gastric cancer and colorectal cancer. Hum Mol Genet 8(4):607–610
16. Park JG et al (2000) Report on the first meeting of the International Collaborative Group on Hereditary Gastric Cancer. J Natl Cancer Inst 92(21):1781–1782
17. Pedrazzani C et al (2007) E-cadherin and hereditary diffuse gastric cancer. Surgery 142(5):645–657
18. Brooks-Wilson AR et al (2004) Germline E-cadherin mutations in hereditary diffuse gastric cancer: assessment of 42 new families and review of genetic screening criteria. J Med Genet 41(7):508–517
19. Oliveira C et al (2009) Germline CDH1 deletions in hereditary diffuse gastric cancer families. Hum Mol Genet 18(9):1545–1555
20. Berx G et al (1995) E-cadherin is a tumour/invasion suppressor gene mutated in human lobular breast cancers. EMBO J 14(24): 6107–6115
21. Grunwald GB (1993) The structural and functional analysis of cadherin calcium-dependent cell adhesion molecules. Curr Opin Cell Biol 5(5):797–805
22. Chan AO (2006) E-cadherin in gastric cancer. World J Gastroenterol 12(2):199–203
23. Becker KF et al (1994) E-cadherin gene mutations provide clues to diffuse type gastric carcinomas. Cancer Res 54(14):3845–3852
24. Grady WM et al (2000) Methylation of the CDH1 promoter as the second genetic hit in hereditary diffuse gastric cancer. Nat Genet 26(1):16–17
25. Keller G et al (1999) Diffuse type gastric and lobular breast carcinoma in a familial gastric cancer patient with an E-cadherin germline mutation. Am J Pathol 155(2):337–342
26. Schrader KA et al (2008) Hereditary diffuse gastric cancer: association with lobular breast cancer. Fam Cancer 7(1):73–82
27. Norton JA et al (2007) CDH1 truncating mutations in the E-cadherin gene: an indication for total gastrectomy to treat hereditary diffuse gastric cancer. Ann Surg 245(6):873–879
28. Birchmeier W (1995) E-cadherin as a tumor (invasion) suppressor gene. Bioessays 17(2):97–99
29. Birchmeier W, Hulsken J, Behrens J (1995) E-cadherin as an invasion suppressor. Ciba Found Symp 189:124–136, discussion 136–141, 174–176
30. Carneiro F et al (1999) E-cadherin changes in gastric carcinoma. Histopathology 35(5):477–478
31. Oliveira C et al (2009) Quantification of epigenetic and genetic second hits in CDH1 during hereditary diffuse gastric cancer syndrome progression. Gastroenterology 136(7):2137–2148.
32. Machado JC et al (2001) E-cadherin gene (CDH1) promoter methylation as the second hit in sporadic diffuse gastric carcinoma. Oncogene 20(12):1525–1528
33. Oliveira C et al (2004) Intragenic deletion of CDH1 as the inactivating mechanism of the wild-type allele in an HDGC tumour. Oncogene 23(12):2236–2240
34. Tamura G et al (2000) E-Cadherin gene promoter hypermethylation in primary human gastric carcinomas. J Natl Cancer Inst 92(7):569–573
35. Graziano F et al (2004) Prognostic analysis of E-cadherin gene promoter hypermethylation in patients with surgically resected, node-positive, diffuse gastric cancer. Clin Cancer Res 10(8): 2784–2789
36. Graziano F et al (2004) Combined analysis of E-cadherin gene (CDH1) promoter hypermethylation and E-cadherin protein expression in patients with gastric cancer: implications for treatment with demethylating drugs. Ann Oncol 15(3):489–492
37. Suriano G et al (2003) E-cadherin germline missense mutations and cell phenotype: evidence for the independence of cell invasion on the motile capabilities of the cells. Hum Mol Genet 12(22): 3007–3016
38. Suriano G et al (2003) The intracellular E-cadherin germline mutation V832 M lacks the ability to mediate cell–cell adhesion and to suppress invasion. Oncogene 22(36):5716–5719
39. Suriano G et al (2005) Beta-catenin (CTNNB1) gene amplification: a new mechanism of protein overexpression in cancer. Genes Chromosomes Cancer 42(3):238–246
40. Oliveira C et al (2004) E-Cadherin (CDH1) and p53 rather than SMAD4 and Caspase-10 germline mutations contribute to genetic predisposition in Portuguese gastric cancer patients. Eur J Cancer 40(12):1897–1903
41. Caldas C et al (1999) Familial gastric cancer: overview and guidelines for management. J Med Genet 36(12):873–880
42. Pharoah PD, Guilford P, Caldas C (2001) Incidence of gastric cancer and breast cancer in CDH1 (E-cadherin) mutation carriers from hereditary diffuse gastric cancer families. Gastroenterology 121(6): 1348–1353
43. Vasen HF et al (1996) Cancer risk in families with hereditary non-polyposis colorectal cancer diagnosed by mutation analysis. Gastroenterology 110(4):1020–1027
44. Aarnio M et al (1997) Features of gastric cancer in hereditary non-polyposis colorectal cancer syndrome. Int J Cancer 74(5):551–555
45. Giardiello FM et al (2000) Very high risk of cancer in familial Peutz-Jeghers syndrome. Gastroenterology 119(6):1447–1453
46. Masciari S et al (2007) Germline E-cadherin mutations in familial lobular breast cancer. J Med Genet 44(11):726–731
47. Oliveira C, Seruca R, Caldas C (2003) Genetic screening for hereditary diffuse gastric cancer. Expert Rev Mol Diagn 3(2):201–215

48. Suriano G et al (2005) Characterization of a recurrent germ line mutation of the E-cadherin gene: implications for genetic testing and clinical management. Clin Cancer Res 11(15):5401–5409

49. Mullins FM et al (2007) Identification of an intronic single nucleotide polymorphism leading to allele dropout during validation of a CDH1 sequencing assay: implications for designing polymerase chain reaction-based assays. Genet Med 9(11):752–760

50. Charlton A et al (2004) Hereditary diffuse gastric cancer: predominance of multiple foci of signet ring cell carcinoma in distal stomach and transitional zone. Gut 53(6):814–820

51. Huntsman DG et al (2001) Early gastric cancer in young, asymptomatic carriers of germ-line E-cadherin mutations. N Engl J Med 344(25):1904–1909

52. Blair V et al (2006) Hereditary diffuse gastric cancer: diagnosis and management. Clin Gastroenterol Hepatol 4(3):262–275

53. Tatsuta M et al (1982) Endoscopic diagnosis of early gastric cancer by the endoscopic Congo red-methylene blue test. Cancer 50(12):2956–2960

54. Iishi H, Tatsuta M, Okuda S (1988) Diagnosis of simultaneous multiple gastric cancers by the endoscopic Congo red-methylene blue test. Endoscopy 20(2):78–82

55. Shaw D et al (2005) Chromoendoscopic surveillance in hereditary diffuse gastric cancer: an alternative to prophylactic gastrectomy? Gut 54(4):461–468

56. Barber ME et al (2008) Histopathological and molecular analysis of gastrectomy specimens from hereditary diffuse gastric cancer patients has implications for endoscopic surveillance of individuals at risk. J Pathol 216(3):286–294

57. van Kouwen MC et al (2004) [18F]Fluoro-2-deoxy-D-glucose positron emission tomography detects gastric carcinoma in an early stage in an asymptomatic E-cadherin mutation carrier. Clin Cancer Res 10(19):6456–6459

58. Yamada A et al (2006) Evaluation of 2-deoxy-2-[18F]fluoro-D-glucose positron emission tomography in gastric carcinoma: relation to histological subtypes, depth of tumor invasion, and glucose transporter-1 expression. Ann Nucl Med 20(9):597–604

59. Chung DC et al (2007) Case records of the Massachusetts General Hospital. Case 22-2007. A woman with a family history of gastric and breast cancer. N Engl J Med 357(3):283–291

60. Chun YS et al (2001) Germline E-cadherin gene mutations: is prophylactic total gastrectomy indicated? Cancer 92(1):181–187

61. Lewis FR et al (2001) Prophylactic total gastrectomy for familial gastric cancer. Surgery 130(4):612–617, discussion 617–619

62. Rogers WM et al (2008) Risk-reducing total gastrectomy for germline mutations in E-cadherin (CDH1): pathologic findings with clinical implications. Am J Surg Pathol 32(6):799–809

63. Hartgrink HH et al (2004) Extended lymph node dissection for gastric cancer: who may benefit? Final results of the randomized Dutch gastric cancer group trial. J Clin Oncol 22(11):2069–2077

64. Park DJ et al (2005) Predictors of operative morbidity and mortality in gastric cancer surgery. Br J Surg 92(9):1099–1102

65. Wanebo HJ et al (1993) Cancer of the stomach. A patient care study by the American College of Surgeons. Ann Surg 218(5):583–592

66. Fujimoto S et al (1991) Stapled or manual suturing in esophagojejunostomy after total gastrectomy: a comparison of outcome in 379 patients. Am J Surg 162(3):256–259

67. Seufert RM, Schmidt-Matthiesen A, Beyer A (1990) Total gastrectomy and oesophagojejunostomy – a prospective randomized trial of hand-sutured versus mechanically stapled anastomoses. Br J Surg 77(1):50–52

68. Hyodo M et al (2007) Minimum leakage rate (0.5%) of stapled esophagojejunostomy with sacrifice of a small part of the jejunum after total gastrectomy in 390 consecutive patients. Dig Surg 24(3):169–172

69. Donovan IA et al (1982) Bile diversion after total gastrectomy. Br J Surg 69(7):389–390

70. Lehnert T, Buhl K (2004) Techniques of reconstruction after total gastrectomy for cancer. Br J Surg 91(5):528–539

71. Fein M et al (2008) Long-term benefits of Roux-en-Y pouch reconstruction after total gastrectomy: a randomized trial. Ann Surg 247(5):759–765

72. Roviello F et al (2007) High incidence of familial gastric cancer in Tuscany, a region in Italy. Oncology 72(3–4):243–247

73. Dulucq JL et al (2005) Completely laparoscopic total and partial gastrectomy for benign and malignant diseases: a single institute's prospective analysis. J Am Coll Surg 200(2):191–197

74. Usui S et al (2005) Laparoscopy-assisted total gastrectomy for early gastric cancer: comparison with conventional open total gastrectomy. Surg Laparosc Endosc Percutan Tech 15(6):309–314

75. Miholic J et al (1990) Nutritional consequences of total gastrectomy: the relationship between mode of reconstruction, postprandial symptoms, and body composition. Surgery 108(3):488–494

76. Francis A et al (2001) The diagnosis of invasive lobular breast carcinoma. Does MRI have a role? Breast 10(1):38–40

Chapter 9
Familial Renal Cell Cancers and Pheochromocytomas

Gayun Chan-Smutko and Othon Iliopoulos

Keywords Von Hippel Lindau (VHL) syndrome • Renal cell cancer • Pheochromocytoma • Hemangioblastoma • VHL gene • mTOR • Hypoxia inducible factor (HIF) • Tuberous sclerosis • TSC1 • TSC2 • Paraganglioma • SDH

Introduction

Clinicians face two main questions when evaluating an individual for the risk of an inheritable form of renal cell carcinoma (RCC). First, what is the likelihood that the individual harbors a germline mutation in one of the genes that predisposes to RCC and, second, which gene is the likely culprit?

Clues to the answer of the first question may be found in the family medical history. In the classic examples of hereditary RCC, several members of the family across two or more generations develop kidney cancer, often at a young age (less than 45 years old). However, germline mutations that predispose to RCC may also predispose to extrarenal tumors or benign lesions, present in the proband or in family members at the time of evaluation. It is therefore possible that no family member is diagnosed with RCC but they may nonetheless be at high risk for developing RCC, as indicated by the presence of typical extrarenal manifestations of an inheritable germline mutation.

The answer to the second question, determining the likely germline mutation placing the proband and the family members at risk, can be greatly facilitated by the histologic type of RCC. The majority of non-inherited (sporadic) tumors consist of clear cell carcinoma (75%). The rest are papillary carcinomas of type 1 or 2 (15%), chromophobe (5%), or oncocytomas (5%) [1]. With the exception of Birt-Hogg-Dube disease, germline mutations in a specific gene predispose to tumors corresponding to one of the histologic types

described above. Therefore, the best entry point into diagnostic testing is provided by the histology of RCC.

The diagnosis of an inherited form of RCC and the underlying mutation allows for the identification of the family members at risk. Such family members can enter surveillance protocols and potentially, in the future, preventive treatment. In addition, germline mutations can serve as biomarkers that help select from the rapidly increasing list of targeted therapies.

In this chapter, we will describe the clinical presentations and molecular genetics of inherited forms of RCC in adult patients, and we will provide an algorithm for the genetic evaluation of the risk for developing RCC. The reader is encouraged to refer to the Online Mendelian Inheritance in Man (OMIM; http://www.ncbi.nlm.nih.gov/omim/) for a detailed and continuously updated description of the diseases and their molecular defects.

Familial RCC with Clear Cell Histology

Von Hippel-Lindau (VHL) Disease (OMIM 193300)

The disease owes its name to the Swedish ophthalmologist Arvin Lindau and the German pathologist Von Hippel who first described the familial occurrence of retinal "angiomas." Prior to the cloning of *VHL* gene, the diagnosis was based on major and minor clinical criteria, comprehensively presented by Melmon and Rose [2]. Cloning of the *VHL* susceptibility gene [3] and the availability of genetic testing led to revision of these "classic" clinical criteria.

Clinical Presentation

VHL is an autosomal dominant condition that affects approximately 1 in 36,000 live births and is the most common cause of familial clear cell renal carcinoma. VHL patients are at high

O. Iliopoulos (✉)
Harvard Medical School, Boston, MA, USA
Familial Renal Carcinoma Clinic, Massachusetts General Hospital
Cancer Center, Boston, MA, USA
e-mail: oiliopoulos@partners.org

risk for developing any of the following lesions: (1) hemangioblastomas (HB) of the central nervous system (CNS), including the retina, (2) multiple and bilateral renal cysts and RCC of clear cell histologic type, (3) pheochromocytomas and occasionally paragangliomas, (4) pancreatic cysts and pancreatic neuroendocrine tumors (PNETs), and (5) papillary cystadenomas of the endolymphatic sac of the ear, the epididymis, the adnexal organs, and the pancreas [4].

The disease is characterized by almost complete penetrance by the sixth decade of life. Typically, signs and symptoms develop during the second to third decade of life, with the exception of pheochromocytomas and retinal hemangioblastomas which may develop in early childhood.

The expressivity of the disease may vary significantly among individuals with the same germline mutation, even among members of the same family. In some cases, young patients present with multiple hemangioblastomas in areas difficult to treat with surgery or radiation and/or multiple renal cancers. On the other hand, the same germline mutation that resulted in an aggressive disease in one patient may lead to a much milder disease course in another. As an example, we established the diagnosis of VHL disease in a 52-year-old asymptomatic male with negative family history, referred to us with a single pancreatic cyst and a single cerebellar hemangioblastoma.

The clinical presentation of VHL disease clusters in two phenotypes. Type 1 patients develop HB and RCC but not pheochromocytoma. In contrast, type 2 patients are at risk for pheochromocytoma and are subdivided in three subtypes. Type 2A patients are at low risk for RCC and type 2B at high risk for RCC. Type 2C patients present as cases of familial pheochromocytoma only, without development of RCC or HB. Germline mutations in the VHL gene consist of large or small deletions, nonsense mutations, missense mutations, or silencing of the gene by methylation [5, 6]. Mutations that result in total protein deletion or its unfolding lead to type 1 disease, whereas missense mutations that are predicted to preserve partial function of the protein lead to type 2 disease [5, 6].

Central Nervous System Hemangioblastomas

The lifetime risks of developing hemangioblastoma of the cerebellum, brainstem, or spinal cord are approximately 44–72, 10–25, and 13–50%, respectively [7]. These are non-metastatic, hypervascular, neoplastic lesions of the CNS. The cell of origin for hemangioblastomas, termed hemangioblast, is of mesenchymal origin, displays hematopoietic and endothelial cell markers and can differentiate along these lineages when cultured under appropriate conditions in vitro [8]. Hemangioblastomas (HB) can present typically in four different forms: (a) as solid tumors of extremely rich vasculature, (b) as a predominant cystic form with a solid eccentric

nidus, (c) as a mixture of solid and cystic components, or (d) as a simple cyst, in which the solid component is not easily discernible. They develop more often in the cerebellum but they frequently present anywhere along the CNS axis, as single or multiple, synchronous or metachronous lesions [9]. Supratentorial hemangioblastomas are almost pathognomonic of VHL disease. Hemangioblastomas are non-metastatic tumors but they are responsible for the major morbidity or even mortality encountered in VHL patients, due to their space-occupying nature and/or syrinx formation in the cord. Symptoms depend on the anatomic location of the hemangioblastoma and range from headaches, vomiting and changes in vision to peripheral motor and sensory symptoms [9].

The frequency of retinal hemangioblastomas (formerly reported as retinal angiomas) is 25–60% and may cause retinal detachment heralded by changes in vision [10]. Hemangioblastomas of the optic nerve may lead to decrease in visual acuity and eventually loss of vision [11, 12].

RCC

VHL patients present typically with multiple and bilateral renal cysts of varying size. They have a ~40% lifetime risk of developing synchronous and/or metachronous RCC, exclusively of clear cell type, arising either in the cysts or from the non-cystic parenchyma [13]. Clear cystic lesions may, within time, develop into complex cysts that harbor a visibly solid RCC component and progress into purely solid RCC. Nevertheless, the cyst is not an obligatory premalignant stage, as the majority of RCCs in the VHL patients develop as solid tumors from non-cystic parenchyma.

Pheochromocytoma

Approximately 10–20% [7] of VHL patients develop pheochromocytomas and very rarely paragangliomas. These lesions are typically limited to the type 2 phenotype. Pheochromocytomas may be present in early childhood, warranting biochemical screening of children at risk for VHL shortly after birth. Pheochromocytomas may release catecholamines and therefore cause symptoms such as sweating, tremor, palpitations, and high blood pressure. In this chapter, we discuss VHL-associated pheochromocytomas and compare them to other inheritable forms of pheochromocytoma and paraganglioma in the section on inheritable pheochromocytomas.

Pancreatic Lesions

VHL patients are not at high risk for classic adenocarcinoma of the pancreas or for premalignant mucinous cystadenoma [7]. However, 35–70% of VHL patients can develop multiple cysts in the pancreas, neuroendocrine tumors, or papillary cystadenomas [7, 14]. These lesions are usually asymptomatic, even when the radiologic presentation is dramatic. We have so far not encountered any patient with symptoms of endocrine or exocrine pancreatic insufficiency in our MGH VHL Clinic over the last 8 years. Neuroendocrine tumors may secrete biologically active peptides and cause corresponding symptoms (such as diarrhea or hypoglycemia). Symptoms of epigastric discomfort are rare. Imaging of the pancreatic lesions is usually sufficiently characteristic to lead to the diagnosis. We reserve biopsy of the neuroendocrine tumors for cases in which surgery is planned [14].

Papillary Cystadenomas

These characteristic lesions may develop in the middle ear (called endolymphatic sac tumors, or ELST), the epididymis or the female adnexal organs. As ELST they may cause tinnitus, decreased hearing, or acute bleeding resulting in hearing loss [15, 16]. Epididymal and adnexal lesions may lead to discomfort or pain during intercourse or at rest [17].

Treatment Considerations

Health care providers caring for VHL patients must identify at-risk family members who should be screened for VHL disease, enroll the VHL patients in surveillance programs, and also select the timing and modality of intervention if lesions progress. We will describe below the principles guiding these choices. Any of these clinical decisions is individualized; nevertheless clinical experience over the last 15 years has formed a consensus approach to VHL patient surveillance and treatment.

Who Should Be Tested for Germline VHL Mutations?

In Table 9.1, we list the criteria used in MGH Familial Renal Cell Carcinoma Clinic for testing patients for VHL germline mutations. As mentioned before, with the availability of genetic testing we have come to appreciate the wide range of disease expressivity and we incorporated this concept in the proposed criteria.

Molecular diagnosis of the disease is made by sequencing the entire gene for point mutations and by evaluating the presence of one or both copies of the gene by Southern blot analysis. The test has an almost 100% sensitivity and specificity in laboratories with professional licensing for the test [18]. Few cases of "classic" VHL disease with negative testing exist; they may be explained by somatic mosaicism or mutations in genes of the hypoxia-HIF-VHL signaling pathway other than VHL itself (see below).

Table 9.1 Criteria for referral to VHL clinic (Massachusetts General Hospital)

1. Any blood relative of an individual diagnosed with VHL disease
2. Any individual with *TWO* VHL-associated lesions[a]
3. Any individual with *ONE* or more of the following
   - CNS hemangioblastoma
   - Pheochromocytoma or paraganglioma
   - Endolymphatic sac tumor (ELST)
   - Epididymal papillary cystadenoma
4. Any individuals with

Clear cell Renal Carcinoma (RCC) diagnosed at a <40 y/o patient

Bilateral and/or multiple clear cell RCC

>1 Pancreatic Serous Cystadenoma

>1 Pancreatic neuroendocrine tumor

Multiple pancreatic cysts + any VHL associated lesion

[a]*VHL associated lesions*: hemangioblastoma (HB), clear cell renal carcinoma (RCC), pheochromocytoma (PHE), endolymphatic sac tumor (ELST), epididymal or adnexal papillary cystadenoma, pancreatic serous cystadenomas, pancreatic neuroendocrine tumors

Specifically, patients with sporadic hemangioblastomas usually have a single lesion, present later in life than VHL patients and have a negative family history and absence of other VHL-associated lesions. Woodward et al. tested a cohort of consecutive patients presenting with such a seemingly sporadic hemangioblastoma and reported germline mutations in 5% of these patients [19]. Moreover, of the ones who tested negative, 5% developed a VHL-related lesion in the ensuing years [19]. We therefore recommend that all patients with a hemangioblastoma be tested for VHL germline mutations, even if the HB is a single lesion. For similar reasons outlined below in the pheochromocytoma section, we recommend VHL testing in every patient with pheochromocytoma.

When to Intervene

Morbidity in VHL patients can be caused by tumor progression or, on the other hand, by over treating the patient. Repeated neurosurgical operations or removal of kidney tumors along with normal parenchyma can lead to permanent neurologic symptoms or renal failure. The current approach to treatment of VHL related lesions pays great attention in minimizing damage of normal parenchyma by selective interventions only when lesions enlarge beyond a safe size. Physicians need to incorporate in their treatment decisions the fact that the growth pattern of any VHL lesion may alternate between periods of variable growth rate and stability. Of course, new symptoms should be evaluated immediately as deemed appropriate.

We and other centers observe RCC until it reaches 3 cm without intervention. It is recommended that removal of larger lesions is done with minimal injury of normal surrounding parenchyma, often just by simple enucleation of the lesion [20, 21]. A laparoscopic approach minimizes operative blood loss and trauma, post-operative pain, and the duration of hospitalization. Radiofrequency ablation (RFA) has been successfully applied to tumors located in accessible positions in the kidney and so far appears a safe alternative to surgery for selected tumors [22, 23].

Hemangioblastomas, like other VHL lesions, follow a variable growth pattern with alternating periods of growth and stability [9]. The definitive treatment is surgery and it is recommended when the growth rate is accelerated or they become symptomatic [10, 24–26]. Lesions no more than 1 cm without a cystic component can be treated with radiosurgery [27, 28]. The cystic component may be treated with radiosurgery (gamma knife or proton beam radiation). The cystic component of HB does not respond to radiation treatment but in cases where open craniotomy needs to be avoided, treatment of the solid component with radiation may delay tumor progression for a while.

Retinal hemangioblastomas can be definitively treated with laser beam, proton beam radiation, or cryotherapy [29]. Recent advances in antiangiogenic therapy may have, in their current form (see following section), some role in treatment of ocular VHL disease [12].

Pancreatic cysts and papillary cystadenomas are very rarely symptomatic and require no intervention. PNETs should be excised before they reach metastatic potential. Blansfield et al. studied predictors of metastasis in VHL patients with PNET and showed that tumors less than 3 cm, with a doubling time >500 days and mutations in exon 1 and 2 have a minimal risk for metastasis and can be observed [30].

Antiangiogenic Agents in VHL Patients

Loss-of-VHL function results in up regulation of the transcription factor Hypoxia Inducible Factor (HIF) activity within cells. HIF activates several secreted growth and angiogenic factors that promote tumor progression and metastasis, among them Vascular Endothelial Growth Factor (VEGF), Platelet-Derived Growth Factor (PDGF), TGFalpha, and erythropoietin. These molecular alterations explain the hypervascular nature of the VHL lesions and render VHL-associated tumors prime candidates for antiangiogenic therapy. Systemic administration of the VEGF receptor tyrosine kinase inhibitor sunitinib in a VHL patient with metastatic pheochromocytoma resulted in significant tumor response [31]. Systemic administration of antiangiogenic agents for retinal HB led to improvement in tissue edema and visual acuity but a limited response in tumor size [32–34]. On the other hand, intravitreal injections of a neutralizing anti-VEGF antibody in VHL patients with retinal hemangioblastoma did not result in significant clinical improvement over time [35]. The reserved use of antiangiogenic agents in VHL patients has been so far based on concerns related to bleeding of CNS hemangioblastomas, although the magnitude of this risk has not been assessed vigorously. Clearly, as the benefits of systemic administration of antiangiogenic agents may outweigh the risks, in selected cases, we will learn more about the role of these agents in the future management of the disease. Protocol-based clinical investigation of these agents is warranted.

Surveillance Considerations

The goal of surveillance is early identification of tumors displaying an aggressive growth pattern from the ones that can be safely observed. Table 9.2 provides details of the MGH protocol for surveillance of VHL patients. Children at risk can be either genetically tested to rule out the disease or, if this elected for a later stage in life, they should undergo retinal examination and biochemical tests to rule out pheochromocytoma. We strongly recommend that every child at risk is tested by the age of 10 years old, a time that more frequent surveillance tests need to be implemented.

Table 9.2 Surveillance guidelines for patients with VHL disease

Any age	Families receive genetic counseling and information about genetic testing.
	Before any type of surgery or childbirth procedures, rule out pheochromocytomas (see description of blood test below).
From birth	Inform pediatrician of family history of VHL
	Eye examinations by Ophthalmologist informed about VHL
Age 2–10	Annual:
	Eye examinations
	Physical examination by Physician informed about VHL
	Blood test for plasma metanephrine, nor-metanephrine, epinephrine, nor-epinephrine (screen for pheochromocytoma)
Ages 11–19	Annual:
	Eye examinations
	Physical examination by Physician informed about VHL (including scrotal exam in males)
	Blood test for plasma metanephrine, nor-metanephrine, epinephrine, nor-epinephrine
	Ultrasound of abdomen (focus on kidneys, pancreas, and adrenals)
	Every 2 years:
	MRI w/ gadolinium of brain and spine (annually at onset of puberty)
Age 20 and beyond	Annual:
	CT scan w/ and w/o contrast of abdomen (focus on kidneys, pancreas, and adrenals) OR MRI of the kidneys and pancreas
	Eye/retinal exam
	Blood test for plasma metanephrine, nor-metanephrine, epinephrine, nor-epinephrine
	MRI w/ gadolinium of brain and spine

Every VHL patient needs to be evaluated for pheochromocytoma prior to surgery, so that the appropriate anesthesia treatment is administered. Type I VHL patients are at extremely low risk for pheochromocytoma. Nevertheless, we do measure blood catecholamines in these patients every 3–4 years and we promptly evaluate any symptoms suggestive of the disease. Blood epinephrine, norepinephrine, metanephrine, normetanephrine, and dopamine have specificity and sensitivity equal or higher than 24 h collection for catecholamines, and it is our preferred method for measurement of catecholamine levels [36]. The combination of those tests with meta-iodobenzylguanidine (MIBG) nuclear scan provides a specificity and sensitivity of 95% for imaging of pheochromocytomas [37].

We strongly prefer abdominal MRI with gadolinium to CT scans for all VHL patients, in order to minimize the cumulative exposure to radiation over the patient's lifetime. We think this is an important issue, given the carcinogenic potential of organs with monoallelic VHL mutation. Moreover, surveillance of the CNS for hemangioblastomas can only be informative with the use of MRIs [38].

VHL patients may suffer from suboptimal kidney function because of repeated surgeries, innumerable cysts, or age-related reasons that are not linked to VHL disease (such as hypertension and diabetes). Administration of gadolinium in patients with glomerular filtration rate (GFR) less than 60 ml/min/1.73 m^2 appears associated with a risk for development of Nephrogenic Systemic Fibrosis (NSF), a systemic disease of skin and parenchymal organ fibrosis that can be lethal [39]. This risk exponentially increases if the GFR is less than 30 ml/min/1.73 m^2. We therefore measure creatinine and creatinine clearance in all patients above 60 or VHL patients of any age at risk for declined kidney function (post-partial nephrectomy or with significant number of cysts). Updated recommendations for administration of contrast agents in relation to kidney function can be found in the web site of American College of Radiology (http://www.acr.org/SecondaryMainMenuCategories/quality_safety/MRSafety.aspx).

Molecular Genetics of VHL Disease

The *VHL* acts as a tumor suppressor gene, conforming to the Knudson "two-hit" model [40]. VHL patients harbor a germline inactivation of the gene; tumor initiation is linked to inactivation of the second, wild-type allele [13, 41]. Similarly, both copies of the gene are inactivated in the majority of sporadic clear cell RCC [42, 43]. The protein encoded by the VHL gene (pVHL) can act as the substrate receptor of an intracellular E3 multiprotein ubiquitin ligase that targets specific substrates for ubiquitination and proteasomal destruction. One of the most established functions of pVHL with a

clear role in RCC formation is its ability to bind to the alpha regulatory subunits of the Hypoxia Inducible Factors (HIF1a, HIF2a) and lead to their ubiquitination and degradation [44–46].

VHL-mediated regulation of HIF1a and HIF2a has been established as a causative link between loss-of-VHL function and development of RCC (Fig. 9.1). HIF is a heterodimeric transcription factor consisting of a hypoxia-regulated (HIF-1a and HIF-2a) and a constitutively expressed (HIF-1b) subunit [47]. It is stabilized by hypoxia [47] and acts as a transcription factor promoting the secretion of numerous pro-angiogenic and tumor growth factors [48]. Loss of VHL function is a molecular hallmark of familial or sporadic clear cell RCC tumors, results in constitutive up regulation of HIF1a/2a and transactivation of hypoxia inducible genes. Experiments using human renal cancer cell lines xenografted in mice showed that regulation of HIF2a by VHL is necessary and sufficient for the ability of VHL to suppress tumor growth [49–52]. Mice engineered to lack *Vhl* in the liver or kidneys develop VHL-associated lesions (cysts and HB) in the targeted organs. Such lesions can be reversed by suppression of HIF function through genetic elimination of the constitutive HIF beta subunit, which is obligatory for HIF activity. Lastly, the risk of VHL patients for RCC inversely correlates with the ability of their germline VHL mutation to bind and degrade HIF2a, in other words Type 2A germline mutations tested in vitro display a relatively stronger binding

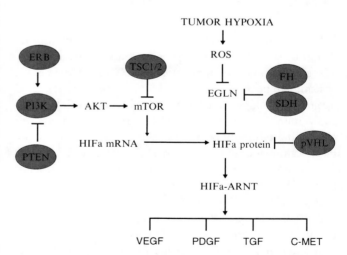

Fig. 9.1 Regulation of HIF1a/2a expression by cellular signaling pathways, which are mutated in human tumors. *ERB* family of ERB transmembrane receptor tyrosine kinases, activated by mutations or gene amplification; *PI3K* phosphatidilinositol-3-Kinase, activated by mutations in several human tumors; *PTEN* phosphatase and Tensin homologue, inhibitor of PI3K, deleted in several human malignancies; *TSC1/2* Tuberous Sclerosis Genes 1 and 2; *mTOR* mammalian target of rapamycin; *pVHL* Von Hippel-Lindau proteins, destabilize HIF regulatory subunits; *SDH* Succinate Dehydrogenases (B, C and D); *FH* fumarate hydratase, FH and SDH inactivating mutations inhibit metabolically the activity of EGLN

to HIF1a/2a, compared to Type 2B mutations [53], while Type 2C mutations (which do not put VHL patients at risk for RCC) retain their ability to bind and degrade HIF1a/2a [54, 55].

It is therefore no surprise that inhibitors of downstream targets of HIF have met with modest but clear clinical success. Antibodies neutralizing the pro-angiogenic VEGF and inhibitors of receptor tyrosine kinases up regulated by HIF (VEGF-R as well as PDGF receptor among others) prolong disease free, and in some cases overall survival, of patients with metastatic, sporadic RCC [56–59]. Combinations of existing targeted therapies have been judiciously tested in selected clinical settings involving VHL patients, as presented above. Novel small molecules targeting HIF2a itself or the VHL signaling pathway are emerging as new therapeutic agents to be tested in inheritable or sporadic, VHL-deficient RCC [60–62].

Other functions attributed to pVHL, likely to be involved in the full phenotype of VHL-associated tumors, include its ability to regulate extracellular fibronectin matrix deposition [63], to promote microtubule assembly and orientation [64] and thus contribute to cilia formation [65], to inhibit beta-catenin activation [66], and to enhance the stability and activity of the tumor suppressor protein p53 [67].

Tuberous Sclerosis Complex (TSC1, OMIM 191100 and TSC2, OMIM 191092)

Tuberous sclerosis complex (TSC) is a multisystem disorder that affects the skin, brain, kidneys, heart, lungs, and eyes. The condition occurs in about 1 in 6,000 live births and is transmitted in an autosomal dominant pattern [68]. TSC demonstrates high variable expressivity between families and within families as well. TSC patients are at risk for developing primarily renal cysts and benign angiomyolipomas, leading often to renal failure and chronic dialysis. Renal disease is a leading cause of mortality in TSC patients, according to some reports [69]. Two genes are associated with the disease: TSC1 (OMIM 191100) on ch.9q34 [70] and TSC2 (OMIM 191092) on ch.16p13.3 [71]. The clinical manifestations derived from mutations in either gene are the same, although TSC1 associated disease is considered to have a milder clinical course [72].

Clinical Presentations

Major and minor features have been proposed for the clinical diagnosis of TSC disease and the revised TSC diagnostic criteria are presented in Table 9.3. Here we will discuss the main features of the disease.

Table 9.3 Diagnostic criteria for TSC

Major features
Facial angiofibromas or forehead plaque
Nontraumatic ungual or periungual fibroma
Hypomelanotic macules (three or more)
Shagreen patch (connective tissue nevus)
Multiple retinal nodular hamartomas
Cortical tuber[a]
Subependymal nodule
Subependymal giant cell astrocytoma
Cardiac rhabdomyoma, single or multiple
Lymphangiomyomatosis[b]
Renal angiomyolipoma[b]

Minor features
Multiple, randomly distributed pits in dental enamel
Hamartomatous rectal polyps[c]
Bone cysts[d]
Cerebral white matter radial migration lines[a,d,e]
Gingival fibromas
Nonrenal hamartoma[c]
Retinal achromic patch
Confetti skin lesions
Multiple renal cysts[c]

Definite TSC: Either two major features or one major feature plus two minor features

Probable TSC: One major plus one minor feature

Possible TSC: Either one major feature or two or more minor features

From Roach ES, Gomez MR, Northrup H (1998) Tuberous sclerosis complex consensus conference: revised clinical diagnostic criteria. J Child Neurol 13(13):624–628, copyright 1998 by SAGE Publications. Reprinted by Permission of SAGE Publications

[a]When cerebral cortical dysplasia and cerebral white matter migration tracts occur together, they should be counted as one rather than two features of tuberous sclerosis

[b]When both lymphangiomyomatosis and renal angiomyolipomas are present, other features of tuberous sclerosis should be present before a definitive diagnosis is assigned

[c]Histological confirmation is suggested

[d]Radiographic confirmation is sufficient

[e]One panel member (M.R.G.) felt strongly that three or more radial migration lines should constitute a major sign

Benign angiomyolipomas represent the most common renal manifestation of TSC, occurring in 70–80% of affected individuals [73]. Angiomyolipomas in children can increase in size and number over time and may become symptomatic (pain) due to hemorrhage into the tumor. Angiomyolipomas should be monitored by MRI or CT to determine their size and growth, as size has been shown to be a good indicator for determining which lesions have a higher potential for hemorrhage. Angiomyolipomas harbor micro- and macro-aneurysms, and it has been reported that the risk of hemorrhage is increased when aneurysms exceed 5 mm in size [74]. Multiple and bilateral cysts with an epithelial lining of hypertrophic/hyperplastic eosinophilic occur in approximately 30% of patients with TSC [73]. More rare histologies of TSC-associated tumors include oncocytoma (<1%), clear cell RCC (<3%), and malignant angiomyolipoma (<1%). The latter two lesions occur at low frequency in patients with TSC compared to other component renal tumors; however, the mortality risk is high, signifying the importance of surveillance of the kidneys of TSC patients [75, 76]. Clear cell RCC has been reported in young patients with TSC, although the lifetime risk for clear cell RCC has not been epidemiologically established so far. It is possible that some of the lesion reported in the past as clear cell RCC may be epithelioid variants of angiomyolipoma [77]. MRI is the method of choice for differential diagnosis between the various kidney tumors, although CT has a very characteristic appearance in the case of angiomyolipomas.

Two causative genes, *TSC1* and *TSC2*, have been cloned in families with TSC. The *TSC2* gene is adjacent to the *PKD1* gene, which is associated with autosomal dominant polycystic kidney disease. Contiguous germ-line deletions of both genes, termed the "contiguous TSC/PKD syndrome" have been reported to result in polycystic kidney disease with earlier onset than in patients with a mutation in *PKD1* gene alone. Very often the kidneys of these patients contain angiomyolipomas as well [78].

Other major clinical criteria for diagnosis of TSC include skin hypomelanotic macules, shagreen patches, facial angiofibromas, and ungual fibromata [79]. Almost all patients with TSC have skin involvement, although none of the skins lesions are considered pathognomonic as they can be seen in isolation within the general population.

CNS lesions in TSC include cortical tubers, calcified subependymal glial nodules, and subependymal giant cell astrocytomas and are the leading cause of morbidity and mortality. Neurologic manifestations of TSC involve epilepsy (infantile spasms), mental retardation/learning disabilities, and behavioral abnormalities. A positive correlation between cortical tuber count and severity of neurologic dysfunction has been suggested by Goodman et al. In their study, patients with greater than seven cortical tubers were more likely to have poorly controlled seizures and cognitive impairment [80]. However, the number of tubers is not predictive of overall clinical severity of TSC [80]. Autism and pervasive developmental disorder are observed in patients with TSC. It is therefore highly recommended that neuropsychological assessment is obtained in early childhood. Neuropsychological therapeutic interventions, combined with seizure control, may be beneficial in improving long-term neurobehavioral outcome [81]. Giant cell astrocytomas may obstruct normal cerebral spinal fluid flow and cause symptoms such as increased intracranial pressure, new focal neurologic deficits, or decreased seizure control. Surgical intervention is generally curative.

Retinal hamartomas and/or mulberry lesions are frequently detected in patients with TSC and are often asymptomatic. Cardiac rhabdomyomas are detected in approximately two thirds of newborns with TSC, and some cases may be evident during prenatal ultrasonography examinations. The lesions are often largest during the neonatal period but they have been shown to regress over time. If cardiac outflow obstruction occurs at birth then surgical intervention is indicated; however, if obstruction does not occur at birth the individual is unlikely to become symptomatic later in life and intervention is not necessary [68, 82].

Pulmonary function may also be affected in patients with TSC and is five times more common in females than males. Lung lesions include lymphangioleiomyomatosis and multifocal micronodular pneumoctye hyperplasia. Symptoms such as spontaneous pneumothorax or respiratory insufficiency usually do not present until the third of fourth decade of life. Furthermore, lung lesions can be detected on CT in asymptomatic adults [68].

Diagnostic Considerations

The consensus diagnostic criteria are an effective standard for identifying affected probands. In contrast to VHL disease (discussed in the previous section), genetic testing for mutations in *TSC1* and *TSC2* genes is reserved for the purposes of molecular confirmation in clinically borderline cases. However, the mutation detection rate for both genes combined is ~80–85%, leaving a moderate number of suspected probands without an identifiable gene mutation but still at risk for developing TSC1/2-associated lesions. Simplex (i.e., no significant family history) or borderline cases with no detectable germline mutation should still be followed on a regular basis, particularly if the initial evaluation occurs in childhood, as additional features of TSC may present later in life.

Genetic testing may also serve the purpose of identifying at-risk family members and for providing prenatal diagnosis and/or pre-implantation genetic diagnosis. The complicating feature in genetic counseling for TSC is the high apparent de novo mutation rate, where two thirds of affected probands represent new mutations.

Patients with de novo TSC mutations are more likely to harbor a germline mutation in the TSC2 gene [83]. In contrast, TSC1 mutations are encountered with higher frequency in familial cases. It is possible, though, that these differences are due to ascertainment bias: TSC2 mutations result in a more severe disease phenotype, especially mental retardation, compared to that from *TSC1* mutations [84, 85]. It is therefore possible that TSC2 mutation carriers might have a reduced reproductive fitness.

Parents may test negative in certain cases that do not constitute true de novo mutations in the offspring. Even when both parents test negative for the proband's mutation, careful examination of all organ systems of the parents for evidence of TSC is necessary, as compelling evidence of somatic mosaicism has been reported [86]. In the case of somatic mosaicism, the parents of an affected child both test negative by peripheral blood analysis; however, upon thorough examination one of the parents is found to be mildly affected and has not previously come to medical attention for having TSC. The recurrence risk to offspring in a parent with somatic mosaicism is 50%.

A few instances have been reported where one parent harbors germline mosaicism for TSC [87]. In this case, both parents of the proband test negative on peripheral blood leukocytes, but, in contrast to the cases of somatic mosaicism, they have no TSC features on exam. Nevertheless, such parents may bear more than one offspring with TSC due to mosaicism in the gametes where a proportion of germ cells contain a mutation while the remaining cells do not. Therefore in the case of TSC, parents that test negative for their child's gene mutation and have no clinical evidence of TSC themselves should be counseled with a 2% recurrence risk to future offspring.

Molecular Genetics of TSC1/2 and Therapeutic Implications

The TSC2 gene consists of 42 exons and encodes a 5.5 kb mRNA [88]. The gene is expressed in all adult human tissues examined so far. Rat [89], mouse [90], and *Drosophila* [91, 92] homologues of TSC2 have been cloned. The TSC1 gene consists of 23 exons and encodes an 8.6 kb mRNA. TSC2 gene encodes for a 1,807 amino acid protein (tuberin, 200 kD) [88] while TSC1 gene encodes for a 1,164 amino acid protein (130 kD, hamartin). Tuberin and hamartin form a heterodimeric complex in vitro and in vivo that mediates the downstream action of these proteins [93].

TSC1/2 act as tumor suppressor genes and inactivation of both alleles is necessary for the formation of TSC-associated lesions. Tsc2 null mice die as embryos. Heterozygous Tsc2+/− or Tsc1+/− mice survive to develop multiple and bilateral renal cystadenomas, liver hemangiomas, and lung adenomas [94–96]. TSC-associated tumors display loss of heterozygosity (LOH) in the TSC1 or TSC2 locus [97, 98]. Sporadic counterparts of TSC-associated tumors, in particular renal angiomyolipomas and pulmonary lymphangiomas also display LOH in the TSC1 or TSC2 locus [98, 99].

Genetic experiments in *Drosophila* and biochemical experiments in mammalian cells showed that loss of TSC1/2 function results in constitutively active mammalian target of rapamycin 1 (TORC1) [100–103]. The reader is referred to scholarly reviews of the signaling interplay between activation of PI3Kinase, Akt, TSC, and mTOR [104].

The well-delineated connections between TSC and regulation of mTOR function suggest that inhibitors of mTORC1 may inhibit the growth of TSC1/2 deficient tumors [105].

Preclinical animal data obtained by treating Tsc+/− mice with systemic administration of rapamycin suggest that mTOR inhibitors may ameliorate the CNS anatomical and functional defects (such as mouse learning deficits and epilepsy) caused by loss-of-TSC function. In addition, animal studies suggested that mTOR inhibitors may reduce the growth of renal tumors [106–110].

Phase I/II clinical trials provided evidence that mTOR inhibition has promising therapeutic value in TSC patients. Topical application of mTOR inhibitors on TSC patients' angiofibroma improved the skin lesions [111]. Systemic administration of temsirolimus in a small cohort of TSC patients led to size reduction of renal angiomyolipomas and significant improvement of their pulmonary function. While there was no detectable improvement in the size of CNS lesions during this specific study [112], other small trials indicate that administration of rapamycin improves the size of subependymal giant cell astrocytomas and reduces the frequency of seizure activity in children with CNS symptoms [113].

These early but clearly promising results with mTOR inhibitors are likely to change the standards of care for TSC patients in the near future.

Constitutive Translocations Involving Chromosome 3

Somatic chromosomal aberrations in sporadic kidney cancer have been systematically catalogued but germline balanced translocations can occur at a relatively low frequency in familial clear cell RCC. These translocations typically involve the short or long arm of chromosome 3 and either chr. 6, 2, or 8.

1. t(3;6)(q13;q25) [114] and (3;6)(q12;q15) [115]
2. t(2 ;3) (q35 ;q21) [116, 117]
3. t(2 ;3) (q33 ;q21) [118]
4. t(3 ;8) (p14 ;q34) [119]

The mechanism(s) linking the translocation with malignant transformation are currently unclear. One possible mechanism invokes loss of the derivative chromosome bearing the short arm of ch.3 (der3) in tumors and therefore loss of one copy of the VHL gene that resides in this arm, while the other allele is mutated [115, 119, 120]. An alternative explanation predicts that the translocation disrupts tumor suppressor genes spanning the specific area. Breaks in ch.3p14 region disrupt the FHIT (Fragile Histidine Triad) gene that encodes for an Ap3A hydrolase [121]. The translocations involving ch.8q24 region disrupt the gene TRC8, and TRC8 mutations have been detected in RCC [122, 123]. In vitro analysis of TRC8 function supports the notion that

TRC8 acts as a tumor suppressor gene, although the mechanism(s) of its function are not currently clear [124, 125]. The 2q33 area and the 3q21 area encode the genes deleted in renal cancer 1 (DIRC1) and DIRC2, respectively. Their function is currently unknown [116, 126]. In summary, the various models proposed as explanations of 3p translocation-associated RCC require further experimental testing but, at a clinical level, detection of these cytogenetic abnormalities may help to evaluate inherited predisposition to RCC.

Succinate Dehydrogenase-Related RCC

There have been reports of patients with clear cell RCC linked to germline mutations in subunits of succinate dehydrogenase B (SDHB), an enzyme of the mitochondrial Krebs cycle. We discuss the full spectrum of clinical presentation of these mutations at the hereditary pheochromocytoma and paraganglioma section of this chapter. The number of RCC cases reported is small and their histology reportedly includes clear cell and non-clear cell tumors, such as chromophobe RCC [127].

Supernumerary Nipple Syndrome

An association between polymastia and RCC has been reported in a Hungarian family [128]. Although a molecular genetic analysis for this family is not yet available, it has been hypothesized that developmental abnormalities affecting the urogenital tract predispose to RCC and also cause supernumerary nipples [129]. We follow such a single, large family in our institution; external ear and kidney abnormalities have been observed as part of the clinical phenotype but so far there has been no evidence of RCC in this family.

Familial RCC with Papillary Histology

Papillary carcinoma comprises approximately 10% of sporadic RCC tumors [1]. Tumors are classified as papillary when >75% of the tumor mass consists of papillary components. Histologically and clinically, papillary cancers are subdivided in type 1 and type 2 [130]. Type 1 tumors are characterized by small cuboidal cells displaying uniform nuclei and small nucleoli. Type 2 tumors are characterized by large eosinophilic cells with pleomorphic nuclei and prominent nucleoli. There is evidence that type 1 tumors have a better clinical prognosis than type 2 [131].

Hereditary Papillary RCC Type 1 (HPRCC1) (OMIM 1447000)

Clinical Presentation

Family members with HPRCC 1 develop multiple and bilateral papillary type 1 RCC at a much younger age than those with sporadic papillary RCC and the disease is inherited in an autosomal dominant fashion. The frequency of HPRCC type 1 is estimated 1 in one million [132]. Linkage analysis mapped the gene responsible for HPRCC 1 to ch.7q31-q34, and later studies identified it as the c-MET proto-oncogene [133]. Approximately 80% of the families presenting with the phenotype of the disease harbor germline mutations in c-MET [133]. As in sporadic papillary RCC tumors, several HPRCC type 1 tumors manifest trisomy of ch.7, with the duplicated ch.7 also harboring a mutation of the c-MET proto-oncogene [134]. No extra-renal clinical manifestations have been described in the HPRCC Type 1 patients so far.

Molecular Genetics of HPRCC1 and Therapeutic Implications

The c-MET proto-oncogene consists of 21 exons, and it is expressed in several adult tissues, including the kidney. The encoded protein is a heterodimeric transmembrane receptor tyrosine kinase stimulated by its cognate ligand, the hepatocyte growth factor/scatter factor (HGF/SF) [135, 136]. The intracellular part of the receptor has a catalytic domain and a C-terminal "multi-docking domain." Ligand induced dimerization of the receptor leads to activation of the PI3K, Grb2/Sos/Ras, Src, and PLC gamma pathways [137]. HPRCC type 1-associated germline mutations map to the catalytic site of the receptor and are predicted to promote phosphorylation of the critical tyrosines [133]. c-MET receptor activation in epithelial cells results in (1) increased proliferation (2) increased motility (3) increased metastatic potential and (4) polarization and tubule formation. Activation of the Ras pathway appears necessary and sufficient for proliferation. Activation of PI3-kinase only appears responsible for increased motility. Activation of both pathways is necessary for acquisition of invasive and metastatic phenotype [138].

Currently, several orally available c-MET inhibitors are in clinical testing and more such compounds are under development and preclinical testing. Patients with hereditary or sporadic forms of papillary RCC Type I harboring c-Met mutations are regarded as prime candidates for such targeted therapy and their involvement in clinical trials with these inhibitors is highly encouraged [139].

Hereditary Leiomyomatosis with RCC (OMIM 150800)

Clinical Presentations

Hereditary Leiomyomatosis with RCC (HLRCC) patients present usually in the third and fourth decade of life with single or multiple leiomyomas of the skin and, in the case of female patients, in the uterus (fibroids) as well as renal cancer [140]. The disease is clinically autosomal dominant with variable expressivity. The majority of the patients may develop cutaneous leiomyomas, although documented HLRCC cases without skin lesions exist; therefore the absence of skin leiomyomas does not exclude the diagnosis. Almost 100% of HLRCC female patients will develop uterine fibroids and the mean of age of onset is a decade earlier than the patients with sporadic fibroids [141]. The majority of renal cell carcinomas in HLRCC patients display characteristic papillary type 2 histology, although rare but well documented cases of collecting duct carcinoma in several members of an HLRCC family have been reported [142]. HLRCC-associated RCCs appear aggressive, with high metastatic potential, and may often present as single unilateral tumors [142]. Papillary RCCs tend to be radiologically isoechoic lesions and they can easily be missed by imaging with ultrasound. Abdominal CT or MRI is the recommended imaging approach. In contrast to VHL-associated RCCs, it is recommended that these tumors are surgically removed independently of their size [143]. HLRCC patients may present, at the time of diagnosis, with any combination and severity of skin or uterine leiomyomas and/or RCC [141]. Recent reports indicate that HLRCC patients may also be at increased risk for breast cancer, bladder cancer, and Leydig (non-germ cell) cancers of the testis [144, 145].

Molecular Genetics of HLRCC

The gene responsible for HLRCC had been mapped by linkage analysis to ch.1q42.3-43 [140, 146] and identified as the Krebs cycle enzyme fumarate hydratase [141]. Germline mutations include missense mutations in or near the catalytic site of the enzyme, but small intragenic or large deletions, insertions and nonsense mutations have been reported [142, 147–150]. All described mutations are predicted to lead to loss-of-FH function and, indeed, direct measurements of the FH enzymatic activity in lymphoblastoid cell lines from affected individuals confirmed marked reduction [147]. Tumors arising in HLRCC patients harbor a second inactivation mutation in or loss of the remaining wild-type allele (LOH). Genotype analysis of HLRCC family members indicates, so far, that the type of mutation does not predict any aspects of the clinical phenotype of the disease, including the risk for developing RCC. The sensitivity of the genetic test for detection of FH mutations has ranged significantly at the hands of different groups between 55 and 93% [145, 149].

FH is a mitochondrial enzyme catalyzing the hydration of fumarate to malate. Loss of FH activity disrupts progression of Krebs cycle and results in increased levels of fumarate and subsequently its precursor succinate, which in turn diffuses into the cytoplasm and competes with 2-oxoxglutarate for binding to EGLN.

Inhibition of EGLN function results in HIF stabilization and overexpression [151]. Gene expression analysis of HLRCC-related fibroids revealed a significant increase in HIF-target genes regulating carbohydrate metabolism, glycolysis, and iron homeostasis [152]. FH mutations may dysregulate other genes beyond HIF and whether inhibition of HIF is sufficient for treatment of HLRCC-related tumors remains to be determined.

Screening and Treatment Recommendations for HLRCC

1. Patients with personal or family history of leiomyomatosis, especially if presented in the second or third decade of life should be tested for germline FH mutations.
2. Patients with personal or family history of type 2 papillary or collecting duct RCC should be tested for germline FH mutations.
3. It is advisable to remove any RCC in HLRCC patients independently of its size.
4. Abdominal MRI or CT are the recommended imaging modalities for surveillance imaging of HLRCC patients.
5. Consider screening HLRCC patients for breast, bladder and testicular tumors.

HPRCC Associated with Papillary Thyroid Cancer (OMIM 605642)

Malchoff et al. described families with multifocal papillary RCC and papillary thyroid carcinoma [153]. The gene responsible for the syndrome was mapped to ch.1q21, but it is currently unknown.

Familial Chromophobe RCC and/or Oncocytoma

Birt-Hogg-Dube Syndrome (OMIM 135150)

Clinical Presentation

Birt, Hogg, and Dube first described an inherited dermatologic condition characterized by multiple fibrofolliculomas, trichodiscomas, and acrochordons in individuals >25 years old [154]. Patients with Birt-Hogg-Dube syndrome (BHD) are at high risk of developing these skin lesions, renal tumors, and spontaneous pneumothorax. Fibrofolliculomas and trichodiscomas are benign hamartomatous tumors of the skin originating from cellular elements of the base of the hair follicle [155]. Clinically they are almost indistinguishable and present as multiple yellowish or skin-colored papules of the face (including oral mucosa), neck, scalp, and upper trunk. Acrochordons have a "skin tag" more than "papular" appearance but are most likely histologic variants of fibrofolliculomas and trichodiscomas. Lipomas and collagenomas are less characteristic, but they have been described in BHD patients.

Members of families affected with BHD syndrome may develop multiple and bilateral renal neoplasms. In contrast to other inherited RCC diseases, BHD disease predisposes individuals to tumors of more than one histologic type, which may coexist in the same individual. In a recent review of a large cohort of BHD families, the predominant histology of renal tumors was chromophobe RCC, followed by chromophobe/oncocytic hybrids, and less frequently, clear or papillary type [156].

In addition to skin and renal lesions BHD patients have lung cysts and suffer from spontaneous pneumothorax [157, 158]. Colonic polyps and the possibility of colon cancer, although initially reported as part of the syndrome, are not currently considered part of the disease [159].

Molecular Genetics of BHD

The BHD gene maps to ch.17p11.2 [160, 161]. The gene generates at least two isoforms of the tumor suppressor protein folliculin through alternative splicing [162]. Germline mutations detected so far are mainly nonsense mutations leading to frame shift and early protein truncation and intragenic or larger deletions. There is only one reported family, at the time that this chapter is written, in which the germline mutation constitutes a missense mutation [156]. Initial studies indicate that folliculin is 57 kDa phosphoprotein that localizes to the nucleus and the cytoplasm and it may be involved, directly or indirectly, in regulating mTOR function [163]. The sensitivity of current genetic testing for mutations in the BHD gene is approximately 85% [162].

Approach to the Patient with Familial RCC

Who Should Be Referred for Testing?

One or several of the reasons listed below may prompt the referral and evaluation of a patient for genetic predisposition to RCC. Physicians and genetic counselors can avoid potential pitfalls by carefully evaluating and accurately documenting any of these reasons. To this end it is paramount to obtain, after consent of the patient or the legal guardian, medical records of the referred patient and, if needed, family members. Figure 9.2 presents a suggested algorithm of approaching patients evaluated for inheritable forms of RCC.

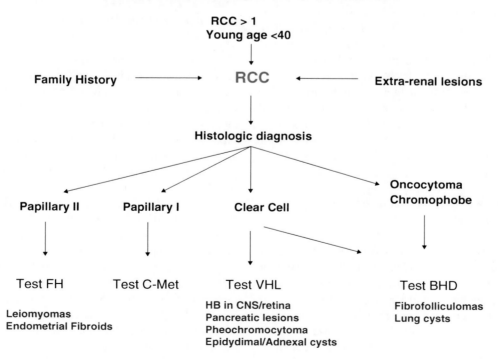

Approach to Diagnosis of Familial RCC

Fig. 9.2 Proposed approach for evaluation and genetic testing of patients with possible familial RCC. Family history, age of tumor onset, and extrarenal lesions guide selection of candidate genes

Referral Because of Positive Family History

The documented occurrence of kidney cancer in two or more members of the family at least in two successive generations raises the possibility of an inherited form of RCC [164]. The accurate interpretation of the family history requires documentation of tumor histology (by obtaining pathology reports), age of onset, site or sites of occurrence, intervals between metachronous presentations, and the presence of non-RCC characteristic lesions that may raise the suspicion of inheritable cancer, in both the index case and family members. Critical also is the investigation for a possible environmental exposure that may explain the occurrence of the disease in multiple family members.

It is very important to emphasize that the absence of family history does not rule out the possibility of inheritable kidney cancer. The likely explanations for a negative family history, in case of an inheritable form of cancer include (a) the presence of de novo mutation that occurred spontaneously during gametogenesis in one of the parents, (b) parental germline mosaicism, or (c) reduced penetrance and/or variable expressivity of the disease in different family members.

Referral Because of Early Onset and/or Multifocal RCC

Diagnosis of RCC during the fourth decade of life or earlier raises the suspicion of a genetic predisposition. One should bear in mind though that the development of RCC may be a late feature in any of the diseases examined in this chapter and that the presence of a suggestive family history alone may be sufficient reason for genetic testing. Multifocal disease, either ipsilateral or contralateral, raises the suspicion of an inheritable form. Patients with localized, sporadic (non-inheritable) RCC are also at risk for local recurrence or development of a second primary in the contra-lateral kidney over at least a period of 10 years. These presentations may simulate metachronous occurrence, and the presence of the second lesion needs to be evaluated in the overall context of the clinical presentation. It should be emphasized that, in particular, patients with HLRCC or HPRCC1 may present with a single lesion.

Referral Because of Extrarenal Lesions and Corresponding Symptoms

Extrarenal lesions may be diagnosed in the index case, or they may be discovered by clinical and radiologic examination. Depending on the expressivity of the disease though they may be absent in the referred patient but present in family members. Their presence therefore has to be considered in the context of the whole family and uncovered through careful family history and reference to medical documentation (Fig. 9.2). It is possible that some of these lesions can only be suspected in family members that passed away, based on clinical manifestations. For example, deceased relatives in families with VHL disease, with the diagnosis of "brain tumor" or "stroke," might have been suffering from cerebellar hemangioblastomas.

Extrarenal lesions for VHL patients include hemangioblastomas of the CNS, including the retina (often referred to as "retinal hemangioma"), pheochromocytomas, pancreatic lesions (cysts, neuroendocrine tumors, papillary cystadenoma), adnexal and epididymal cysts or papillary cystadenomas, and endolymphatic sac tumors of the middle ear. Symptoms in the personal or family history corresponding to these lesions may provide clues regarding the presence of an inherited form.

Patients with HLRCC often provide a personal or family history of skin and/or uterine leiomyomas. A personal or family history of lower abdominal pain, heavy menstruation, menorrhagia or hysterectomy at young age may provide clues for uterine leiomyomatosis. Similarly patients with BHD disease may provide a personal or family history of spontaneous pneumothorax or "skin lesions."

We cannot emphasize enough that the combination of the type and severity of lesions and symptoms can vary widely among patients, even members of the same family. The availability of genetic testing has expanded the clinical spectrum of documented inheritable RCC diseases, particularly in milder forms that would go otherwise undiagnosed on clinical grounds alone.

The Genetic Test Is Negative: Does the Patient Have the Disease?

The genetic testing for VHL disease has an almost perfect sensitivity and specificity. Nevertheless, we and other centers care for rare families with a typical presentation of VHL disease for which genetic testing identifies no mutation. As mentioned above, one of the possible explanations is germline mosaicism. Alternatively, mutations in genetic regulatory elements not examined by the available genetic testing or in other members of the VHL-HIF pathway may account for this presentation. Such families undergo surveillance imaging and therapeutic recommendations identical to the families with identifiable mutations.

The case of a negative genetic test in the context of a suggestive clinical picture presents a diagnostic and management challenge, particular in the cases of HPRCC, HLRCC and BHD disease, where the sensitivity of the corresponding genetic tests range from 55 to 85%. It is also complicated by the fact that the referred patient is likely of young age and we are just beginning to appreciate the full spectrum of the natural history of these diseases. The type and frequency of surveillance should correspond to the degree of clinical suspicion and it should consider patient age and preferences. Generally we recommend periodic surveillance with MRI of the kidney at intervals longer than cases with a documented mutation, particularly if the clinical suspicion is moderate.

Familial Pheochromocytoma and Paraganglioma

In the 2004 WHO classification, a pheochromocytoma is a rare tumor of the adrenal gland arising from the chromaffin cells of the adrenal medulla [165]. Pheochromocytomas are most often catecholamine-secreting. Paragangliomas arise from extra-adrenal chromaffin cells of the sympathetic nervous system and parasympathetic ganglia. Sympathetic paragangliomas tend to be catecholamine-secreting, whereas parasympathetic paragangliomas usually are not.

The prevalence of pheochromocytoma/paraganglioma (Pheo/PG) is not known; however, the incidence is estimated to be about one in 300,000/year (geneclinics.org). The tumors tend to come to medical attention due to signs and symptoms associated with hypertension due to excess secretion of catecholamines. Additionally, Pheo/PG may present due to mass effects from the tumor, or as incidental findings on imaging studies. Although the clinical presentation of Pheo/PG is similar in both sporadic and familial cases, the latter tend to present at younger ages and are more likely to be multifocal, bilateral or demonstrate multiple synchronous tumors.

Clinical Presentation

Due to the rarity of Pheo/PG, an inherited genetic susceptibility should always be considered regardless of age at diagnosis, and a complete family medical history should be obtained. Even in apparently isolated cases of Pheo/PG (i.e., negative family history), a significant proportion of patients harbor a germline mutation in a susceptibility gene [166]. As previously described in this chapter, pheochromocytoma and paraganglioma are component tumors of von Hippel-Lindau disease. A positive personal or family history of other VHL-related tumors warrants discussion of *VHL* germline testing of the affected individual (see algorithm). However, in the absence of other VHL-related findings, other hereditary conditions should be considered in the differential diagnosis, including Neurofibromatosis type 1 (NF1), Multiple Endocrine Neoplasia type 2 (MEN2), and the more recently described Hereditary Paraganglioma-Pheochromocytoma syndromes (HPGL).

Von Hippel-Lindau Disease

Type 2 germline VHL mutations predispose to pheochromocytoma. VHL-related pheochromocytomas are more likely to be norepinephrine-secreting, compared to MEN2-related pheochromocytomas, which tend to be epinephrine-secreting [167]. However, such a biochemical comparison should be interpreted with great caution, since it is possible that it reflects biases in founder effects or errors due to a relatively small sample size.

Neurofibromatosis Type 1 (See Chap. 13: Neurofibromatosis)

The clinical features of NF1 include multiple café-au-lait spots, axillary and inguinal freckling, and neurofibromas. Pheochromocytoma may also occur in a small proportion of patients with NF1. Germline mutations in the *NF1* tumor-suppressor gene have been identified in patients meeting clinical diagnostic criteria for NF1. A careful physical exam for NF1 stigmata is warranted to rule out this condition.

Multiple Endocrine Neoplasia Type 2 (See Chap. 11: MEN Syndromes)

Mutations in the *RET* proto-oncogene have been identified in patients with MEN2. MEN2 is characterized by an increased risk for medullary thyroid cancer, and approximately 50% of individuals with MEN Type 2A or 2B develop pheochromocytoma [168]. Additionally, pheochromocytomas in individuals with MEN2 tend to be metanephrine/epinephrine secreting tumors that are often bilateral. Paragangliomas have not been observed in patients with MEN2 [169].

Hereditary Paraganglioma-Pheochromocytoma Syndromes

Germline mutations in three genes, *SDHD*, *SDHB*, and *SDHC*, have been identified in HPGL families to date and are inherited in an autosomal dominant manner [170–172]. Additional genes are likely, but have not yet been cloned. *SDHD*, *SDHB*, and *SDHC* encode three of the four subunits of the mitochondrial succinate dehydrogenase complex. Loss of succinate activity due to inactivating mutations leads to inhibition of the Krebs' cycle and the cytoplasmic accumulation of succinate, which in turn may inhibit cytoplasmic prolyl-hydroxylase and aberrantly stabilize HIF [173].

Although germline mutations in each *SDHx* (*SDHB*, *SDHD*, and *SDHC*) gene contributes to an increased risk for developing Pheo/PG, some observed differences may apply and prove useful in guiding targeted genetic analysis [174]. Again, caution should be exercised here, since these are observations based on small patient cohorts: (1) *SDHB* and *SDHD* germline mutation carriers have a corresponding 77 and 86% risk of developing a Pheo/PG by age 50, (2) An *SDHB* mutation is strongly associated with extra-adrenal sympathetic paraganglioma, particularly in the abdomen or thorax, (3) A larger proportion of *SDHB* related tumors are malignant at diagnosis compared to *SDHD* or *SDHC* mutation carriers and, (4) *SDHD* and *SDHC* associated tumors are more frequently parasympathetic paraganglioma of the head and neck compared to *SDHB*.

Tumors other than Pheo/PG have been associated with SDHx germline mutations. An association with RCC and papillary thyroid cancer has been reported in some germline *SDHx* mutation carriers [127, 175]. Some families with Carney-Stratakis syndrome, characterized by a dyad of paraganglioma and gastrointestinal stromal tumors, have been reported to harbor mutations in the SDHx genes [176]. Additionally, Ying Ni et al. recently reported a small subset of individuals with phenotypic features suggestive of Cowden syndrome (see Chap. 3) with germline mutations in *SDHD/SDHB* [177]. These patients were also germline *PTEN* negative and had a significantly increased frequency of breast, thyroid, and RCC compared to patients with *PTEN* mutations. The clinical significance of these findings involving non-paraganglioma neoplasms is unclear.

Treatment of pheochromocytoma/paraganglioma in HPGL is similar to that of sporadic cases. Patients with secreting tumors should be treated for catecholamine excess prior to surgical removal of the tumor. Surgery is also the treatment of choice for nonsecreting tumors.

Currently, no strategies are available for the prevention of pheochromocytoma or paragangliomas. However, studies involving antiangiogenic and anti-VEGF agents are currently underway. Avoidance of cigarette smoking which predisposes to lung disease and situations involving prolonged hypoxic conditions (such as high-altitudes) are reasonable for patients to consider.

Diagnostic Considerations and Recommendations for Genetic Testing

Any patient presenting with the clinical diagnosis of pheochromocytoma (and in particular if the proband is younger than 50 years old) should be considered for genetic testing. The decision is reinforced if there is a documented positive family history for pheochromocytoma, if the proband presents with multiple synchronous or metachronous tumors, or if the patient has lesions consistent with VHL, MEN2 or NF1 which can be detected by clinical examination or by imaging. It is worth emphasizing that given the variable penetrance and expressivity of the pheochromocytoma associated genes, almost every individual with documented pheochromocytoma should be regarded as a candidate for genetic testing. For example, up to 50% of malignant, extra-adrenal paraganglioma have an *SDHB* mutation [178]. Furthermore, the cumulative frequency of germline mutations in *VHL*, *MEN2*, *SDHD*, and *SDHB* are estimated to be in the range of 7.4–24% of apparently sporadic pheochromocytoma/paragangliomas [179]. Although the reported frequencies have been based on different populations and as a result may involve ascertainment bias and founder effects, the probability of a mutation is significant enough to warrant genetic testing.

Several genetic testing algorithms have been proposed [157, 179] and do not demonstrate much variability. The algorithm in Fig. 9.3 has been adapted from Bornstein et al., based on the conclusions of the International Symposium on Pheochromocytoma (ISP2005) and does not include *SDHC* testing due to the infrequency of finding a causative mutation in the gene. This algorithm was tested on a French cohort of 314 patients with good fidelity; however, may require updating as more data is published on larger study populations.

Surveillance Recommendations

Early detection is a key component to reducing morbidity and mortality in HPGL families. Although there is no standard guideline specifying the age at which to begin screening, pheochromocytoma/paraganglioma have been known to manifest in childhood in some families. Thus, screening should begin by age 10 or at least 10 years earlier than the youngest age of disease manifestation for any individual who carries an *SDHx* gene mutation or has a personal or family history consistent with HPGL. This includes HPGL families in which a disease-causing mutation has not been found in an affected family member, as well as at-risk relatives of mutation carriers who have not yet elected to pursue pre-symptomatic DNA testing. The following screening guidelines are suggested for monitoring tumor recurrence and for early detection of new lesions:

1. Annual biochemical screening with plasma catecholamine measurement.
2. For *SDHD* and *SDHC* mutation carriers, MRI or CT of the head and neck every 1–2 years and MRI or CT and ^{123}I-MIBG scintigraphy of the body every 3–4 years.
3. For *SDHB* mutation carriers, MRI or CT of the abdomen, pelvis, and thorax every 1–2 years. Additionally, ^{123}I-MIBG scintigraphy every 3–4 years for detection of paragangliomas or metastatic disease that may be missed on MRI or CT.

Fig. 9.3 Proposed approach for genetic testing in pheochromocytoma and paragangliomas. Biochemical pattern may help to prioritize VHL testing versus RET testing*. The algorithm is intended as a guide for cost-effective prioritization; however, some patients may warrant further genetic testing

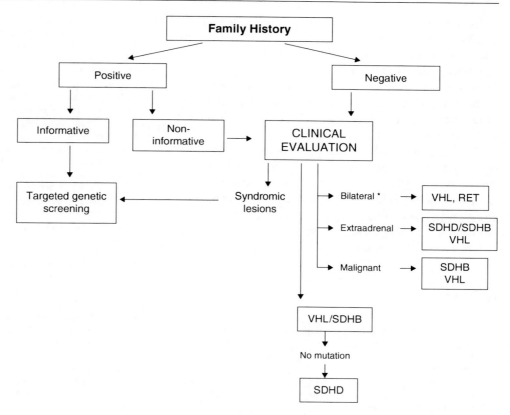

Approach to the Patient with Hereditary Pheochromocytoma

The principles of cancer genetic counseling are thoroughly discussed in Chap. 2. However, a few additional points should be considered when counseling families with HPGL.

Genetic Testing of At-Risk Family Members

Genetic testing should be offered to first-degree relatives of the proband by the age of 10 or a minimum of 10 years earlier that the youngest age of diagnosis of a pheochromocytoma/paraganglioma in the family.

Most mutation carriers have a family history consistent with HPGL, and careful examination of the family history will demonstrate which side of the family is transmitting the disease. However, given that there is variable expressivity and incomplete penetrance in HPGL, confirmation through genetic testing of parents is warranted. Genetic testing can then be offered to the appropriate side of the family. Examples have been reported where both parents of the proband are negative for the proband's mutation. Possible explanations include germline mosaicism in one parent or the proband is a de novo mutation carrier.

If a parent of the proband is identified as a mutation carrier, then each sibling of the proband has a 50% chance of also carrying the mutation. If neither parent is a carrier, siblings should also be offered genetic testing in the event that one parent has germline mosaicism.

A parent of origin effect has been observed in *SDHD* families, where a disease causing mutation inherited from a male carrier confers an increased risk for developing disease. A maternally inherited *SDHD* gene mutation does not cause disease, although exceptions have been reported. It is important to note that an individual who inherited the *SDHD* mutation from his/her mother still has a 50% chance of transmitting the mutation to each offspring.

The Genetic Test Is Negative: Does the Patient Have the Disease?

It is possible that the family history is consistent with HPGL (with two or more cases of pheochromocytoma or paraganglioma on one side of the family) but no mutation is identified. In this case, the members of the family at risk should be offered biochemical surveillance and imaging for early-detection. We should emphasize that there are well documented cases of HPGL syndrome for which the responsible germline mutations have not been identified.

If the proband has a negative family history and all reasonable genetic tests have turned up negative, then there are three possible explanations: (1) the proband truly represents a sporadic case (i.e., no inherited susceptibility), (2) the proband carries a mutation in a gene or gene(s) that has not yet been discovered, or (3) the proband carries a mutation in one of the five susceptibility genes that cannot be identified with current methodologies.

When the proband's clinical presentation is compelling (i.e., bilateral or multifocal tumors, other manifestations consistent with VHL, MEN2, or NF1) and no mutation is identified, the proband should continue to be monitored for disease recurrence and development of new lesions. Periodic biochemical screening for pheochromocytoma/paraganglioma in first-degree relatives should also be considered.

References

1. Reuter VE, Presti JC (2000) Contemporary approach to the classification of renal epithelial tumors. Semin Oncol 27(2):124–137
2. Melmon K, Rosen S (1964) Lindau's disease. Am J Med 36:595–617
3. Latif F, Tory K, Gnarra J et al (1993) Identification of the von Hippel-Lindau disease tumor suppressor gene. Science 260:1317–1320
4. Iliopoulos O (2001) von Hippel-Lindau disease: genetic and clinical observations. Front Horm Res 28:131–166
5. Crossey PA, Richards FM, Foster K et al (1994) Identification of intragenic mutations in the von Hippel-Lindau disease tumour suppressor gene and correlation with disease phenotype. Hum Mol Genet 3(8):1303–1308
6. Chen F, Kishida T, Yao M et al (1995) Germline mutations in the von hippel-lindau disease tumor suppressor gene: correlations with phenotype. Hum Mutat 5:66–75
7. Lonser RR, Glenn GM, McClellan W et al (2003) von Hippel-Lindau disease. Lancet 361:2059–2067
8. Park DM, Zhuang Z, Chen L et al (2007) von Hippel-Lindau disease-associated hemangioblastomas are derived from embryologic multipotent cells. PLoS Med 4(2):e60
9. Wanebo JE, Lonser RR, Glenn GM, Oldfield EH (2003) The natural history of hemangioblastomas of the central nervous system in patients with von Hippel-Lindau disease. J Neurosurg 98(1):82–94
10. Lonser RR, Weil RJ, Wanebo JE, DeVroom HL, Oldfield EH (2003) Surgical management of spinal cord hemangioblastomas in patients with von Hippel-Lindau disease. J Neurosurg 98(1):106–116
11. Wong WT, Agron E, Coleman HR et al (2007) Genotype-phenotype correlation in von Hippel-Lindau disease with retinal angiomatosis. Arch Ophthalmol 125(2):239–245
12. Wong WT, Chew EY (2008) Ocular von Hippel-Lindau disease: clinical update and emerging treatments. Curr Opin Ophthalmol 19(3):213–217
13. Lubensky IA, Gnarra JR, Bertheau P, Walther MM, Linehan WM, Zhuang Z (1996) Allelic deletions of the VHL gene detected in multiple microscopic clear cell renal lesions in von Hippel-Lindau disease patients. Am J Pathol 149:2089–2094
14. Choyke PL, Glenn GM, Walther MM, Patronas NJ, Linehan WM, Zbar B (1995) von Hippel-Lindau disease: genetic, clinical and imaging features. Radiology 194:629–642
15. Manski TJ, Heffner DK, Glenn GM et al (1997) Endolymphatic sac tumors. A source of morbid hearing loss in von Hippel-Lindau disease. JAMA 277(18):1461–1466
16. Kim HJ, Butman JA, Brewer C et al (2005) Tumors of the endolymphatic sac in patients with von Hippel-Lindau disease: implications for their natural history, diagnosis, and treatment. J Neurosurg 102(3):503–512
17. Choyke PL, Glenn GM, Wagner JP et al (1997) Epididymal cystadenomas in von Hippel-Lindau disease. Urology 49(6):926–931
18. Stolle C, Glenn G, Zbar B et al (1998) Improved detection of germline mutations in the von Hippel-Lindau disease tumor suppressor gene. Hum Mutat 12(6):417–423
19. Woodward ER, Wall K, Forsyth J, Macdonald F, Maher ER (2007) VHL mutation analysis in patients with isolated central nervous system haemangioblastoma. Brain 130(Pt 3):836–842
20. Grubb RL 3rd, Choyke PL, Pinto PA, Linehan WM, Walther MM (2005) Management of von Hippel-Lindau-associated kidney cancer. Nat Clin Pract Urol 2(5):248–255
21. Duffey BG, Choyke PL, Glenn G et al (2004) The relationship between renal tumor size and metastases in patients with von Hippel-Lindau disease. J Urol 172(1):63–65
22. Gervais DA, Arellano RS, McGovern FJ, McDougal WS, Mueller PR (2005) Radiofrequency ablation of renal cell carcinoma: part 2, Lessons learned with ablation of 100 tumors. AJR Am J Roentgenol 185(1):72–80
23. Gervais DA, McGovern FJ, Arellano RS, McDougal WS, Mueller PR (2005) Radiofrequency ablation of renal cell carcinoma: part 1, Indications, results, and role in patient management over a 6-year period and ablation of 100 tumors. AJR Am J Roentgenol 185(1):64–71
24. Jagannathan J, Lonser RR, Smith R, DeVroom HL, Oldfield EH (2008) Surgical management of cerebellar hemangioblastomas in patients with von Hippel-Lindau disease. J Neurosurg 108(2): 210–222
25. Lonser RR, Oldfield EH (2006) Spinal cord hemangioblastomas. Neurosurg Clin N Am 17(1):37–44
26. Weil RJ, Lonser RR, DeVroom HL, Wanebo JE, Oldfield EH (2003) Surgical management of brainstem hemangioblastomas in patients with von Hippel-Lindau disease. J Neurosurg 98(1):95–105
27. Chang SD, Meisel JA, Hancock SL, Martin DP, McManus M, Adler JR (1998) Treatment of hemangioblastomas in von Hippel-Lindau disease with linear accelerator-based radiosurgery. Neurosurgery 43(1):28–34
28. Kano H, Niranjan A, Mongia S, Kondziolka D, Flickinger JC, Lunsford LD (2008) The role of stereotactic radiosurgery for intracranial hemangioblastomas. Neurosurgery 63(3):443–450, discussion 450–441
29. Wittebol-Post D, Lips CJM, Hes FJ (1998) The eye in von Hippel-Lindau disease. Long term follow up of screening and treatment recommendations. J Intern Med 243:555–561
30. Blansfield JA, Choyke L, Morita SY et al (2007) Clinical, genetic and radiographic analysis of 108 patients with von Hippel-Lindau disease (VHL) manifested by pancreatic neuroendocrine neoplasms (PNETs). Surgery 142(6):814–818, discussion 818, e811–e812
31. Jimenez C, Cabanillas ME, Santarpia L et al (2009) Use of the tyrosine kinase inhibitor sunitinib in a patient with von Hippel-Lindau disease: targeting angiogenic factors in pheochromocytoma and other von Hippel-Lindau disease-related tumors. J Clin Endocrinol Metab 94(2):386–391
32. Aiello LP, George DJ, Cahill MT et al (2002) Rapid and durable recovery of visual function in a patient with von hippel-lindau syndrome after systemic therapy with vascular endothelial growth factor receptor inhibitor su5416. Ophthalmology 109(9):1745–1751
33. Girmens JF, Erginay A, Massin P, Scigalla P, Gaudric A, Richard S (2003) Treatment of von Hippel-Lindau retinal hemangioblastoma by the vascular endothelial growth factor receptor inhibitor SU5416 is more effective for associated macular edema than for hemangioblastomas. Am J Ophthalmol 136(1):194–196

34. Madhusudan S, Deplanque G, Braybrooke JP et al (2004) Antiangiogenic therapy for von Hippel-Lindau disease. JAMA 291(8):943–944

35. Wong WT, Liang KJ, Hammel K, Coleman HR, Chew EY (2008) Intravitreal ranibizumab therapy for retinal capillary hemangioblastoma related to von Hippel-Lindau disease. Ophthalmology 115(11):1957–1964

36. Eisenhofer G, Lenders JW, Linehan WM, Walther MM, Goldstein DS, Keiser HR (1999) Plasma normetanephrine and metanephrine for detecting pheochromocytoma in von Hippel-Lindau disease and multiple endocrine neoplasia type 2. N Engl J Med 340(24):1872–1879

37. Iliopoulos O, Eng C (2000) Genetic and clinical aspects of familial renal neoplasms. Semin Oncol 27(2):138–149

38. Choyke PL, Glenn GM, Walther MM, Zbar B, Linehan WM (2003) Hereditary renal cancers. Radiology 226(1):33–46

39. Kribben A, Witzke O, Hillen U, Barkhausen J, Daul AE, Erbel R (2009) Nephrogenic systemic fibrosis: pathogenesis, diagnosis, and therapy. J Am Coll Cardiol 53(18):1621–1628

40. Knudson AG Jr (1971) Mutation and cancer: statistical study of retinoblastoma. Proc Natl Acad Sci U S A 68:820–823

41. Lubensky IA, Pack S, Ault D et al (1998) Multiple neuroendocrine tumors of the pancreas in von Hippel-Lindau disease patients: histopathological and molecular genetic analysis. Am J Pathol 153(1):223–231

42. Shuin T, Kondo K, Torigoe S et al (1994) Frequent somatic mutations and loss of heterozygosity of the von Hippel-Lindau tumor suppressor gene in primary human renal cell carcinomas. Cancer Res 54(11):2852–2855

43. Gnarra JR, Tory K, Weng Y et al (1994) Mutations of the VHL tumour suppressor gene in renal carcinoma. Nat Genet 7:85–90

44. Maxwell PH, Wiesener MS, Chang GW et al (1999) The tumour suppressor protein VHL targets hypoxia-inducible factors for oxygen-dependent proteolysis. Nature 399(6733):271–275

45. Ivan M, Kondo K, Yang H et al (2001) HIF1a targeted for VHL-mediated destruction by proline hydroxylation: implications for oxygen sensing. Science 292(5516):464–468

46. Jaakkola P, Mole D, Tian YM et al (2001) Targeting of HIF-alpha to the von Hippel-Lindau ubiquitylation complex by O2-regulated prolyl hydroxylation. Science 292(5516):468–472

47. Semenza GL (2000) HIF-1: mediator of physiological and pathophysiological responses to hypoxia. J Appl Physiol 88(4):1747–1480

48. Maxwell PH, Pugh CW, Ratcliffe PJ (2001) Activation of the HIF pathway in cancer. Curr Opin Genet Dev 11:293–299

49. Zimmer M, Doucette D, Siddiqui N, Iliopoulos O (2004) Inhibition of hypoxia-inducible factor is sufficient for growth suppression of VHL-/- tumors. Mol Cancer Res 2(2):89–95

50. Kondo K, Kim WY, Lechpammer M, Kaelin WG (2003) Inhibition of HIF2alpha Is Sufficient to Suppress pVHL-Defective Tumor Growth. PLoS Biol 1(3):83

51. Maranchie JK, Vasselli JR, Riss J, Bonifacino JS, Linehan WM, Klausner RD (2002) The contribution of VHL substrate binding and HIF1-alpha to the phenotype of VHL loss in renal cell carcinoma. Cancer Cell 1(3):247–255

52. Kondo K, Klco J, Nakamura E, Lechpammer M, Kaelin WG (2002) Inhibition of HIF is necessary for tumor suppression by the von Hippel-Lindau protein. Cancer Cell 1(3):237–246

53. Knauth K, Bex C, Jemth P, Buchberger A (2006) Renal cell carcinoma risk in type 2 von Hippel-Lindau disease correlates with defects in pVHL stability and HIF-1alpha interactions. Oncogene 25(3):370–377

54. Hoffman MA, Ohh M, Yang H, Klco JM, Ivan M, Kaelin WG (2001) Von Hippel-Lindau protein mutants linked to type 2C VHL disease preserve the ability to downregulate HIF. Hum Mol Genet 10(10):1019–1027

55. Clifford SC, Cockman ME, Smallwood A et al (2001) Contrasting effects on HIF1a regulation by disease-causing pVHL mutations correlate with patterns of tumorigenesis in von Hippel-Lindau disease. Hum Mol Genet 10(10):1029–1038

56. Yang JC, Haworth L, Sherry RM et al (2003) A randomized trial of bevacizumab, an anti-vascular endothelial growth factor antibody, for metastatic renal cancer. N Engl J Med 349(5):427–434

57. Motzer RJ, Bukowski RM (2006) Targeted therapy for metastatic renal cell carcinoma. J Clin Oncol 24(35):5601–5608

58. Motzer RJ, Hutson TE, Tomczak P et al (2007) Sunitinib versus interferon alfa in metastatic renal-cell carcinoma. N Engl J Med 356(2):115–124

59. Escudier B, Eisen T, Stadler WM et al (2007) Sorafenib in advanced clear-cell renal-cell carcinoma. N Engl J Med 356(2):125–134

60. Turcotte S, Chan DA, Sutphin PD, Hay MP, Denny WA, Giaccia AJ (2008) A molecule targeting VHL-deficient renal cell carcinoma that induces autophagy. Cancer Cell 14(1):90–102

61. Sutphin PD, Chan DA, Li JM, Turcotte S, Krieg AJ, Giaccia AJ (2007) Targeting the loss of the von Hippel-Lindau tumor suppressor gene in renal cell carcinoma cells. Cancer Res 67(12):5896–5905

62. Zimmer M, Ebert BL, Neil C et al (2008) Small-molecule inhibitors of HIF-2a translation link its 5'UTR iron-responsive element to oxygen sensing. Mol Cell 32(6):838–848

63. Ohh M, Yauch RL, Lonergan KM et al (1998) The von Hippel-Lindau tumor suppressor protein is required for proper assembly of an extracellular fibronectin matrix. Mol Cell 1(7):959–968

64. Hergovich A, Lisztwan J, Barry R, Ballschmieter P, Krek W (2003) Regulation of microtubule stability by the von Hippel-Lindau tumour suppressor protein pVHL. Nat Cell Biol 5(1):64–70

65. Schermer B, Ghenoiu C, Bartram M et al (2006) The von Hippel-Lindau tumor suppressor protein controls ciliogenesis by orienting microtubule growth. J Cell Biol 175(4):547–554

66. Chitalia VC, Foy RL, Bachschmid MM et al (2008) Jade-1 inhibits Wnt signalling by ubiquitylating beta-catenin and mediates Wnt pathway inhibition by pVHL. Nat Cell Biol 10(10):1208–1216

67. Roe JS, Kim H, Lee SM, Kim ST, Cho EJ, Youn HD (2006) p53 stabilization and transactivation by a von Hippel-Lindau protein. Mol Cell 22(3):395–405

68. Crino PB, Nathanson KL, Henske EP (2006) The tuberous sclerosis complex. N Engl J Med 355(13):1345–1356

69. Shepherd CW, Gomez MR, Lie JT, Crowson CS (1991) Causes of death in patients with tuberous sclerosis. Mayo Clin Proc 66(8):792–796

70. Consortium (1997) Identification of the TSC1 gene on chromosome 9q34. Science 277:805–808

71. European Consortium on Tuberous Sclerosis (1993) Identification and characterization of the tuberous sclerosis gene on chromosome 16. Cell 75:1305–1315

72. Niida Y, Lawrence-Smith N, Banwell A et al (1999) Analysis of both TSC1 and TSC2 for germline mutations in 126 unrelated patients with tuberous sclerosis. Hum Mutat 14(5):412–422

73. Stillwell TJ, Gomez MR, Kelalis PP (1987) Renal lesions in tuberous sclerosis. J Urol 138(3):477–481

74. Yamakado K, Tanaka N, Nakagawa T, Kobayashi S, Yanagawa M, Takeda K (2002) Renal angiomyolipoma: relationships between tumor size, aneurysm formation, and rupture. Radiology 225(1):78–82

75. Patel U, Simpson E, Kingswood JC, Saggar-Malik AK (2005) Tuberose sclerosis complex: analysis of growth rates aids differentiation of renal cell carcinoma from atypical or minimal-fat-containing angiomyolipoma. Clin Radiol 60(6):665–673, discussion 663–664

76. Cook JA, Oliver K, Mueller RF, Sampson J (1996) A cross sectional study of renal involvement in tuberous sclerosis. J Med Genet 33(6):480–484

77. Saito K, Fujii Y, Kasahara I, Kobayashi N, Kasuga T, Kihara K (2002) Malignant clear cell "sugar" tumor of the kidney: clear cell variant of epithelioid angiomyolipoma. J Urol 168(6):2533–2534

78. Martignoni G, Bonetti F, Pea M, Tardanico R, Brunelli M, Eble JN (2002) Renal disease in adults with TSC2/PKD1 contiguous gene syndrome. Am J Surg Pathol 26(2):198–205

79. Siegel DH, Howard R (2002) Molecular advances in genetic skin diseases. Curr Opin Pediatr 14(4):419–425

80. Goodman M, Lamm SH, Engel A, Shepherd CW, Houser OW, Gomez MR (1997) Cortical tuber count: a biomarker indicating neurologic severity of tuberous sclerosis complex. J Child Neurol 12(2):85–90

81. Zaroff CM, Devinsky O, Miles D, Barr WB (2004) Cognitive and behavioral correlates of tuberous sclerosis complex. J Child Neurol 19(11):847–852

82. Verhaaren HA, Vanakker O, De Wolf D, Suys B, Francois K, Matthys D (2003) Left ventricular outflow obstruction in rhabdomyoma of infancy: meta-analysis of the literature. J Pediatr 143(2):258–263

83. MacCollin M, Kwiatkowski D (2001) Molecular genetic aspects of the phakomatoses: tuberous sclerosis complex and neurofibromatosis 1. Curr Opin Neurol 14(2):163–169

84. Dabora SL, Jozwiak S, Franz DN et al (2001) Mutational analysis in a cohort of 224 tuberous sclerosis patients indicates increased severity of TSC2, compared with TSC1, disease in multiple organs. Am J Hum Genet 68(1):64–80

85. Langkau N, Martin N, Brandt R et al (2002) TSC1 and TSC2 mutations in tuberous sclerosis, the associated phenotypes and a model to explain observed TSC1/TSC2 frequency ratios. Eur J Pediatr 161(7):393–402

86. Verhoef S, Bakker L, Tempelaars AM et al (1999) High rate of mosaicism in tuberous sclerosis complex. Am J Hum Genet 64(6):1632–1637

87. Rose VM, Au KS, Pollom G, Roach ES, Prashner HR, Northrup H (1999) Germ-line mosaicism in tuberous sclerosis: how common? Am J Hum Genet 64(4):986–992

88. Consortium. European Consostrium on Tuberous Sclerosis (1993) Identification and characterization of the tuberous sclerosis gene on chromosome 16. Cell 75:1305–1315

89. Yeung RS, Xiao G-H, Jin F, Lee W-C, Testa JR, Knudson AG (1994) Predisposition to renal carcinoma in the Eker rat is determined by germ-line mutation of the tuberous sclerosis 2 (TSC2) gene. Proc Natl Acad Sci U S A 91:11413–11416

90. Rennebeck G, Kleymenova EV, Anderson R, Yeung RS, Artzt K, Walker CL (1998) Loss of function of the tuberous sclerosis 2 tumor suppressor gene results in embryonic lethality characterized by disrupted neuroepithelial growth and development. Proc Natl Acad Sci U S A 95(26):15629–15634

91. Ito N, Rubin GM (1999) Gigas, a Drosophila homolog of tuberous sclerosis gene product-2, regulates the cell cycle. Cell 96(4):529–539

92. Tapon N, Ito N, Dickson BJ, Treisman JE, Hariharan IK (2001) The Drosophila tuberous sclerosis complex gene homologs restrict cell growth and cell proliferation. Cell 105(3):345–355

93. Van Slegtenhorst M, Nellist M, Nagelkerken B et al (1998) Interaction between hamartin and tuberin, TSC1 and TSC2 gene products. Hum Mol Genet 7(6):1053–1057

94. Kobayashi T, Minowa O, Kuno J, Mitani H, Hino O, Noda T (1999) Renal carcinogenesis, hepatic hemangiomatosis, and embryonic lethality caused by a germ-line Tsc2 mutation in mice. Cancer Res 59(6):1206–1211

95. Kobayashi T, Minowa O, Sugitani Y et al (2001) A germ-line Tsc1 mutation causes tumor development and embryonic lethality that are similar, but not identical to, those caused by Tsc2 mutation in mice. Proc Natl Acad Sci U S A 98(15):8762–8767

96. Onda H, Lueck A, Marks PW, Warren HB, Kwiatkowski DJ (1999) Tsc2(+/-) mice develop tumors in multiple sites that express gelsolin

and are influenced by genetic background. J Clin Invest 104(6):687–695

97. Sepp T, Yates JR, Green AJ (1996) Loss of heterozygosity in tuberous sclerosis hamartomas. J Med Genet 33(11):962–964

98. Carsillo T, Astrinidis A, Henske EP (2000) Mutations in the tuberous sclerosis complex gene TSC2 are a cause of sporadic pulmonary lymphangioleiomyomatosis. Proc Natl Acad Sci U S A 97(11):6085–6090

99. Henske EP, Neumann HP, Scheithauer BW, Herbst EW, Short MP, Kwiatkowski DJ (1995) Loss of heterozygosity in the tuberous sclerosis (TSC2) region of chromosome band 16p13 occurs in sporadic as well as TSC-associated renal angiomyolipomas. Genes Chromosomes Cancer 13(4):295–298

100. Gao X, Zhang Y, Arrazola P et al (2002) Tsc tumour suppressor proteins antagonize amino-acid-TOR signalling. Nat Cell Biol 4(9):699–704

101. Inoki K, Li Y, Zhu T, Wu J, Guan KL (2002) TSC2 is phosphorylated and inhibited by Akt and suppresses mTOR signalling. Nat Cell Biol 4(9):648–657

102. Potter CJ, Pedraza LG, Xu T (2002) Akt regulates growth by directly phosphorylating Tsc2. Nat Cell Biol 4(9):658–665

103. Inoki K, Corradetti MN, Guan KL (2005) Dysregulation of the TSC-mTOR pathway in human disease. Nat Genet 37(1):19–24

104. Yuan TL, Cantley LC (2008) PI3K pathway alterations in cancer: variations on a theme. Oncogene 27(41):5497–5510

105. Sampson JR (2009) Therapeutic targeting of mTOR in tuberous sclerosis. Biochem Soc Trans 37(Pt 1):259–264

106. Meikle L, Pollizzi K, Egnor A et al (2008) Response of a neuronal model of tuberous sclerosis to mammalian target of rapamycin (mTOR) inhibitors: effects on mTORC1 and Akt signaling lead to improved survival and function. J Neurosci 28(21):5422–5432

107. Lee N, Woodrum CL, Nobil AM, Rauktys AE, Messina MP, Dabora SL (2009) Rapamycin weekly maintenance dosing and the potential efficacy of combination sorafenib plus rapamycin but not atorvastatin or doxycycline in tuberous sclerosis preclinical models. BMC Pharmacol 9:8

108. Rauktys A, Lee N, Lee L, Dabora SL (2008) Topical rapamycin inhibits tuberous sclerosis tumor growth in a nude mouse model. BMC Dermatol 8:1

109. Ehninger D, Han S, Shilyansky C et al (2008) Reversal of learning deficits in a Tsc2+/- mouse model of tuberous sclerosis. Nat Med 14(8):843–848

110. Zeng LH, Xu L, Gutmann DH, Wong M (2008) Rapamycin prevents epilepsy in a mouse model of tuberous sclerosis complex. Ann Neurol 63(4):444–453

111. Hofbauer GF, Marcollo-Pini A, Corsenca A et al (2008) The mTOR inhibitor rapamycin significantly improves facial angiofibroma lesions in a patient with tuberous sclerosis. Br J Dermatol 159(2):473–475

112. Bissler JJ, McCormack FX, Young LR et al (2008) Sirolimus for angiomyolipoma in tuberous sclerosis complex or lymphangioleiomyomatosis. N Engl J Med 358(2):140–151

113. Koenig MK, Butler IJ, Northrup H (2008) Regression of subependymal giant cell astrocytoma with rapamycin in tuberous sclerosis complex. J Child Neurol 23(10):1238–1239

114. Kovacs G, Brusa P, De Riese W (1989) Tissue-specific expression of a constitutional 3;6 translocation: development of multiple bilateral renal-cell carcinomas. Int J Cancer 43(3):422–427

115. Eleveld MJ, Bodmer D, Merkx G et al (2001) Molecular analysis of a familial case of renal cell cancer and a t(3;6)(q12;q15). Genes Chromosomes Cancer 31(1):23–32

116. Bodmer D, Eleveld M, Kater-Baats E et al (2002) Disruption of a novel MFS transporter gene, DIRC2, by a familial renal cell carcinoma-associated t(2;3)(q35;q21). Hum Mol Genet 11(6):641–649

117. Bodmer D, Eleveld M, Ligtenberg M et al (2002) Cytogenetic and molecular analysis of early stage renal cell carcinomas in a family

with a translocation (2;3)(q35;q21). Cancer Genet Cytogenet 134(1):6–12

118. Podolski J, Byrski T, Zajaczek S et al (2001) Characterization of a familial RCC-associated t(2;3)(q33;q21) chromosome translocation. J Hum Genet 46(12):685–693

119. Li FP, Decker HJ, Zbar B et al (1993) Clinical and genetic studies of renal cell carcinomas in a family with a constitutional chromosome 3;8 translocation. Genetics of familial renal carcinoma. Ann Intern Med 118(2):106–111

120. Schmidt L, Li F, Brown RS et al (1995) Mechanism of tumorigenesis of renal carcinomas associated with the constitutional chromosome 3;8 translocation. Cancer J Sci Am 1(3):191–195

121. Ohta M, Inoue H, Cotticelli MG et al (1996) The FHIT gene, spanning the chromosome 3p14.2 fragile site and renal carcinoma-associated t(3;8) breakpoint, is abnormal in digestive tract cancers. Cell 84(4):587–597

122. Gemmill RM, West JD, Boldog F et al (1998) The hereditary renal cell carcinoma 3;8 translocation fuses FHIT to a patched-related gene, TRC8. Proc Natl Acad Sci U S A 95(16):9572–9577

123. Poland KS, Azim M, Folsom M et al (2007) A constitutional balanced t(3;8)(p14;q24.1) translocation results in disruption of the TRC8 gene and predisposition to clear cell renal cell carcinoma. Genes Chromosomes Cancer 46(9):805–812

124. Brauweiler A, Lorick KL, Lee JP et al (2007) RING-dependent tumor suppression and G2/M arrest induced by the TRC8 hereditary kidney cancer gene. Oncogene 26(16):2263–2271

125. Gemmill RM, Lee JP, Chamovitz DA, Segal D, Hooper JE, Drabkin HA (2005) Growth suppression induced by the TRC8 hereditary kidney cancer gene is dependent upon JAB1/CSN5. Oncogene 24(21):3503–3511

126. Druck T, Podolski J, Byrski T et al (2001) The DIRC1 gene at chromosome 2q33 spans a familial RCC-associated t(2;3)(q33;q21) chromosome translocation. J Hum Genet 46(10):583–589

127. Ricketts C, Woodward ER, Killick P et al (2008) Germline SDHB mutations and familial renal cell carcinoma. J Natl Cancer Inst 100(17):1260–1262

128. Goedert JJ, McKeen EA, Fraumeni JF (1981) Polymastia and renal adenocarcinoma. Ann Intern Med 95(2):182–184

129. Mehes K (1996) Familial association of supernumerary nipple with renal cancer. Cancer Genet Cytogenet 86(2):129–130

130. Kovacs G, Akhtar M, Beckwith BJ et al (1997) The Heidelberg classification of renal cell tumours. J Pathol 183(2):131–133

131. Pignot G, Elie C, Conquy S et al (2007) Survival analysis of 130 patients with papillary renal cell carcinoma: prognostic utility of type 1 and type 2 subclassification. Urology 69(2):230–235

132. Zbar B (2000) Inherited epithelial tumors of the kidney: old and new diseases. Semin Cancer Biol 10(4):313–318

133. Schmidt L, Duh FM, Chen F et al (1997) Germline and somatic mutations in the tyrosine kinase domain of the MET proto-oncogene in papillary renal carcinomas. Nat Genet 16:68–73

134. Zhuang Z, Park WS, Pack S et al (1998) Trisomy 7-harbouring non-random duplication of the mutant MET allele in hereditary papillary renal carcinomas. Nat Genet 20(1):66–69

135. Bottaro DP, Rubin JS, Faletto DL et al (1991) Identification of the hepatocyte growth factor receptor as the c-met proto-oncogene product. Science 251(4995):802–804

136. Ponzetto C, Bardelli A, Zhen Z et al (1994) A multifunctional docking site mediates signaling and transformation by the hepatocyte growth factor/scatter factor receptor family. Cell 77(2):261–271

137. Boccaccio C, Comoglio PM (2006) Invasive growth: a MET-driven genetic programme for cancer and stem cells. Nat Rev Cancer 6(8):637–645

138. Giordano S, Zhen Z, Medico E, Gaudino G, Galimi F, Comoglio PM (1993) Transfer of mitogenic and invasive response to scatter factor/hepatocyte growth factor by transfection of human MET protooncogene. Proc Natl Acad Sci U S A 90(2):649–653

139. Comoglio PM, Giordano S, Trusolino L (2008) Drug development of MET inhibitors: targeting oncogene addiction and expedience. Nat Rev Drug Discov 7(6):504–516

140. Launonen V, Vierimaa O, Kiuru M et al (2001) Inherited susceptibility to uterine leiomyomas and renal cell cancer. Proc Natl Acad Sci U S A 98(6):3387–3392

141. Consortium TML (2002) Germline mutations in FH predispose to dominantly inherited uterine fibroids, skin leiomyomata and papillary renal cell cancer. Nat Genet 30(4):306–310

142. Toro JR, Nickerson ML, Wei MH et al (2003) Mutations in the fumarate hydratase gene cause hereditary leiomyomatosis and renal cell cancer in families in North America. Am J Hum Genet 73(1):95–106

143. Sudarshan S, Pinto PA, Neckers L, Linehan WM (2007) Mechanisms of disease: hereditary leiomyomatosis and renal cell cancer – a distinct form of hereditary kidney cancer. Nat Clin Pract Urol 4(2):104–110

144. Carvajal-Carmona LG, Alam NA, Pollard PJ et al (2006) Adult leydig cell tumors of the testis caused by germline fumarate hydratase mutations. J Clin Endocrinol Metab 91(8):3071–3075

145. Lehtonen HJ, Kiuru M, Ylisaukko-Oja SK et al (2006) Increased risk of cancer in patients with fumarate hydratase germline mutation. J Med Genet 43(6):523–526

146. Alam NA, Bevan S, Churchman M (2001) Localization of a gene (MCUL1) for multiple cutaneous leiomyomata and uterine fibroids to chromosome 1q42.3-q43. Am J Hum Genet 68(5):1264–1269

147. Alam NA, Rowan AJ, Wortham NC et al (2003) Genetic and functional analyses of FH mutations in multiple cutaneous and uterine leiomyomatosis, hereditary leiomyomatosis and renal cancer, and fumarate hydratase deficiency. Hum Mol Genet 12(11):1241–1252

148. Alam NA, Olpin S, Leigh IM (2005) Fumarate hydratase mutations and predisposition to cutaneous leiomyomas, uterine leiomyomas and renal cancer. Br J Dermatol 153(1):11–17

149. Wei MH, Toure O, Glenn GM et al (2006) Novel mutations in FH and expansion of the spectrum of phenotypes expressed in families with hereditary leiomyomatosis and renal cancer. J Med Genet 43(1):18–27

150. Stewart L, Glenn GM, Stratton P et al (2008) Association of germline mutations in the fumarate hydratase gene and uterine fibroids in women with hereditary leiomyomatosis and renal cell cancer. Arch Dermatol 144(12):1584–1592

151. Isaacs JS, Jung YJ, Mole DR et al (2005) HIF overexpression correlates with biallelic loss of fumarate hydratase in renal cancer: novel role of fumarate in regulation of HIF stability. Cancer Cell 8(2):143–153

152. Vanharanta S, Pollard PJ, Lehtonen HJ et al (2006) Distinct expression profile in fumarate-hydratase-deficient uterine fibroids. Hum Mol Genet 15(1):97–103

153. Malchoff CD, Sarfarazi M, Tendler B et al (2000) Papillary thyroid carcinoma associated with papillary renal neoplasia: genetic linkage analysis of a distinct heritable tumor syndrome. J Clin Endocrinol Metab 85(5):1758–1764

154. Birt AR, Hogg GR, Dube WJ (1977) Hereditary multiple fibrofolliculomas with trichodiscomas and acrochordons. Arch Dermatol 113:1674–1677

155. Scalvenzi M, Argenziano G, Sammarco E, Delfino M (1998) Hereditary multiple fibrofolliculomas, trichodiscomas and acrochordons: syndrome of Birt-Hogg-Dube. J Eur Acad Dermatol Venereol 11(1):45–47

156. Toro JR, Wei MH, Glenn GM et al (2008) BHD mutations, clinical and molecular genetic investigations of Birt-Hogg-Dube syndrome: a new series of 50 families and a review of published reports. J Med Genet 45(6):321–331

157. Ayo DS, Aughenbaugh GL, Yi ES, Hand JL, Ryu JH (2007) Cystic lung disease in Birt-Hogg-Dube syndrome. Chest 132(2):679–684

158. Toro JR, Pautler SE, Stewart L et al (2007) Lung cysts, spontaneous pneumothorax, and genetic associations in 89 families with Birt-Hogg-Dube syndrome. Am J Respir Crit Care Med 175(10):1044–1053

159. Zbar B, Alvord WG, Glenn G et al (2002) Risk of renal and colonic neoplasms and spontaneous pneumothorax in the Birt-Hogg-Dube syndrome. Cancer Epidemiol Biomarkers Prev 11(4):393–400

160. Khoo SK, Bradley M, Wong FK, Hedblad MA, Nordenskjold M, Teh BT (2001) Birt-Hogg-Dube syndrome: mapping of a novel hereditary neoplasia gene to chromosome 17p12-q11.2. Oncogene 20(37):5239–5242

161. Schmidt LS, Warren MB, Nickerson ML et al (2001) Birt-Hogg-Dube syndrome, a genodermatosis associated with spontaneous pneumothorax and kidney neoplasia, maps to chromosome 17p11.2. Am J Hum Genet 69(4):876–882

162. Nickerson ML, Warren MB, Toro JR et al (2002) Mutations in a novel gene lead to kidney tumors, lung wall defects, and benign tumors of the hair follicle in patients with the Birt-Hogg-Dube syndrome. Cancer Cell 2(2):157–164

163. Baba M, Hong SB, Sharma N et al (2006) Folliculin encoded by the BHD gene interacts with a binding protein, FNIP1, and AMPK, and is involved in AMPK and mTOR signaling. Proc Natl Acad Sci U S A 103(42):15552–15557

164. Clague J, Lin J, Cassidy A et al (2009) Family history and risk of renal cell carcinoma: results from a case-control study and systematic meta-analysis. Cancer Epidemiol Biomarkers Prev 18(3):801–807

165. Bravo EL, Tagle R (2003) Pheochromocytoma: state-of-the-art and future prospects. Endocr Rev 24(4):539–553

166. Neumann HP, Bausch B (2002) McWhinney SRea. Germ-line mutations in nonsyndromic pheochromocytoma. N Engl J Med 346(19):1459–1466

167. Neumann H, Bausch B, McWhinney SR et al (2002) Germ-line mutations in nonsyndromic pheochromocytoma. N Engl J Med 346(19):1459–1466

168. Eng C, Clayton D, Schuffenecker I et al (1996) The relationship between specific RET proto-oncogene mutations and disease phenotype in multiple endocrine neoplasia type 2. International RET mutation consortium analysis. JAMA 276(19):1575–1579

169. Eisenhofer G, Walther MM, Huynh TT et al (2001) Pheochromocytomas in von Hippel-Lindau syndrome and multiple endocrine neoplasia type 2 display distinct biochemical and clinical phenotypes. J Clin Endocrinol Metab 86(5):1999–2008

170. Baysal BE, Ferrell RE, Willett-Brozick JE et al (2000) Mutations in SDHD, a mitochondrial complex II gene, in hereditary paraganglioma. Science 287(5454):848–851

171. Niemann S, Müller U (2000) Mutations in SDHC cause autosomal dominant paraganglioma, type 3. Nat Genet 26:268–270

172. Astuti D, Douglas F, Lennard TW et al (2001) Germline SDHD mutation in familial phaeochromocytoma. Lancet 357:1181–1182

173. Selak MA, Armour SM, MacKenzie ED et al (2005) Succinate links TCA cycle dysfunction to oncogenesis by inhibiting HIF-alpha prolyl hydroxylase. Cancer Cell 7(1):77–85

174. Neumann HP, Pawlu C, Peczkowska M et al (2004) Distinct clinical features of paraganglioma syndromes associated with SDHB and SDHD gene mutations. JAMA 292(8):943–951

175. Vanharanta S, Buchta M, McWhinney SR et al (2004) Early-onset renal cell carcinoma as a novel extraparagangial component of SDHB-associated heritable paraganglioma. Am J Hum Genet 74(1):153–159

176. Pasini B, McWhinney SR, Bei T et al (2008) Clinical and molecular genetics of patients with the Carney-Stratakis syndrome and germline mutations of the genes coding for the succinate dehydrogenase subunits SDHB, SDHC, and SDHD. Eur J Hum Genet 16(1):79–88

177. Ni Y, Zbuk KM, Sadler T et al (2008) Germline mutations and variants in the succinate dehydrogenase genes in Cowden and Cowden-like syndromes. Am J Hum Genet 83(2):261–268

178. Brouwers FM, Eisenhofer G, Tao JJ et al (2006) High frequency of SDHB germline mutations in patients with malignant catecholamine-producing paragangliomas: implications for genetic testing. J Clin Endocrinol Metab 91(11):4505–4509

179. Brouwers FM, Elkahloun AG, Munson PJ et al (2006) Gene expression profiling of benign and malignant pheochromocytoma. Ann N Y Acad Sci 1073:541–556

Chapter 10
Familial Atypical Mole Melanoma (FAMM) Syndrome

Elizabeth D. Chao, Michele J. Gabree, and Hensin Tsao

Keywords Melanoma • Atypical mole • p16 gene • CDKN2 gene • Cell cycle

Introduction

The incidence of cutaneous melanoma continues to increase rapidly worldwide. In the United States alone, the incidence of melanoma has been roughly doubling each decade, and according to the most recent projections by the American Cancer Society and the National Cancer Institute Surveillance, Epidemiology, and End Results (SEER), it was estimated that 1 in 41 Americans would develop melanoma in their lifetime. In 2009, 68,720 new cases of melanoma were diagnosed, with 8,650 deaths attributable to the disease [1].

Approximately 5–12% of all melanoma cases are hereditary [2–6]. The familial atypical mole-melanoma (FAMM) syndrome is a form of hereditary melanoma that can be recognized by the presence of a strong familial predisposition to cutaneous melanoma and by large numbers of clinically and pathologically confirmed atypical nevi. The origin of the FAMM syndrome can be traced back to 1820, when William Norris documented the first case of familial melanoma associated with unusual mole patterns and a "strong tendency to hereditary predisposition." He observed that both the father and son had melanoma and other family members had large numbers of atypical moles [7, 8]. Accumulating evidence for the co-occurrence of multiple atypical nevi in families predisposed to melanoma [9, 10] culminated in its designation as the familial atypical multiple mole melanoma (FAMMM) or the "B-K mole syndrome" [7, 11, 12]. Historically, other eponyms such as [11], "dysplastic nevus syndrome" (DNS) [13] and "classical atypical mole syndrome" [14] have also

been used. However, the current designation is the familial atypical mole-melanoma (FAMM) syndrome [15].

In this chapter, we further elaborate on the clinical and molecular aspects of the FAMM syndrome and its associated noncutaneous malignancies, as well as some basic guidelines for genetic testing, management, and prevention.

Clinical Features

The clinical features defining the FAMM syndrome continue to evolve, but generally include the presence of a strong familial predisposition to cutaneous melanoma and large numbers of clinically and pathologically confirmed atypical nevi. The National Institutes of Health (NIH) Consensus Conference on Diagnosis and Treatment of Early Melanoma in 1992 proposed a more specific definition of the FAMM syndrome, which is gradually gaining acceptance and includes (1) the occurrence of malignant melanoma in a proband in addition to one or more first- or second-degree relatives; (2) a large number of melanocytic nevi, often more than 50, some of which are atypical and often variable in size, and (3) melanocytic nevi that demonstrate certain histological features [15] (Table 10.1).

While no universally accepted criteria exist for the FAMM syndrome, the MGH Melanoma and Pigmented Lesion Center (PLC) uses the following criteria for defining hereditary melanoma irrespective of mole phenotype:

1. An individual affected with melanoma and one or more first-degree relatives with melanoma on the same side of the family.
2. Affected or unaffected individuals with two or more affected relatives on the same side of the family regardless of degree.
3. One individual with three or more cases of primary cutaneous melanoma, regardless of family history.
4. Personal and/or family history of melanoma and pancreatic cancer in one individual or in multiple individuals on the same side of the family.

H. Tsao (✉)
MGH Melanoma and Pigmented Lesion Center, MGH Melanoma Genetics Program, Wellman Center for Photomedicine, Massachusetts General Hospital, Boston, MA, USA

D.C. Chung and D.A. Haber (eds.), *Principles of Clinical Cancer Genetics: A Handbook from the Massachusetts General Hospital*,
DOI 10.1007/978-0-387-93846-2_10, © Springer Science+Business Media, LLC 2010

Table 10.1 Histopathological criteria for diagnosis of atypical (dysplastic) nevus

	Features
Architectural features	Disordered intraepidermal melanocytic proliferation (lentiginous patterns)[a]
	Variation in size, shape, location of junctional nests with bridging or confluence[a]
	Lack of cellular cohension within nests
	"Shoulder" phenomenon (lateral extension of junctional component)
	Asymmetry
	Poor circumscription of intraepidermal component
Cytologic features	Nuclear atypia (i.e., pleomorphism, enlargement, hyperchromasia, prominent nucleoli)[a]
	Spindle cell or epithelioid cell pattern
	Prominent pale or dusty cytoplasm
	Large melanin granules
	Mitotic figures absent or very rare
Host response[b]	Mononuclear cell/lymphocytic infiltrates
	Fibroplasia (concentric eosinophilic or lamellar pattern)
	Prominent vascularity

[a]Major criteria, essential for diagnosis

[b]Strongly supportive of diagnosis

Adapted from Barnhill RL, Mihm MC Jr (1998) Histopathology and precursor lesions. In: Balch CM, Houghton AN, Sober AJ, Soong S (eds) Cutaneous melanoma. Quality Medical, St. Louis, MO; Piepkorn M, Barnill RL (2004) Common acquired and atypical (dysplastic) melanocytic nevi. In: Barnill RL, Piepkorn M, Busam KI (eds) Pathology of melanocytic nevi and malignant melanoma. Springer, New York

Our definition of hereditary melanoma shifts the focus away from atypical nevi to melanoma. The clinical and histological imprecision with which atypical moles have been described presents a considerable challenge in the diagnosis of FAMM syndrome. The lack of consensus in the descriptive features of atypical moles, to distinguish them from other pigmented lesions and melanoma, has thus resulted in confusing nosology. Numerous terms such as "Clark's nevus," "B-K mole," "nevus with architectural disorder and cytologic atypia," and "dysplastic nevus" have been used interchangeably with "atypical nevi."

Even though "dysplastic nevus (DN)" is probably the most common appellation, there is still considerable controversy since DN can be used as both a clinical and a histological descriptor. To some, the term "dysplastic" denoted the developmental anomaly as a precursor to melanoma [16–23], while to others, the term described architectural and cytologic atypical melanocytes that identified individuals at increased risk for development of melanomas [24–32]. Thus, weakness in the criteria used to define the "dysplastic nevus" created remarkable difficulties in the ability to reproduce, interpret, and compare the results of various studies, and even resulted in a tenfold discrepancy in estimates of the frequency of these lesions. In an effort to resolve the controversy, the NIH Consensus Development Panel on Early Melanoma [15] suggested that the term "dysplastic nevus" "be avoided."

At the MGH PLC, we use "clinically atypical moles or nevi (CAM or CAN)" to describe the clinical lesion and "DN with varying degrees of atypia" to describe the pathological features. CAN grossly differ from "typical" benign nevi in that they possess asymmetry, poorly circumscribed borders/margins, irregularity in contour, variegated pigmentation, and a larger size (>5 mm); individuals with CAN often harbor hundreds of lesions (Fig. 10.1a). A characteristic presentation of a CAN is a pigmented papule of one color surrounded by a macular collar of pigmentation of a different shade, also referred to as a "fried-egg" or "target-shaped" nevus (Fig. 10.1b). The nevi are often pigment gradations of tan and pink, with a surface that is variable and complex, containing macular and/or papular components. Atypical nevi vary in size and are often larger than benign nevi, and have borders that are irregular and indistinct, often fading into the surrounding skin.

Histologically, DN exhibit architectural disorder and varying degrees of melanocytic nuclear atypia (Table 10.1). The 1992 NIH Consensus Conference designated the following histological criteria for the evaluation of dysplastic nevi: architectural disorder with asymmetry, subepidermal (concentric eosinophilic and/or lamellar) fibroplasia of the papillary dermis, and lentiginous melanocytic hyperplasia with spindle or epithelioid melanocytes aggregating in junctional nests of variable size and forming bridges between adjacent rete ridges. Melanocytic atypia may be present to a variable degree. In addition, there may be dermal infiltration with lymphocytes, as well as the "shoulder" phenomenon (intraepidermal melanocytes extending singly or in nests laterally beyond the main dermal component). Interestingly, none of the histological criteria, when taken alone, can define an atypical mole, since many of the features are shared to varying degrees by early melanoma. Thus, it is the constellation of histological features, in addition to the lack of superficial pagetoid spread, absence of mitotic activity, or lack of

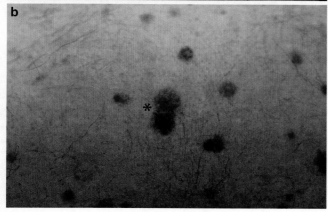

Fig. 10.1 A FAMM syndrome patient. (a) The striking feature is the large number of melanocytic nevi (>70) on his upper back and the heterogeneity of his moles in terms of diameter, shape, and color. (b) An enlarged, close-up view of a clinically atypical nevus (CAN) (asterisk, from boxed area in (a)) on the patient's back, surrounded by smaller atypical and "typical" benign nevi. CAN exhibit prominent border irregularity and asymmetry, variegated pigmentation, and a larger size (>5 mm); individuals with CAN often harbor hundreds of lesions. A characteristic presentation of a CAN is a pigmented papule of one color (i.e., brown) surrounded by a macular collar of pigmentation of a different shade (pink)

effacement of the dermoepidermal junctions, that help to distinguish atypical moles histologically from melanomas [33].

Although correlations exist between CAN and DN, the actual concordance between clinical and histological features of atypical nevi is weak; clinically atypical nevi are frequently found to lack histological atypia, and vice versa [34–39]. Thus, the low predictive value of clinical criteria in detecting histologically atypical nevi has raised concerns about the existence of the atypical nevus as a distinct clinicopathological entity [34]. Despite the controversy, a large majority of dermatologists accept the atypical nevus as a legitimate entity that confers an increased risk for the development of melanoma [40].

There exists significant diagnostic heterogeneity and inconsistency because the clinical criteria used to define FAMM is incomplete and replete with ambiguity. In addition to the uncertainty surrounding the diagnosis of CAN and DN, the minimum size or number of total moles and/or atypical moles required for a diagnosis of FAMM syndrome has not yet been established, although an arbitrary standard of 50–100 nevi has been proposed [35, 41]. However, individuals with FAMM have been found to have anywhere from one to several hundred CAN. Another issue is the distribution of atypical nevi on affected individuals and its unexplained primary predilection for the trunk and secondary propensity for the scalp, breasts, buttocks, and feet. The impact of nongenetic factors on the FAMM syndrome is also an important consideration, since the number of moles, for instance, increases with age and solar exposure [33].

Ultimately, the diagnosis of the FAMM syndrome is a clinical impression, necessitating the consideration of all the various aspects of phenotype such as total mole count, distribution, clinical appearance of the moles, the age of onset, site, and number of melanomas.

Distinguishing Sporadic From Hereditary Forms of the FAMM Syndrome

Since hereditary melanoma can account for up to 12% of all cases of melanomas [2–6, 42, 43], the remaining cases are attributable to sporadic, or "nonfamilial," events. Atypical moles, which have largely been described in familial melanoma settings thus far, also occur in individuals with no familial predisposition to melanoma or without already preexisting atypical moles. It has been estimated that the incidence of having five or more atypical nevi in the general population is 6% [44].

Atypical moles that arise in a sporadic setting cannot be distinguished clinically or histologically from those that develop in the setting of the FAMM syndrome. In the general population, a continuum of clinically and histologically atypical moles exists and thus the degree of susceptibility to melanoma can be viewed as a spectrum. At one extreme, an individual can belong to classic FAMM kindred, where multiple members have atypical moles and/or melanoma. At the other extreme, an individual may have only a few atypical moles without any personal or family history of melanoma. This situation would be viewed as a "nonfamilial" or "sporadic" case, and the risk of developing melanoma is reduced compared to someone with the FAMM syndrome although the magnitude of this risk reduction has not been precisely calculated.

A more formal and operational classification of the FAMM phenotype that has been used to assess risk for melanoma in FAMM individuals is based on five classes of kindred, designated A through D-2, who are stratified according to their

Table 10.2 Classification of kindreds with the FAMM syndrome (dysplastic nevus syndrome)

Class	Name	Description
A	Sporadic dysplastic nevus	One family member with dysplastic nevus; no melanoma
B	Familial dysplastic nevus	Two or more family members with dysplastic nevus; no melanoma
C	Sporadic dysplastic nevus and melanoma	One family member with both dysplastic nevus and melanoma
Dl	Familial dysplastic nevus and melanoma	Two or more family members with dysplastic nevus; one member with both dysplastic nevus and melanoma
D2	Familial dysplastic nevus and melanoma	Two or more family members with both dysplastic nevus and melanoma

family and individual histories of atypical nevi and melanoma (Table 10.2). The original classifications formulated by Kenneth Kraemer in 1983 utilized the term "dysplastic nevus" before the current NIH recommended the use of the "atypical mole" terminology. Type A represents patients with sporadic DNS who did not have melanoma; type B, persons with the familial DNS who did not have melanoma; type C, individuals who had both dysplastic nevi and melanoma but no familial disposition toward either DN or melanoma; type D-1, persons with one family member having melanoma plus DN; and type D-2, persons with at least two relatives having melanoma plus DN. While those in kindred type A have the lowest risk of developing melanoma, which is still 26 times greater than that for the general population [45], those in the type D-2 class have the highest risk. For individuals in the type D-2 class, the projected cumulative lifetime risk of melanoma was 100% by the age of 75 [46], which is 148 times greater than that in the general Caucasian population [5]. The addition of a personal history of melanoma would increase the relative risk of developing a second melanoma by 500- to 1,000-fold.

Genetics and Genotype/Phenotype Correlations

Approximately 5–12% of all malignant melanoma cases occur in individuals who have one or more first-degree relatives with melanoma [2–6, 42, 43]. An early report estimated that 69% of melanomas arising in the familial context occur with an atypical nevus in contiguity with the melanoma; this suggested that 5.5% of all melanomas are likely to be attributed to FAMM syndrome [45].

Although the FAMM syndrome was recognized over 30 years ago, a full genetic explanation of the disease remains elusive. This has largely been attributable to the difficulty in establishing a clear genetic association between the two key defining features of FAMM: malignant melanoma and atypical nevi. While compelling evidence support a link between the presence of atypical moles and an increased risk for cutaneous melanoma [25, 29, 47–51], the widespread variability in the mole phenotype among melanoma-prone family members has made it difficult to isolate the genetic locus(i) responsible for the phenotype.

Despite the phenotypic variation of atypical moles, genetic factors do play a substantial, permissive role in the development of nevi, such as controlling the numbers of nevi that may develop as a result of early childhood sun exposure [52]. The genetic control of nevi is reflected in the strong concordance of the atypical nevus phenotype in monozygotic twins [53], as well as in data collected from segregation analysis [54–56]. However, the interplay of nongenetic factors, such as sun exposure, affects the development and progression of atypical nevi, and hamper attempts to determine a simple pattern of Mendelian inheritance. Thus, the atypical mole phenotype may best be described as a continuous, quantitative trait, in contrast to melanoma, which, like most cancers, is considered a dichotomous characteristic [33]. Consequently, the precise inheritance pattern of the FAMM syndrome remains as a source of dispute [57] although more modern insights into the role of modifier genes and the environment may supplant the notion of a fixed inheritance pattern.

Ultimately, the identification of the major locus for melanoma susceptibility became clear after the confounding influences introduced by the concept of the dysplastic nevus were set aside. The first hints for the localization of a melanoma susceptibility gene came from molecular cytogenetic studies and loss of heterozygosity (LOH) analysis of melanoma cell lines [58]. Linkage analysis narrowed the region to the 9p13-22 locus [59–62], and a combination of tumor deletion studies, recombination mapping, and positional cloning identified the *CDKN2A* locus, which was later found to encode a previously identified inhibitor of cyclin-dependent kinase 4, called p16 [63–66] and found to cosegregate with melanoma susceptibility in several melanoma families, thus establishing *CDKN2A* as a major melanoma susceptibility locus in familial melanoma [67]. Since its discovery, *CDKN2A* has been known by a plethora of other names, such as *CDKN2*, *p16*, *p16INK4*, *MTS1*, *INK4A*, and *CDK4I*. However, the Human Genome Organization nomenclature committee officially assigned the designation of *CDKN2A* to minimize confusion.

The gene structure of the *CDKN2A* (Cyclin-dependent kinase inhibitor 2A) locus is unusual in that it encodes for two structurally distinct proteins, p16[INK4A] and p14[ARF], through the

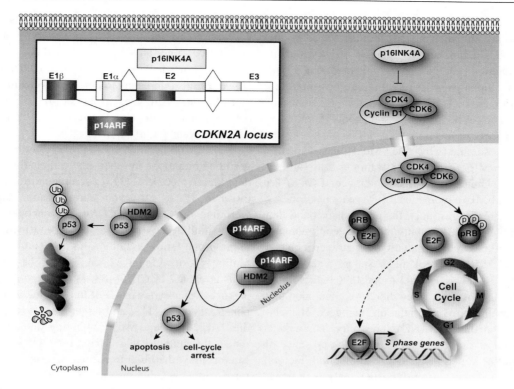

Fig. 10.2 Structure and function of the *CDKN2A* gene. Inset: The cyclin-dependent kinase inhibitor 2A (*CDKN2A*) locus on chromosome 9p21. Through alternative splicing, this gene encodes two distinct proteins: p16INK4A and p14ARF. p16INK4A is encoded by exons 1α, 2, and 3 (yellow), whereas p14ARF is encoded by exons 1β, 2, and 3 (blue). Pathway: p16INK4A blocks cell cycle entry at the G1-S checkpoint by inhibiting the cyclin-dependent kinases, CDK4 and CDK6. Ordinarily, these two kinases, CDK4 and CDK6, function as part of a complex with D-type cyclins (Cyclin D1) and drive the cell cycle by phosphorylating the retinoblastoma protein (pRb), releasing it from its inhibitory interaction with the E2F transcription factor, and thereby allowing the expression of E2F-related genes and progression from G1 to S. In a separate pathway, p14ARF participates in the core regulatory process that controls levels of protein 53 (p53). Usually in response to DNA damage, the human homolog of mouse double minute 2 (HDM2) protein binds to the transcriptional activation domain of p53, blocking p53-mediated gene regulation while simultaneously leading to p53 ubiquitination, nuclear export, and proteosomal degradation. p14ARF opposes this action by sequestering HDM2 in the nucleolus. Disruption of the HDM2–p53 interaction stabilizes p53 and enables it to either activate DNA repair and cell-cycle arrest or induce apoptosis

utilization of alternative promoters and first exons [68, 69] (Fig. 10.2, inset). Although structurally dissimilar, both proteins act as tumor suppressors by negatively regulating cell cycle progression [70–74] (Fig. 10.2, pathway). The first *CDKN2A* protein product, p16[INK4A], is encoded by exons 1α, 2, and 3, and negatively regulates cell cycle progression by inhibiting the catalytic activity of the cyclin D1-cyclin-dependent kinase complex, CDK4/CDK6. Inhibition of CDK4/CDK6 prevents phosphorylation of the retinoblastoma protein (pRB), which enables pRB to sequester the E2F transcription factor and prevent it from initiating the G1-to-S transition into the cell cycle [75]. The second protein product, p14[ARF] (ARF, for alternative reading frame), is encoded by exons 1β, 2, and 3. p14[ARF] exerts its inhibitory effect on the cell cycle by directly sequestering the human homolog of murine double minute 2 (Hdm2), an E3 ubiquitin ligase that catalyzes the ubiquitin-mediated proteasomal degradation of the tumor suppressor p53. One of the main functions of p53 is to sense DNA damage and either halt the cell cycle to initiate DNA repair or activate an apoptotic program to clear irreparably damaged cells. Therefore, genetic or epigenetic changes resulting in a functional loss of either p16[INK4A] or p14[ARF] ultimately lead to uninhibited cellular growth and proliferation.

It is estimated that germline mutations in the *CDKN2A* locus contribute to 20–50% of all hereditary melanoma cases [76, 77] and 1–3% of all sporadic malignant melanoma cases [78], although smaller population studies of *CDKN2A* mutations in patients with sporadic multiple primary melanomas have shown higher rates of up to 16% [79–85]. In addition, somatic mutations in *CDKN2A* have been reported in up to 30–70% of sporadic melanomas. The majority of *CDKN2A* mutations have been reported in exon 1α and exon 2 [86], with a preferential affect on the protein product, p16[INK4A]. Mutations in effecting p14[ARF] alone are much rarer [87–89], suggesting that it is p16[INK4A], and not p14[ARF], that plays the critical role in melanoma predisposition. Founder mutations have been reported across various ethnic groups, such as the Dutch [90], Swedish [91, 92], British [93–96], Celtic [79], and Slovenian [97] populations. The two most notable founder mutations include the methionine-53-isoleucine mutation ("Scottish") [98] and the glycine-101-tryptophan ("Ligurian") mutation [99]. Not only do the nature and type of *CDKN2A* mutations vary across ethnic groups, but their prevalence varies as well. For example, the prevalence of *CDKN2A* mutations among Israeli melanoma families is lower than Northern European kindreds [100, 101].

From data assembled by the Melanoma Genetics Consortium (GenoMEL) examining 80 families from Europe, Australia, and the United States, the penetrance of *CDKN2A* was estimated to be 0.30 by the age of 50 years and 0.67 by the age of 80 years. Interestingly, the group also found that the penetrance of *CDKN2A* mutations varied geographically [102]: by age 50, *CDKN2A* mutation penetrance reached 0.13 in Europe, 0.50 in the United States, and 0.32 in Australia; by age 80, it was 0.58 in Europe, 0.76 in the United States, and 0.91 in Australia. They therefore concluded that the same factors that affect population incidence of melanoma might also mediate *CDKN2A* penetrance. These studies strongly support an interaction between the presence of germline *CDKNA* mutations and environmental factors, such as sunlight and UV exposure. Earlier analysis of melanoma kindreds had also found variable penetrance from 53 to 100% [63, 103], further substantiating the critical role for additional genetic and/or environmental factors. However, if melanoma cases were ascertained through the general population rather than through families, the estimated *CDKN2A* penetrance is much lower [78]: 14% (95% CI=8–22%) by age 50 years, 24% (95% CI=15–34%) by age 70 years, and 28% (95% CI=18–40%) by age 80 years. Thus, it is quite likely that familial ascertainment coselects for other risk-enhancing modifiers and thus contributes to the higher calculated penetrance.

Mutations in the melanocortin-1-receptor gene (*MC1R*), which encodes a seven-transmembrane G protein-coupled receptor expressed on the surface of melanocytes, have been shown to increase the penetrance of *CDKN2A,* as well as reduce the age at onset of melanoma [104]. An allele-dose dependent increase in melanoma risk for carriers of variant *MC1R* alleles, with an elevated risk among familial melanoma patients with atypical nevi, was observed compared to sporadic patients [105]. In contrast to the highly penetrant *CDKN2A* gene, *MC1R* is a low penetrance susceptibility locus for melanoma [106, 107]. It encodes a receptor for α-melanocyte stimulating hormone (α-MSH) and its antagonist, the agouti signaling protein (ASIP) [108, 109]. The binding of α-MSH to Mc1r leads to an induction in intracellular cAMP and a biochemical switch in melanin from the red/yellow pheomelanin pigments to the brown/black eumelanins [110]. Thus, functional variants in *MC1R* are highly polymorphic and the presence of one or more variant alleles is strongly associated with red hair, fair skin (skin type I), and freckling [107, 111, 112]. The discovery that *MC1R*

variants were associated with an increased risk of melanoma was therefore not surprising, given its association with melanoma-prone fair skin type individuals, especially those with red hair, inability to tan, and tendency to freckle. However, it is interesting to note that even after adjusting for hair color and skin type, carriers of *MC1R* variants who had darker skin and were able to tan still had the same degree of risk for melanoma [107].

The remaining melanoma-prone families likely harbor germline mutations in other genes, including cyclin-dependent kinase 4 (*CDK4*) [113] and unidentified genes on chromosome 1p22 [114] and chromosome 20q11.22 [115]. Germline mutations of *CDK4*, the oncogenic pRb-kinase that is inhibited by p16[INK4A], have been identified in melanoma-prone families. Only a limited number of melanoma families worldwide have been found to be carriers of mutations in exon 2 of *CDK4* [88, 116]. These mutations, which are an extremely rare cause of familial melanoma, are highly penetrant (63%) [113] and target a conserved arginine residue (Arg24) in the p16[INK4A]-binding domain of Cdk4 and render the mutant Cdk4 protein resistant to inhibition [89]. Interestingly, the binding partner of Cdk4 in the retinoblastoma pathway, Cdk6, has not been found to contribute significantly to melanoma predisposition. Despite the sequence and functional homology between *CDK4* and *CDK6*, germline mutations in *CDK6* in melanoma-prone families have not yet been detected [117]. Since *CDK4* and *CDKN2A* alterations together account for only 20–50% of hereditary melanoma, the critical role of other genetic loci is likely. A genome-wide screen of microsatellite markers in 49 melanoma families yielded a significant linkage to a marker on chromosome 1p22 [114]. LOH studies have indicated that a tumor suppressor may be present at this locus [118], and most recently, it was proposed that microRNA-137 may function in that role by regulating the expression of micropthalmia-associated transcription factor (MITF), a master regulator of melanocyte development that plays a key role in melanoma [119]. In addition, another linkage analysis of Danish kindreds yielded a suggested linkage to markers on chromosome 9q21.32, although the responsible gene has also not been determined [120].

Associated Malignancies

Individuals with the FAMM syndrome are at increased risk of developing other malignancies, most commonly pancreatic carcinoma (PC) [2, 121–128]. Although the cumulative risk of pancreatic cancer in FAMM individuals is unclear, it has been proposed in one study that individuals harboring certain mutations in the *CDKN2A* gene have a cumulative risk of 17% by age 75, with a mean age at diagnosis of 58 years [129]. In 1968, Lynch and Krush were the first to report a co-occurrence of PC and malignant melanoma in a family [130], and subsequent studies confirmed the clinical association between PC and cutaneous melanoma in families with the FAMM syndrome. In 1995, Whelan et al. identified a *CDKN2A* germline mutation in a family with an excess of PC and malignant melanoma, and thus provided the first evidence linking the predisposition to PC in kindreds with the FAMM syndrome to an inherited mutation in the *CDKN2A* gene [131]. These observations were further substantiated by other documented cases of families with FAMM and PC with the *CDKN2A* Dutch p16Leiden mutation [90, 129], the Mediterranean p.G101W mutation [124, 132, 133], the Swedish pR112_L113insR founder mutations [123, 134], and the Australian and United Kingdom Met53Ile mutation [124, 134]. An example of a family with the Met53Ile mutation is illustrated in Fig. 10.3. In contrast, *CDKN2A* mutations were rarely found in non-FAMM kindreds with PC or familial PC (FPC) [135].

The frequent co-occurrence of PC, cutaneous melanoma, and atypical nevi phenotypes, in concert with *CDKN2A* mutations, became collectively referred to as a "new" hereditary carcinoma syndrome, FAMMM-PC (familial atypical multiple mole melanoma and PC) [136]. A large study of families from North America, Europe, Asia, and Australia from GenoMEL demonstrated a strong association between PC and *CDKN2A* mutations ($P < 0.0001$) that exhibited

differences between mutations and also between geographical regions [134]. While the association of pancreatic cancer with *CDKN2A* mutations is well known, the prevalence of pancreatic cancer has not been observed consistently in all *CDKN2A* mutation carrier families [2, 90, 123, 129, 135–141]. It has been proposed that other genetic or environmental factors may modify the risk of pancreatic cancer in *CDKN2A* families [116]. For example, a prospective study examining melanoma-prone families found that only mutations in *CDKN2A* that impaired the function of the p16INK4A protein (p16M alleles) increased the risk of pancreatic cancer by 22-fold over the general population risk. By contrast, no cases of pancreatic cancer were found in kindreds with *CDKN2A* mutations that did not alter the function of the p16INK4A protein (p16W alleles) [2].

A number of studies have also suggested that patients with FAMM are at higher risk for the development of other noncutaneous malignancies, such as neural system tumors (NSTs), ocular melanoma (OM), and breast cancer, though the associations are not as strong as the association observed for FAMMM-PC. Mutations in *CDKN2A* that affect p14ARF have been reported to be associated with an increased risk of central nervous system tumors, including gliomas [134, 142–146]. In smaller studies, such as one that examined families with clustering of melanomas, neurofibromas, and multiple atypical nevi with large genomic deletions spanning the *CDKN2A* locus, novel splice site mutations were found in these families that resulted in the absence of exon 2, which encodes a substantial portion of both p16INK4A and p14ARF proteins [144]. The largest study to date documenting the association between germline *CDKN2A* mutations and NSTs found that only mutations that affected the p14ARF transcript were significant, thus lending support for a credible relationship between germline mutations affecting p14ARF, NSTs, and familial melanoma [134].

The co-occurrence of OMs and the FAMM syndrome have also been examined extensively [147–158], although the direct association between OMs and atypical/dysplastic nevi is still debatable [159]. The most common primary intraocular malignancy in adults in the US, OMs have an average annual incidence of six cases per million and approximately 1,200 new cases diagnosed each year. The visual loss, local tissue destruction in the eye, and the propensity for metastasis of OMs result in significant patient morbidity and mortality [150]. Interestingly, however, unlike the association between the FAMM syndrome and PC, the link between the FAMM syndrome and OM is not through the presence of mutations in *CDKN2A* [160]. One potential candidate, the oculocutaneous albinism 2 gene (*OCA2*), was recently implicated as a potential low-risk melanoma gene [161, 162], and may account for the increased risk of OMs in FAMM kindreds. *OCA2* encodes a melanosomal transmembrane protein involved in the determination of eye color as well as in the most common form of human oculocutaneous

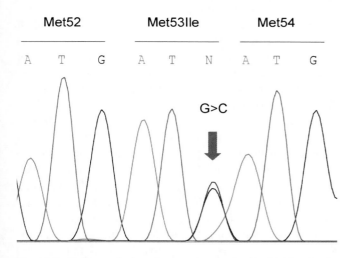

Fig. 10.3 Pedigree of a hereditary melanoma family. (a) Nine family members, including the proband (arrow), were affected by cutaneous malignant melanoma (colored upper right quadrant). The median age of diagnosis of melanoma was 41 years (range 28–78); seven of the affected family members were younger than 50 years of age at diagnosis. Four of the affected family members developed multiple primary melanomas; the father and brother of the proband developed three primary melanomas, with the first melanoma diagnosed before the age of 50. Two of the affected family members, now deceased, also developed pancreatic cancer (colored lower right quadrant). (b) Pedigree legend. (c) DNA chromatogram of the Met53Ile germline missense mutation in *CDKN2A*. In this family, a G-to-C transversion at nucleotide position 159 leading to an amino acid change from Met to Ile at codon 53 in exon 2 of *CDKN2A* was detected in both the index proband and his brother (+)

albinism, a human genetic disorder characterized by fair pigmentation and susceptibility to skin cancer.

Finally, breast cancer has also been reported to occur at increased frequency in several studies of families with *CDKN2A* mutations; for example, a study of *CDKN2A*-associated melanoma families in Sweden identified a 113insArg founder mutation that not only conferred an increased risk of multiple melanomas and pancreatic cancer, but also of breast cancer [123]. However, large-scale confirmatory investigations are still needed to demonstrate a significant association.

Genetic Counseling and Testing

Predictive genetic testing for FAMM remains controversial. The identification of *CDKN2A*, a dominantly inherited melanoma susceptibility gene that appears to be responsible for nearly half of hereditary melanomas worldwide, has lead to the development of a commercially available test for *CDKN2A* mutations. However, both the American Society of Clinical Oncology (ASCO) and the Melanoma Genetics Consortium do not recommend testing for *CDKN2A* mutations outside of defined research protocols [163, 164]. This recommendation remains under review, and family members should still be counseled regarding the advantages and disadvantages of genetic testing.

While early intervention, psychological reassurance, and increased compliance to preventative measures are clearly associated with the benefits of genetic testing, there are also limitations to genetic testing. First, even with a strong family history of melanoma, the prevalence of a germline mutation in the *CDKN2A* gene is only 20–50%; therefore, many melanoma families lack identifiable germline mutations in known high-risk genes. Second, knowledge of the risk of melanoma and other cancers in individuals who have germline mutations is still incomplete, making the implications of a positive test result imprecise. Third, individuals who do not carry a mutation in *CDKN2A* can still develop melanoma; thus, a negative test result could lead to false reassurance. Fourth, unlike other types of cancer where knowledge of genetic status can guide specific management options, including prophylactic surgeries, the genetic status of a hereditary melanoma family may have a limited impact on medical management. Finally, testing performed on healthy individuals may provoke various psychological and emotional issues, undue anxiety, as well a lower threshold for biopsies and surgical excisions.

At the MGH, a Center for Cancer Risk Assessment is present at the Cancer Center, which offers patient services, such as genetic counseling, genetic testing, and surveillance. Increased vigilance and surveillance has been shown to benefit patients, reducing not only anxiety, but also morbidity and mortality from the disease. A typical genetic counseling session should include [165]: (a) elicitation of a three- to four-generation pedigree, with specific attention to cancer diagnoses and ages of onset within the family; (b) provision of probability estimates for the FAMM syndrome; (c) description of the population incidence and causes of the FAMM syndrome; (d) education regarding basic genetics principles and the genetic causes of the FAMM syndrome; (e) discussion of risks and possible benefits of genetic testing, including the sensitivity and specificity of the test; (f) assessment of the relevance (if any) for medical management of the patient and family members; and (g) description of the genetic testing process and possible outcomes. Based on this comprehensive consultation, patients should be well informed about the issues related to provision of genetic testing for the FAMM syndrome.

Genetic testing for germline *CDKN2A* mutations should be offered only in conjunction with qualified genetic counseling and education and be performed when there is a reasonable likelihood of finding a positive result. Although there are geographic variations, the likelihood of the presence of a hereditary *CDKN2A* mutation increases with (1) the number of first-degree relatives on one side of the family with melanoma; (2) the number of cases of primary cutaneous melanoma in an individual; (3) early age of onset of initial primary cutaneous melanoma; (4) two or more affected relatives on one side of the family regardless of degree; and (5) an incidence of PC. Of these features, the family history of cutaneous melanoma has been suggested to be the most consistent predictor of *CDKN2A* mutations [166]. A pedigree of a family that fulfills these criteria is illustrated in Fig. 10.3. In this family, a total of nine family members, spanning across all four generations, were affected by cutaneous melanoma, with a median age of diagnosis of 41 years (range 28–78). The proband and his brother harbor germline Met53Ile mutations in the *CDKN2A* locus, a commonly reported missense mutation in exon 2 that compromises the ability of p16INK4 to bind to the Cdk4/Cdk6 complex. Both the father and brother of the proband developed three primary melanomas, with the first melanoma diagnosed before the age of 50, and two of the affected family members, now deceased, developed pancreatic cancer.

A recent algorithm, MELPREDICT, aims to estimate the *CDKN2A* carrier probability of probands given a limited set of clinical parameters [166]. Using a cohort of familial cutaneous melanoma patients evaluated over a 4-year period at the MGH PLC, germline *CDKN2A* mutation status were associated with various clinical features and used to build a multiple logistic regression model to predict the *CDKN2A* carrier probability. Although regression models are useful models given their simplicity in design, more sophisticated models that incorporate biological information (i.e. "genetic models") have been constructed to provide more refined estimates of carrier probability; BRCAPRO is the first of such models. Recently, a genetic model for melanoma, termed MelaPRO, has also been created and has been shown to better approximate carrier probability [167]. *CDKN2A* testing is not usually meaningful in patients who have single sporadic cutaneous melanoma without a family history of melanoma, even if the melanoma has occurred at an early age, due to the low frequency (2–3%) of mutations [168, 169]. For the same reason, testing is often not informative in patients who have multiple primary melanomas in the absence of a family history, as the likelihood for these individuals to harbor a *CDKN2A* mutation is estimated to be only 10–15% [78, 80, 82–84, 95]. *CDKN2A* mutations are more prevalent in the setting of familial melanomas. In families with three or more first-degree relatives affected with melanoma, the estimated probability of detecting a *CDKN2A* mutation is 20–50% [164, 170]. The likelihood of detecting a mutation is significantly reduced for individuals with only two affected family members, and is estimated to be less than 5% [170].

The interpretation of the test result and subsequent screening recommendations are dependent upon the individual's personal and family history of cancer. Genetic testing by sequencing of the *CDKN2A* gene may yield either a positive, negative, or inconclusive result. A positive test result indicates a mutation is found that alters gene function. As previously discussed, individuals who carry a *CDKN2A* gene mutation have a significantly increased lifetime risk for developing melanoma, and in some families, also have an increased risk for developing pancreatic cancer. This risk has been shown to vary with environmental exposures and ethnicity. Because of the increased risk for cancer, these individuals should be monitored carefully and educated about risk-reducing behaviors. A positive result has implications for other family members, both affected and unaffected, who are at increased risk to carry the familial mutation. Testing may provide these individuals with more information regarding their genetic status, cancer risks, and subsequent screening recommendations.

On the other hand, the interpretation of a negative result depends on the *CDKN2A* status of other family members, as well as the personal and family history of the proband. If a mutation in the family has been identified, a negative result indicates that the individual did not inherit the familial mutation. Although these individuals do not carry the familial *CDKN2A* mutation, studies indicate that these individuals are still at increased risk for melanoma due to shared environmental factors, and should be screened accordingly; however, the risk for melanoma is significantly lower than the cancer risk individuals who test positive for the familial mutation [102]. Alternatively, a negative result in which no familial mutation has been identified provides limited information on cancer risk. In this case, testing other affected family members may clarify the implications of this result. However, a negative test result for one family member does not exclude the possibility of a *CDKN2A* mutation in other affected family members, due to the possibility of a phenocopy. Other explanations for a

negative result include: (1) a mutation is present in the *CDNK2A* gene that is unidentifiable through current technology; or (2) a mutation is present in a different gene or genes associated with melanoma susceptibility; or 3) the melanoma is sporadic and not do to hereditary factors. Nonetheless, individuals and family members who have a personal and family history of melanoma with no identifiable mutation should continue to be classified as high-risk patients and should be screened accordingly. *CDKN2A* testing may also yield variants that have an unknown effect on gene function. In this case, no additional information regarding the significance of the specific sequence alteration or associated risks can be provided. Thus, until sufficient data is available, individuals or family members should continue to be screened as indicated by personal and family history.

Clinical genetic testing for melanoma susceptibility can have a significant psychological impact not only on the individuals tested, but also on their family members. Ideally, the clarification of melanoma risk through genetic testing should enable physicians to tailor screening measures based on an individual's risk of developing cancer and allow them to encourage high-risk individuals to engage in risk-reducing behaviors, skin self-examinations, and routine clinical screening [171]. These measures could lead to the prevention and/or earlier detection of melanoma. However, without established screening guidelines, the clinical utility of *CDKN2A* testing remains under investigation.

Genetic testing also has been shown to impact the psychosocial issues surrounding screening compliance. Although individuals with an identified genetic predisposition may be motivated to follow screening guidelines, individuals who obtain a negative test result may develop a false sense of security regarding melanoma risk. In one study of an Australian cohort, individuals who were noncarriers or who had an unknown genetic status maintained suboptimal levels of clinical skin exam compliance, while individuals found to carry a *CDKN2A* mutation reported a significantly greater frequency of clinical exams after learning about their mutation status [172]. The authors concluded that mutation-positive individuals use the additional information as justification for adherence to enhanced screening recommendations. In contrast, two other studies of *CDKN2A* carriers, one of which assessed self-skin examination compliance [173] and the other which investigated sun-related behaviors [174], concluded that screening compliance and risk-reducing behaviors were not influenced by mutation status. Genetic testing may also impact family dynamics, anxiety surrounding cancer risks, and concern for other issues associated with genetic testing, such as insurance discrimination.

The final aspect of genetic testing of FAMM individuals involves the consideration to also include pancreatic cancer screening. Given the known risk of pancreatic cancer among some *CDKN2A* mutation carriers as previously described [134], a referral to a gastroenterologist should be considered for individuals who are found to carry a *CDKN2A* mutation and have a family history of pancreatic cancer, to discuss the benefits and limitations of pancreatic cancer screening. Although no standard guidelines exist, generally it is recommended to consult with a gastroenterologist by age 25–30 or 10 years younger than the earliest pancreatic cancer diagnosis in the family; however, this recommendation may vary based on personal factors and family history [175]. The efficacy of pancreatic screening remains uncertain; however, for individuals who are at increased risk based on mutation status and family history, a discussion regarding the option of screening is indicated [128, 176]. Multiple techniques and research protocols are under investigation to screen individuals at increased risk for pancreatic cancer. These screening techniques include: spiral computed tomography, endoscopic ultrasound, serum cancer antigen CA 19-9, magnetic resonance cholangiopancreatography, and endoscopic retrograde cholangiopancreatography. Prophylactic pancreatectomy is also an option for individuals at increased risk for pancreatic cancer; however, this option requires careful consideration because of the serious medical implications [177].

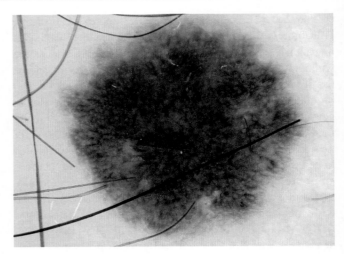

Fig. 10.4 Dermatoscopic view of a clinically atypical nevus on the left lateral calf of a 25-year old man. The pathological diagnosis was that of a lentiginous compound dysplastic nevus with moderate cytological atypia. The lack of surface reflectance permits visualization of the pigment network. Although there is overall symmetry, it is also clear that the nevus exhibits focal areas of irregularity. There is greater central pigmentation and some hints of bluish coloration, which is due to dermal pigmentation from the deeper components of the compound nevus

Management and Prevention

While management protocols vary across the country, current recommendations at the MGH PLC for patients with FAMM syndrome include (1) obtaining a detailed personal and family history for atypical nevi and cutaneous melanoma; (2) performing a thorough examination of the skin; (3) regular follow-up visits for professional mole surveillance; (4) the use of diagnostic aids for early melanoma detection such as dermoscopy; (5) biopsy of suspicious lesions; and (6) prophylactic sun-protection, strict avoidance of excessive sun exposure, and skin self-examination. Due to the hereditary nature of FAMM, first-degree relatives are also recommended for routine examination to facilitate early diagnosis and treatment [178–180]. To further inform patients and their families, pamphlets describing the clinical features of melanoma and atypical nevi are provided during the visit.

During a routine skin examination, patients undergo a full visualization of the cutaneous surface including careful inspection of all lesions. For patients with many atypical moles, the use of dermoscopy (epiluminescence) is recommended. With this visual adjunct, surface reflectance is minimized and pigment features are magnified for detail (Fig. 10.4). Although the actual theory behind dermoscopy is beyond the scope of this article, dermoscopy has been found to increase the accuracy of melanoma diagnosis by approximately 10–27% compared to examination with the naked eye [181–183]. Moreover, it has been found to substantially decrease unnecessary excisions in patients, while also increasing early detection of melanomas [184–186].

Any clinically concerning nevi are excised expeditiously. Any atypical nevi identified in locations that are inaccessible to self-examination or repeatedly irritated from trauma and shaving should also be excised with narrow margins of 2–3 mm, which is typically adequate to accommodate the lateral spread of 0.4–1.2 mm beyond the margins for atypical nevi. All specimens are submitted to a dermatopathologist who is trained in the subtleties of pigmented lesions.

Although some patients with atypical nevi may experience tremendous anxiety about the lesion as well as other lesions on their body, extensive prophylactic removal of all nevi is generally not recommended for the following reasons: most atypical nevi do not progress to melanomas, individuals will continue to develop moles throughout their lifetime, and melanomas often occur de novo on normal skin. Thus, systematic removal of nevi is not only an ineffective method for preventing melanoma, but can also falsely reassure the patient and lead to inadequate follow-up care.

Depending on the number of nevi and their degree of atypia, in addition to a personal or family history of melanoma, physicians typically examine patients routinely every 3–12 months. It is also helpful to offer urgent access tracks to patients who self-detect changes or suspicious moles. Patients with multiple melanomas require increased vigilance and may be seen at shorter intervals. Shorter intervals between visits are also recommended during periods where nevi may change rapidly, such as pregnancy.

Between clinical visits, patients are instructed on periodic 1–2 month skin self-examination (SSE), a careful, deliberate, and purposeful examination of the skin [187]. Though whole-body SSE in the general population is controversial according to the US Preventative Services Task Force [188], several melanoma population studies, including one study specifically focused on individuals from families with FAMM, have found that SSE both reduces the risk of melanoma incidence and increases survival of melanoma through earlier detection [173, 187]. A hand-held mirror used in conjunction with a wall mirror and bright lighting to illuminate the areas being examined usually provides adequate visualization, and family members should be encouraged to participate in patient monitoring. Questionable moles with changes in size, shape, color, pigmentation pattern, and/or elevation, necessitate immediate attention. Monitoring may also be accomplished in the home by documenting moles with photographs. At MGH, selective lesional photography has been valuable in assisting with management decisions.

Summary

The FAMM syndrome is a complex disease requiring careful management. We have attempted to provide a review of the clinical features of FAMM, including the genetic, molecular, and environmental factors that increase risk for the disease. In doing so, we hope we have helped to disentangle the highly confusing and controversial history of the disease as well as its nosology. We have also elaborated on the highly penetrant melanoma susceptibility locus, *CDKN2A*, and its implication in the FAMM syndrome. Since *CDKN2A* mutations only account for 20–50% of hereditary melanomas, intense research efforts are currently underway to elucidate the genetic etiology underlying the disease through the identification of novel melanoma-predisposing genes. Parallel efforts are also in progress to clarify the interplay of nongenetic factors, such as ethnicity, geographical location, and UV sunlight exposure. Finally, we have also provided basic clinical guidelines used by the MGH PLC to perform genetic testing and develop management protocols for patients and their families. While genetic testing of individuals for mutations in *CDKN2A* currently remains under review, exceptions are considered if combined with adequate information and counseling. However, there is a need for improved methods of surveillance of pancreatic cancer in families with germline *CDKN2A* mutations. Ultimately, FAMM individuals and their family members, given their increased risk of melanoma and other noncutaneous malignancies, should be educated regarding sun protection, skin self-examinations, and routine clinical monitoring to reduce their risk.

References

1. Jemal A, Siegel R, Ward E, Hao Y, Xu J, Thun MJ (2009) Cancer statistics, 2009. CA Cancer J Clin 59(4):225–249
2. Goldstein AM, Fraser MC, Struewing JP, Hussussian CJ, Ranade K, Zametkin DP, Fontaine LS, Organic SM, Dracopoli NC, Clark WH Jr et al (1995) Increased risk of pancreatic cancer in melanoma-prone kindreds with p16INK4 mutations. N Engl J Med 333:970–974
3. Goldstein AM, Tucker MA (1995) Genetic epidemiology of familial melanoma. Dermatol Clin 13:605–612
4. Goldstein AM, Tucker MA (2001) Genetic epidemiology of cutaneous melanoma: a global perspective. Arch Dermatol 137:1493–1496
5. Greene MH, Clark WH Jr, Tucker MA, Kraemer KH, Elder DE, Fraser MC (1985) High risk of malignant melanoma in melanoma-prone families with dysplastic nevi. Ann Intern Med 102:458–465
6. Lynch HT, Fusaro RM, Lynch J (1995) Hereditary cancer in adults. Cancer Detect Prev 19:219–233
7. Norris W (1820) Case of Fungoid Disease. Edinb Med Surg J 16:562–565
8. Norris W (1857) Eight cases of melanosis with pathological and therapeutical remarks on that disease, vol 1.   Longman, Brown, Green, Longmans, and Roberts, London
9. Cawley EP, Kruse WT, Pinkus HK (1952) Genetic aspects of malignant melanoma. AMA Arch Derm Syphilol 65:440–450
10. Frichot BC 3rd, Lynch HT, Guirgis HA, Harris RE, Lynch JF (1977) New cutaneous phenotype in familial malignant melanoma. Lancet 1:864–865
11. Clark WH Jr, Reimer RR, Greene M, Ainsworth AM, Mastrangelo MJ (1978) Origin of familial malignant melanomas from heritable melanocytic lesions. 'The B-K mole syndrome'. Arch Dermatol 114:732–738
12. Lynch HT, Frichot BC 3rd, Lynch JF (1978) Familial atypical multiple mole-melanoma syndrome. J Med Genet 15:352–356
13. Clark WH Jr (1988) The dysplastic nevus syndrome. Arch Dermatol 124:1207–1210
14. Kopf AW, Friedman RJ, Rigel DS (1990) Atypical mole syndrome. J Am Acad Dermatol 22:117–118
15. NIH Consensus Development Conference Panel on Early Melanoma (1992) Diagnosis and treatment of early melanoma. In: Consens Statement, January 27–29, 1992, 1–25
16. Ackerman AB (1988) What naevus is dysplastic, a syndrome and the commonest precursor of malignant melanoma? A riddle and an answer. Histopathology 13:241–256
17. Clark WH Jr, Elder DE, Guerry D, Epstein MN, Greene MH, Van Horn M (1984) A study of tumor progression: the precursor lesions of superficial spreading and nodular melanoma. Hum Pathol 15:1147–1165
18. Duray PH, Ernstoff MS (1987) Dysplastic nevus in histologic contiguity with acquired nonfamilial melanoma. Clinicopathologic experience in a 100-bed hospital. Arch Dermatol 123:80–84
19. Greene MH, Clark WH Jr, Tucker MA, Elder DE, Kraemer KH, Guerry D, Witmer WK, Thompson J, Matozzo I, Fraser MC (1985) Acquired precursors of cutaneous melanoma The familial dysplastic nevus syndrome. N Engl J Med 312:91–97
20. Greene MH, Fraser MC, Clark WH Jr, Elder DE, Guerry D, Kraemer KH (1984) For the record: the history of precursors to malignant melanoma. Arch Dermatol 120:18–21
21. Rhodes AR, Harrist TJ, Day CL, Mihm MC Jr, Fitzpatrick TB, Sober AJ (1983) Dysplastic melanocytic nevi in histologic association with 234 primary cutaneous melanomas. J Am Acad Dermatol 9:563–574
22. Rivers JK, Kopf AW, Vinokur AF, Rigel DS, Friedman RJ, Heilman ER, Levenstein M (1990) Clinical characteristics of malignant melanomas developing in persons with dysplastic nevi. Cancer 65:1232–1236

23. Skender-Kalnenas TM, English DR, Heenan PJ (1995) Benign melanocytic lesions: risk markers or precursors of cutaneous melanoma? J Am Acad Dermatol 33:1000–1007

24. Greene MH (1999) The genetics of hereditary melanoma and nevi. 1998 update. Cancer 86:2464–2477

25. Halpern AC, Guerry D, Elder DE, Clark WH Jr, Synnestvedt M, Norman S, Ayerle R (1991) Dysplastic nevi as risk markers of sporadic (nonfamilial) melanoma. A case-control study. Arch Dermatol 127:995–999

26. Holly EA, Kelly JW, Shpall SN, Chiu SH (1987) Number of melanocytic nevi as a major risk factor for malignant melanoma. J Am Acad Dermatol 17:459–468

27. Rigel DS, Rivers JK, Kopf AW, Friedman RJ, Vinokur AF, Heilman ER, Levenstein M (1989) Dysplastic nevi. Markers for increased risk for melanoma. Cancer 63:386–389

28. Roush GC, Nordlund JJ, Forget B, Gruber SB, Kirkwood JM (1988) Independence of dysplastic nevi from total nevi in determining risk for nonfamilial melanoma. Prev Med 17:273–279

29. Slade J, Marghoob AA, Salopek TG, Rigel DS, Kopf AW, Bart RS (1995) Atypical mole syndrome: risk factor for cutaneous melanoma and implications for management. J Am Acad Dermatol 32:479–494

30. Swerdlow AJ, English J, MacKie RM, O'Doherty CJ, Hunter JA, Clark J (1984) Benign naevi associated with high risk of melanoma. Lancet 2:168

31. Swerdlow AJ, English J, MacKie RM, O'Doherty CJ, Hunter JA, Clark J, Hole DJ (1986) Benign melanocytic naevi as a risk factor for malignant melanoma. Br Med J (Clin Res Ed) 292:1555–1559

32. Titus-Ernstoff L, Duray PH, Ernstoff MS, Barnhill RL, Horn PL, Kirkwood JM (1988) Dysplastic nevi in association with multiple primary melanoma. Cancer Res 48:1016–1018

33. Tsao H, Sober AJ, Niendorf KB, Zembowicz A (2004) Case records of the Massachusetts General Hospital. Weekly clinicopathological exercises. Case 7-2004. A 48-year-old woman with multiple pigmented lesions and a personal and family history of melanoma. N Engl J Med 350:924–932

34. Annessi G, Cattaruzza MS, Abeni D, Baliva G, Laurenza M, Macchini V, Melchi F, Ruatti P, Puddu P, Faraggiana T (2001) Correlation between clinical atypia and histologic dysplasia in acquired melanocytic nevi. J Am Acad Dermatol 45:77–85

35. Barnhill RL (1991) Current status of the dysplastic melanocytic nevus. J Cutan Pathol 18:147–159

36. Barnhill RL (2004) Pathology of melanocytic nevi and malignant melanoma. Springer, New York

37. Barnhill RL, Roush GC, Ernstoff MS, Kirkwood JM (1992) Interclinician agreement on the recognition of selected gross morphologic features of pigmented lesions. Studies of melanocytic nevi V. J Am Acad Dermatol 26:185–190

38. Grob JJ, Andrac L, Romano MH, Davin D, Collet-Villette AM, Munoz MH, Bonerandi JJ (1988) Dysplastic naevus in non-familial melanoma. A clinicopathological study of 101 cases. Br J Dermatol 118:745–752

39. Meyer LJ, Piepkorn M, Goldgar DE, Lewis CM, Cannon-Albright LA, Zone JJ, Skolnick MH (1996) Interobserver concordance in discriminating clinical atypia of melanocytic nevi, and correlations with histologic atypia. J Am Acad Dermatol 34:618–625

40. Tripp JM, Kopf AW, Marghoob AA, Bart RS (2002) Management of dysplastic nevi: a survey of fellows of the American Academy of Dermatology. J Am Acad Dermatol 46:674–682

41. Williams ML, Sagebiel RW (1994) Melanoma risk factors and atypical moles. West J Med 160:343–350

42. Florell SR, Boucher KM, Garibotti G, Astle J, Kerber R, Mineau G, Wiggins C, Noyes RD, Tsodikov A, Cannon-Albright LA et al (2005) Population-based analysis of prognostic factors and survival in familial melanoma. J Clin Oncol 23:7168–7177

43. Platz A, Ringborg U, Hansson J (2000) Hereditary cutaneous melanoma. Semin Cancer Biol 10:319–326

44. de Snoo FA, Kroon MW, Bergman W, ter Huurne JA, Houwing-Duistermaat JJ, van Mourik L, Snels DG, Breuning MH, Willemze R, Frants RR et al (2007) From sporadic atypical nevi to familial melanoma: risk analysis for melanoma in sporadic atypical nevus patients. J Am Acad Dermatol 56:748–752

45. Kraemer KH, Greene MH, Tarone R, Elder DE, Clark WH Jr, Guerry D (1983) Dysplastic naevi and cutaneous melanoma risk. Lancet 2:1076–1077

46. Kraemer KH, Tucker M, Tarone R, Elder DE, Clark WH Jr (1986) Risk of cutaneous melanoma in dysplastic nevus syndrome types A and B. N Engl J Med 315:1615–1616

47. Garbe C, Buttner P, Weiss J, Soyer HP, Stocker U, Kruger S, Roser M, Weckbecker J, Panizzon R, Bahmer F et al (1994) Risk factors for developing cutaneous melanoma and criteria for identifying persons at risk: multicenter case-control study of the Central Malignant Melanoma Registry of the German Dermatological Society. J Invest Dermatol 102:695–699

48. Garbe C, Kruger S, Stadler R, Guggenmoos-Holzmann I, Orfanos CE (1989) Markers and relative risk in a German population for developing malignant melanoma. Int J Dermatol 28:517–523

49. Grob JJ, Gouvernet J, Aymar D, Mostaque A, Romano MH, Collet AM, Noe MC, Diconstanzo MP, Bonerandi JJ (1990) Count of benign melanocytic nevi as a major indicator of risk for nonfamilial nodular and superficial spreading melanoma. Cancer 66:387–395

50. Slade J, Salopek TG, Marghoob AA, Kopf AW, Rigel DS (1995) Risk of developing cutaneous melanoma in atypical-mole syndrome: New York University experience and literature review. Recent Results Cancer Res 139:87–104

51. Tucker MA, Halpern A, Holly EA, Hartge P, Elder DE, Sagebiel RW, Guerry D, Clark WH Jr (1997) Clinically recognized dysplastic nevi. A central risk factor for cutaneous melanoma. JAMA 277:1439–1444

52. Armstrong BK, de Klerk NH, Holman CD (1986) Etiology of common acquired melanocytic nevi: constitutional variables, sun exposure, and diet. J Natl Cancer Inst 77:329–335

53. Piepkorn MW (1994) Genetic basis of susceptibility to melanoma. J Am Acad Dermatol 31:1022–1039

54. Goldgar DE, Cannon-Albright LA, Meyer LJ, Piepkorn MW, Zone JJ, Skolnick MH (1991) Inheritance of nevus number and size in melanoma and dysplastic nevus syndrome kindreds. J Natl Cancer Inst 83:1726–1733

55. Goldgar DE, Cannon-Albright LA, Meyer LJ, Piepkorn MW, Zone JJ, Skolnick MH (1992) Inheritance of nevus number and size in melanoma/DNS kindreds. Cytogenet Cell Genet 59:200–202

56. Meyer LJ, Goldgar DE, Cannon-Albright LA, Piepkorn MW, Zone JJ, Risman MB, Skolnick MH (1992) Number, size, and histopathology of nevi in Utah kindreds. Cytogenet Cell Genet 59:167–169

57. Cannon-Albright LA, Kamb A, Skolnick M (1996) A review of inherited predisposition to melanoma. Semin Oncol 23:667–672

58. Dracopoli NC, Houghton AN, Old LJ (1985) Loss of polymorphic restriction fragments in malignant melanoma: implications for tumor heterogeneity. Proc Natl Acad Sci U S A 82:1470–1474

59. Nancarrow DJ, Mann GJ, Holland EA, Walker GJ, Beaton SC, Walters MK, Luxford C, Palmer JM, Donald JA, Weber JL et al (1993) Confirmation of chromosome 9p linkage in familial melanoma. Am J Hum Genet 53:936–942

60. MacGeoch C, Bishop JA, Bataille V, Bishop DT, Frischauf AM, Meloni R, Cuzick J, Pinney E, Spurr NK (1994) Genetic heterogeneity in familial malignant melanoma. Hum Mol Genet 3:2195–2200

61. Cannon-Albright LA, Goldgar DE, Meyer LJ, Lewis CM, Anderson DE, Fountain JW, Hegi ME, Wiseman RW, Petty EM,

Bale AE et al (1992) Assignment of a locus for familial melanoma, MLM, to chromosome 9p13-p22.   Science 258:1148–1152

62. Gruis NA, Sandkuijl LA, Weber JL, van der Zee A, Borgstein AM, Bergman W, Frants RR (1993) Linkage analysis in Dutch familial atypical multiple mole-melanoma (FAMMM) syndrome families. Effect of naevus count. Melanoma Res 3:271–277

63. Cannon-Albright LA, Meyer LJ, Goldgar DE, Lewis CM, McWhorter WP, Jost M, Harrison D, Anderson DE, Zone JJ, Skolnick MH (1994) Penetrance and expressivity of the chromosome 9p melanoma susceptibility locus (MLM). Cancer Res 54:6041–6044

64. Kamb A, Gruis NA, Weaver-Feldhaus J, Liu Q, Harshman K, Tavtigian SV, Stockert E, Day RS 3rd, Johnson BE, Skolnick MH (1994) A cell cycle regulator potentially involved in genesis of many tumor types. Science 264:436–440

65. Kamb A, Shattuck-Eidens D, Eeles R, Liu Q, Gruis NA, Ding W, Hussey C, Tran T, Miki Y, Weaver-Feldhaus J et al (1994) Analysis of the p16 gene (CDKN2) as a candidate for the chromosome 9p melanoma susceptibility locus. Nat Genet 8:23–26

66. Meyer LJ, Zone JH (1994) Genetics of cutaneous melanoma. J Invest Dermatol 103:112S–116S

67. Hussussian CJ, Struewing JP, Goldstein AM, Higgins PA, Ally DS, Sheahan MD, Clark WH Jr, Tucker MA, Dracopoli NC (1994) Germline p16 mutations in familial melanoma. Nat Genet 8:15–21

68. Nobori T, Miura K, Wu DJ, Lois A, Takabayashi K, Carson DA (1994) Deletions of the cyclin-dependent kinase-4 inhibitor gene in multiple human cancers. Nature 368:753–756

69. Serrano M, Hannon GJ, Beach D (1993) A new regulatory motif in cell-cycle control causing specific inhibition of cyclin D/CDK4. Nature 366:704–707

70. Motokura T, Arnold A (1993) Cyclin D and oncogenesis. Curr Opin Genet Dev 3:5–10

71. Nigg EA (1993) Targets of cyclin-dependent protein kinases. Curr Opin Cell Biol 5:187–193

72. Sharpless NE, Kannan K, Xu J, Bosenberg MW, Chin L (2003) Both products of the mouse Ink4a/Arf locus suppress melanoma formation in vivo. Oncogene 22:5055–5059

73. Sherr CJ (1993) Mammalian G1 cyclins. Cell 73:1059–1065

74. Solomon MJ (1993) Activation of the various cyclin/cdc2 protein kinases. Curr Opin Cell Biol 5:180–186

75. Ewen ME, Sluss HK, Sherr CJ, Matsushime H, Kato J, Livingston DM (1993) Functional interactions of the retinoblastoma protein with mammalian D-type cyclins. Cell 73:487–497

76. Eliason MJ, Larson AA, Florell SR, Zone JJ, Cannon-Albright LA, Samlowski WE, Leachman SA (2006) Population-based prevalence of CDKN2A mutations in Utah melanoma families. J Invest Dermatol 126:660–666

77. Goldstein AM, Chan M, Harland M, Hayward NK, Demenais F, Bishop DT, Azizi E, Bergman W, Bianchi-Scarra G, Bruno W et al (2007) Features associated with germline CDKN2A mutations: a GenoMEL study of melanoma-prone families from three continents. J Med Genet 44:99–106

78. Begg CB, Orlow I, Hummer AJ, Armstrong BK, Kricker A, Marrett LD, Millikan RC, Gruber SB, Anton-Culver H, Zanetti R et al (2005) Lifetime risk of melanoma in CDKN2A mutation carriers in a population-based sample. J Natl Cancer Inst 97:1507–1515

79. Aitken J, Welch J, Duffy D, Milligan A, Green A, Martin N, Hayward N (1999) CDKN2A variants in a population-based sample of Queensland families with melanoma. J Natl Cancer Inst 91:446–452

80. Auroy S, Avril MF, Chompret A, Pham D, Goldstein AM, Bianchi-Scarra G, Frebourg T, Joly P, Spatz A, Rubino C et al (2001) Sporadic multiple primary melanoma cases: CDKN2A germline mutations with a founder effect. Genes Chromosomes Cancer 32:195–202

81. Blackwood MA, Holmes R, Synnestvedt M, Young M, George C, Yang H, Elder DE, Schuchter LM, Guerry D, Ganguly A (2002) Multiple primary melanoma revisited. Cancer 94:2248–2255

82. Hashemi J, Platz A, Ueno T, Stierner U, Ringborg U, Hansson J (2000) CDKN2A germ-line mutations in individuals with multiple cutaneous melanomas. Cancer Res 60:6864–6867

83. Helsing P, Nymoen DA, Ariansen S, Steine SJ, Maehle L, Aamdal S, Langmark F, Loeb M, Akslen LA, Molven A et al (2008) Population-based prevalence of CDKN2A and CDK4 mutations in patients with multiple primary melanomas. Genes Chromosomes Cancer 47:175–184

84. Monzon J, Liu L, Brill H, Goldstein AM, Tucker MA, From L, McLaughlin J, Hogg D, Lassam NJ (1998) CDKN2A mutations in multiple primary melanomas. N Engl J Med 338:879–887

85. Puig S, Malvehy J, Badenas C, Ruiz A, Jimenez D, Cuellar F, Azon A, Gonzalez U, Castel T, Campoy A et al (2005) Role of the CDKN2A locus in patients with multiple primary melanomas. J Clin Oncol 23:3043–3051

86. Orlow I, Begg CB, Cotignola J, Roy P, Hummer AJ, Clas BA, Mujumdar U, Canchola R, Armstrong BK, Kricker A et al (2007) CDKN2A germline mutations in individuals with cutaneous melanoma. J Invest Dermatol 127:1234–1243

87. Harland M, Taylor CF, Chambers PA, Kukalizch K, Randerson-Moor JA, Gruis NA, de Snoo FA, ter Huurne JA, Goldstein AM, Tucker MA et al (2005) A mutation hotspot at the p14ARF splice site. Oncogene 24:4604–4608

88. Soufir N, Avril MF, Chompret A, Demenais F, Bombled J, Spatz A, Stoppa-Lyonnet D, Benard J, Bressac-de Paillerets B (1998) Prevalence of p16 and CDK4 germline mutations in 48 melanoma-prone families in France. The French Familial Melanoma Study Group. Hum Mol Genet 7:209–216

89. Zuo L, Weger J, Yang Q, Goldstein AM, Tucker MA, Walker GJ, Hayward N, Dracopoli NC (1996) Germline mutations in the p16INK4a binding domain of CDK4 in familial melanoma. Nat Genet 12:97–99

90. Gruis NA, Sandkuijl LA, van der Velden PA, Bergman W, Frants RR (1995) CDKN2 explains part of the clinical phenotype in Dutch familial atypical multiple-mole melanoma (FAMMM) syndrome families. Melanoma Res 5:169–177

91. Borg A, Johannsson U, Johannsson O, Hakansson S, Westerdahl J, Masback A, Olsson H, Ingvar C (1996) Novel germline p16 mutation in familial malignant melanoma in southern Sweden. Cancer Res 56:2497–2500

92. Hashemi J, Bendahl PO, Sandberg T, Platz A, Linder S, Stierner U, Olsson H, Ingvar C, Hansson J, Borg A (2001) Haplotype analysis and age estimation of the 113insR CDKN2A founder mutation in Swedish melanoma families. Genes Chromosomes Cancer 31:107–116

93. Harland M, Meloni R, Gruis N, Pinney E, Brookes S, Spurr NK, Frischauf AM, Bataille V, Peters G, Cuzick J et al (1997) Germline mutations of the CDKN2 gene in UK melanoma families. Hum Mol Genet 6:2061–2067

94. Liu L, Dilworth D, Gao L, Monzon J, Summers A, Lassam N, Hogg D (1999) Mutation of the CDKN2A 5′ UTR creates an aberrant initiation codon and predisposes to melanoma. Nat Genet 21:128–132

95. MacKie RM, Andrew N, Lanyon WG, Connor JM (1998) CDKN2A germline mutations in U.K. patients with familial melanoma and multiple primary melanomas. J Invest Dermatol 111:269–272

96. Mistry SH, Taylor C, Randerson-Moor JA, Harland M, Turner F, Barrett JH, Whitaker L, Jenkins RB, Knowles MA, Bishop JA et al (2005) Prevalence of 9p21 deletions in UK melanoma families. Genes Chromosomes Cancer 44:292–300

97. Peric B, Cerkovnik P, Novakovic S, Zgajnar J, Besic N, Hocevar M (2008) Prevalence of variations in melanoma susceptibility genes among Slovenian melanoma families. BMC Med Genet 9:86

98. Pollock PM, Spurr N, Bishop T, Newton-Bishop J, Gruis N, van der Velden PA, Goldstein AM, Tucker MA, Foulkes WD, Barnhill R et al (1998) Haplotype analysis of two recurrent CDKN2A mutations in 10 melanoma families: evidence for common founders and independent mutations. Hum Mutat 11:424–431

99. Ciotti P, Struewing JP, Mantelli M, Chompret A, Avril MF, Santi PL, Tucker MA, Bianchi-Scarra G, Bressac-de Paillerets B, Goldstein AM (2000) A single genetic origin for the G101W CDKN2A mutation in 20 melanoma-prone families. Am J Hum Genet 67:311–319

100. Yakobson E, Shemesh P, Azizi E, Winkler E, Lassam N, Hogg D, Brookes S, Peters G, Lotem M, Zlotogorski A et al (2000) Two p16 (CDKN2A) germline mutations in 30 Israeli melanoma families. Eur J Hum Genet 8:590–596

101. Yakobson EA, Zlotogorski A, Shafir R, Cohen M, Icekson M, Landau M, Brenner S, Usher S, Peretz H (1998) Screening for tumour suppressor p16(CDKN2A) germline mutations in Israeli melanoma families. Clin Chem Lab Med 36:645–648

102. Bishop DT, Demenais F, Goldstein AM, Bergman W, Bishop JN, Bressac-de Paillerets B, Chompret A, Ghiorzo P, Gruis N, Hansson J et al (2002) Geographical variation in the penetrance of CDKN2A mutations for melanoma. J Natl Cancer Inst 94:894–903

103. Walker GJ, Hussussian CJ, Flores JF, Glendening JM, Haluska FG, Dracopoli NC, Hayward NK, Fountain JW (1995) Mutations of the CDKN2/p16INK4 gene in Australian melanoma kindreds. Hum Mol Genet 4:1845–1852

104. Box NF, Duffy DL, Chen W, Stark M, Martin NG, Sturm RA, Hayward NK (2001) MC1R genotype modifies risk of melanoma in families segregating CDKN2A mutations. Am J Hum Genet 69:765–773

105. Hoiom V, Tuominen R, Kaller M, Linden D, Ahmadian A, Mansson-Brahme E, Egyhazi S, Sjoberg K, Lundeberg J, Hansson J (2009) MC1R variation and melanoma risk in the Swedish population in relation to clinical and pathological parameters. Pigment Cell Melanoma Res 22:196–204

106. Kennedy C, ter Huurne J, Berkhout M, Gruis N, Bastiaens M, Bergman W, Willemze R, Bavinck JN (2001) Melanocortin 1 receptor (MC1R) gene variants are associated with an increased risk for cutaneous melanoma which is largely independent of skin type and hair color. J Invest Dermatol 117:294–300

107. Palmer JS, Duffy DL, Box NF, Aitken JF, O'Gorman LE, Green AC, Hayward NK, Martin NG, Sturm RA (2000) Melanocortin-1 receptor polymorphisms and risk of melanoma: is the association explained solely by pigmentation phenotype? Am J Hum Genet 66:176–186

108. Blanchard SG, Harris CO, Ittoop OR, Nichols JS, Parks DJ, Truesdale AT, Wilkison WO (1995) Agouti antagonism of melanocortin binding and action in the B16F10 murine melanoma cell line. Biochemistry 34:10406–10411

109. Voisey J, Kelly G, Van Daal A (2003) Agouti signal protein regulation in human melanoma cells. Pigment Cell Res 16:65–71

110. Rouzaud F, Kadekaro AL, Abdel-Malek ZA, Hearing VJ (2005) MC1R and the response of melanocytes to ultraviolet radiation. Mutat Res 571:133–152

111. Box NF, Wyeth JR, O'Gorman LE, Martin NG, Sturm RA (1997) Characterization of melanocyte stimulating hormone receptor variant alleles in twins with red hair. Hum Mol Genet 6:1891–1897

112. Valverde P, Healy E, Jackson I, Rees JL, Thody AJ (1995) Variants of the melanocyte-stimulating hormone receptor gene are associated with red hair and fair skin in humans. Nat Genet 11:328–330

113. Goldstein AM, Chidambaram A, Halpern A, Holly EA, Guerry ID, Sagebiel R, Elder DE, Tucker MA (2002) Rarity of CDK4 germline mutations in familial melanoma. Melanoma Res 12:51–55

114. Gillanders E, Juo SH, Holland EA, Jones M, Nancarrow D, Freas-Lutz D, Sood R, Park N, Faruque M, Markey C et al (2003) Localization of a novel melanoma susceptibility locus to 1p22. Am J Hum Genet 73:301–313

115. Brown KM, Macgregor S, Montgomery GW, Craig DW, Zhao ZZ, Iyadurai K, Henders AK, Homer N, Campbell MJ, Stark M et al (2008) Common sequence variants on 20q11.22 confer melanoma susceptibility. Nat Genet 40:838–840

116. Goldstein AM, Struewing JP, Chidambaram A, Fraser MC, Tucker MA (2000) Genotype-phenotype relationships in U.S. melanoma-prone families with CDKN2A and CDK4 mutations. J Natl Cancer Inst 92:1006–1010

117. Shennan MG, Badin AC, Walsh S, Summers A, From L, McKenzie M, Goldstein AM, Tucker MA, Hogg D, Lassam N (2000) Lack of germline CDK6 mutations in familial melanoma. Oncogene 19:1849–1852

118. Walker GJ, Indsto JO, Sood R, Faruque MU, Hu P, Pollock PM, Duray P, Holland EA, Brown K, Kefford RF et al (2004) Deletion mapping suggests that the 1p22 melanoma susceptibility gene is a tumor suppressor localized to a 9-Mb interval. Genes Chromosomes Cancer 41:56–64

119. Bemis LT, Chen R, Amato CM, Classen EH, Robinson SE, Coffey DG, Erickson PF, Shellman YG, Robinson WA (2008) MicroRNA-137 targets microphthalmia-associated transcription factor in melanoma cell lines. Cancer Res 68:1362–1368

120. Jonsson G, Bendahl PO, Sandberg T, Kurbasic A, Staaf J, Sunde L, Cruger DG, Ingvar C, Olsson H, Borg A (2005) Mapping of a novel ocular and cutaneous melanoma susceptibility locus to chromosome 9q21.32. J Natl Cancer Inst 97:1377–1382

121. Bergman W, Gruis N (1996) Familial melanoma and pancreatic cancer. N Engl J Med 334:471–472

122. Bergman W, Watson P, de Jong J, Lynch HT, Fusaro RM (1990) Systemic cancer and the FAMMM syndrome. Br J Cancer 61:932–936

123. Borg A, Sandberg T, Nilsson K, Johannsson O, Klinker M, Masback A, Westerdahl J, Olsson H, Ingvar C (2000) High frequency of multiple melanomas and breast and pancreas carcinomas in CDKN2A mutation-positive melanoma families. J Natl Cancer Inst 92:1260–1266

124. Goldstein AM (2004) Familial melanoma, pancreatic cancer and germline CDKN2A mutations. Hum Mutat 23:630

125. Hruban RH, Petersen GM, Goggins M, Tersmette AC, Offerhaus GJ, Falatko F, Yeo CJ, Kern SE (1999) Familial pancreatic cancer. Ann Oncol 10(Suppl 4):69–73

126. Landi S (2009) Genetic predisposition and environmental risk factors to pancreatic cancer: A review of the literature. Mutat Res 681:299–307

127. Lynch HT, Fusaro RM (1991) Pancreatic cancer and the familial atypical multiple mole melanoma (FAMMM) syndrome. Pancreas 6:127–131

128. Parker JF, Florell SR, Alexander A, DiSario JA, Shami PJ, Leachman SA (2003) Pancreatic carcinoma surveillance in patients with familial melanoma. Arch Dermatol 139:1019–1025

129. Vasen HF, Gruis NA, Frants RR, van Der Velden PA, Hille ET, Bergman W (2000) Risk of developing pancreatic cancer in families with familial atypical multiple mole melanoma associated with a specific 19 deletion of p16 (p16-Leiden). Int J Cancer 87:809–811

130. Lynch HT, Krush AJ (1968) Heredity and malignant melanoma: implications for early cancer detection. Can Med Assoc J 99:17–21

131. Whelan AJ, Bartsch D, Goodfellow PJ (1995) Brief report: a familial syndrome of pancreatic cancer and melanoma with a mutation in the CDKN2 tumor-suppressor gene. N Engl J Med 333:975–977

132. Mantelli M, Barile M, Ciotti P, Ghiorzo P, Lantieri F, Pastorino L, Catricala C, Torre GD, Folco U, Grammatico P et al (2002) High prevalence of the G101W germline mutation in the CDKN2A (P16(ink4a)) gene in 62 Italian malignant melanoma families. Am J Med Genet 107:214–221

133. Mantelli M, Pastorino L, Ghiorzo P, Barile M, Bruno W, Gargiulo S, Sormani MP, Gliori S, Vecchio S, Ciotti P et al (2004) Early onset may predict G101W CDKN2A founder mutation carrier status in Ligurian melanoma patients. Melanoma Res 14:443–448

134. Goldstein AM, Chan M, Harland M, Gillanders EM, Hayward NK, Avril MF, Azizi E, Bianchi-Scarra G, Bishop DT, Bressac-de Paillerets B et al (2006) High-risk melanoma susceptibility genes and pancreatic cancer, neural system tumors, and uveal melanoma across GenoMEL. Cancer Res 66:9818–9828

135. Bartsch DK, Sina-Frey M, Lang S, Wild A, Gerdes B, Barth P, Kress R, Grutzmann R, Colombo-Benkmann M, Ziegler A et al (2002) CDKN2A germline mutations in familial pancreatic cancer. Ann Surg 236:730–737

136. Lynch HT, Brand RE, Hogg D, Deters CA, Fusaro RM, Lynch JF, Liu L, Knezetic J, Lassam NJ, Goggins M et al (2002) Phenotypic variation in eight extended CDKN2A germline mutation familial atypical multiple mole melanoma-pancreatic carcinoma-prone families: the familial atypical multiple mole melanoma-pancreatic carcinoma syndrome. Cancer 94:84–96

137. Ciotti P, Strigini P, Bianchi-Scarra G (1996) Familial melanoma and pancreatic cancer. Ligurian Skin Tumor Study Group. N Engl J Med 334:469–470; author reply 471–462

138. Ghiorzo P, Ciotti P, Mantelli M, Heouaine A, Queirolo P, Rainero ML, Ferrari C, Santi PL, De Marchi R, Farris A et al (1999) Characterization of ligurian melanoma families and risk of occurrence of other neoplasia. Int J Cancer 83:441–448

139. Lal G, Liu G, Schmocker B, Kaurah P, Ozcelik H, Narod SA, Redston M, Gallinger S (2000) Inherited predisposition to pancreatic adenocarcinoma: role of family history and germ-line p16, BRCA1, and BRCA2 mutations. Cancer Res 60:409–416

140. Lal G, Liu L, Hogg D, Lassam NJ, Redston MS, Gallinger S (2000) Patients with both pancreatic adenocarcinoma and melanoma may harbor germline CDKN2A mutations. Genes Chromosomes Cancer 27:358–361

141. Moskaluk CA, Hruban H, Lietman A, Smyrk T, Fusaro L, Fusaro R, Lynch J, Yeo CJ, Jackson CE, Lynch HT et al (1998) Novel germline p16(INK4) allele (Asp145Cys) in a family with multiple pancreatic carcinomas. Mutations in brief no. 148. Online. Hum Mutat 12:70

142. Bahuau M, Vidaud D, Jenkins RB, Bieche I, Kimmel DW, Assouline B, Smith JS, Alderete B, Cayuela JM, Harpey JP et al (1998) Germ-line deletion involving the INK4 locus in familial proneness to melanoma and nervous system tumors. Cancer Res 58:2298–2303

143. Hewitt C, Lee Wu C, Evans G, Howell A, Elles RG, Jordan R, Sloan P, Read AP, Thakker N (2002) Germline mutation of ARF in a melanoma kindred. Hum Mol Genet 11:1273–1279

144. Petronzelli F, Sollima D, Coppola G, Martini-Neri ME, Neri G, Genuardi M (2001) CDKN2A germline splicing mutation affecting both p16(ink4) and p14(arf) RNA processing in a melanoma/neurofibroma kindred. Genes Chromosomes Cancer 31:398–401

145. Randerson-Moor JA, Harland M, Williams S, Cuthbert-Heavens D, Sheridan E, Aveyard J, Sibley K, Whitaker L, Knowles M, Bishop JN et al (2001) A germline deletion of p14(ARF) but not CDKN2A in a melanoma-neural system tumour syndrome family. Hum Mol Genet 10:55–62

146. Rizos H, Puig S, Badenas C, Malvehy J, Darmanian AP, Jimenez L, Mila M, Kefford RF (2001) A melanoma-associated germline mutation in exon 1beta inactivates p14ARF. Oncogene 20:5543–5547

147. Bataille V, Pinney E, Hungerford JL, Cuzick J, Bishop DT, Newton JA (1993) Five cases of coexistent primary ocular and cutaneous melanoma. Arch Dermatol 129:198–201

148. Bellet RE, Shields JA, Soll DB, Bernardino EA (1980) Primary choroidal and cutaneous melanomas occurring in a patient with the B-K mole syndrome phenotype. Am J Ophthalmol 89:567–570

149. Greene MH, Sanders RJ, Chu FC, Clark WH Jr, Elder DE, Cogan DG (1983) The familial occurrence of cutaneous melanoma, intraocular melanoma, and the dysplastic nevus syndrome. Am J Ophthalmol 96:238–245

150. Hurst EA, Harbour JW, Cornelius LA (2003) Ocular melanoma: a review and the relationship to cutaneous melanoma. Arch Dermatol 139:1067–1073

151. Richtig E, Langmann G, Mullner K, Smolle J (2004) Ocular melanoma: epidemiology, clinical presentation and relationship with dysplastic nevi. Ophthalmologica 218:111–114

152. Rodriguez-Sains RS (1986) Ocular findings in patients with dysplastic nevus syndrome. Ophthalmology 93:661–665

153. Singh AD, Shields CL, Shields JA, Eagle RC, De Potter P (1995) Uveal melanoma and familial atypical mole and melanoma (FAM-M) syndrome. Ophthalmic Genet 16:53–61

154. Singh AD, Shields JA, Eagle RC, Shields CL, Marmor M, De Potter P (1994) Iris melanoma in a ten-year-old boy with familial atypical mole-melanoma (FAM-M) syndrome. Ophthalmic Genet 15:145–149

155. Smith JH, Padnick-Silver L, Newlin A, Rhodes K, Rubinstein WS (2007) Genetic study of familial uveal melanoma: association of uveal and cutaneous melanoma with cutaneous and ocular nevi. Ophthalmology 114:774–779

156. Vajdic CM, Kricker A, Giblin M, McKenzie J, Aitken J, Giles GG, Armstrong BK (2001) Eye color and cutaneous nevi predict risk of ocular melanoma in Australia. Int J Cancer 92:906–912

157. van Hees CL, Jager MJ, Bleeker JC, Kemme H, Bergman W (1998) Occurrence of cutaneous and uveal melanoma in patients with uveal melanoma and their first degree relatives. Melanoma Res 8:175–180

158. Vink J, Crijns MB, Mooy CM, Bergman W, Oosterhuis JA, Went LN (1990) Ocular melanoma in families with dysplastic nevus syndrome. J Am Acad Dermatol 23:858–862

159. Taylor MR, Guerry D, Bondi EE, Shields JA, Augsburger JJ, Lusk EJ, Elder DE, Clark WH Jr, Van Horn M (1984) Lack of association between intraocular melanoma and cutaneous dysplastic nevi. Am J Ophthalmol 98:478–482

160. Wang X, Egan KM, Gragoudas ES, Kelsey KT (1996) Constitutional alterations in p16 in patients with uveal melanoma. Melanoma Res 6:405–410

161. Duffy DL, Box NF, Chen W, Palmer JS, Montgomery GW, James MR, Hayward NK, Martin NG, Sturm RA (2004) Interactive effects of MC1R and OCA2 on melanoma risk phenotypes. Hum Mol Genet 13:447–461

162. Jannot AS, Meziani R, Bertrand G, Gerard B, Descamps V, Archimbaud A, Picard C, Ollivaud L, Basset-Seguin N, Kerob D et al (2005) Allele variations in the OCA2 gene (pink-eyed-dilution locus) are associated with genetic susceptibility to melanoma. Eur J Hum Genet 13:913–920

163. Kefford R, Bishop JN, Tucker M, Bressac-de Paillerets B, Bianchi-Scarra G, Bergman W, Goldstein A, Puig S, Mackie R, Elder D et al (2002) Genetic testing for melanoma. Lancet Oncol 3:653–654

164. Kefford RF, Newton Bishop JA, Bergman W, Tucker MA (1999) Counseling and DNA testing for individuals perceived to be genetically predisposed to melanoma: A consensus statement of the Melanoma Genetics Consortium. J Clin Oncol 17:3245–3251

165. Niendorf KB, Tsao H (2006) Cutaneous melanoma: family screening and genetic testing. Dermatol Ther 19:1–8

166. Niendorf KB, Goggins W, Yang G, Tsai KY, Shennan M, Bell DW, Sober AJ, Hogg D, Tsao H (2006) MELPREDICT: a logistic regression model to estimate CDKN2A carrier probability. J Med Genet 43:501–506

167. Wang W, Niendorf KB, Patel D, Blackford A, Marroni F, Sober AJ, Parmigiani G, Tsao H (2010) Estimating CDKN2A carrier probability and personalizing cancer risk assessments in hereditary melanoma using MelaPRO. Cancer Res 70:552–559

168. Berg P, Wennberg AM, Tuominen R, Sander B, Rozell BL, Platz A, Hansson J (2004) Germline CDKN2A mutations are rare in child and adolescent cutaneous melanoma. Melanoma Res 14:251–255

169. Tsao H, Zhang X, Kwitkiwski K, Finkelstein DM, Sober AJ, Haluska FG (2000) Low prevalence of germline CDKN2A and CDK4 mutations in patients with early-onset melanoma. Arch Dermatol 136:1118–1122

170. Holland EA, Schmid H, Kefford RF, Mann GJ (1999) CDKN2A (P16(INK4a)) and CDK4 mutation analysis in 131 Australian melanoma probands: effect of family history and multiple primary melanomas. Genes Chromosomes Cancer 25:339–348

171. Tsao H, Niendorf K (2004) Genetic testing in hereditary melanoma. J Am Acad Dermatol 51:803–808

172. Kasparian NA, Meiser B, Butow PN, Simpson JM, Mann GJ (2009) Genetic testing for melanoma risk: a prospective cohort study of uptake and outcomes among Australian families. Genet Med 11:265–278

173. Mesters I, Jonkman L, Vasen H, de Vries H (2009) Skin self-examination of persons from families with familial atypical multiple mole melanoma (FAMMM). Patient Educ Couns 75:251–255

174. Bergenmar M, Hansson J, Brandberg Y (2009) Family members' perceptions of genetic testing for malignant melanoma – a prospective interview study. Eur J Oncol Nurs 13:74–80

175. Kimmey MB, Bronner MP, Byrd DR, Brentnall TA (2002) Screening and surveillance for hereditary pancreatic cancer. Gastrointest Endosc 56:S82–S86

176. Rulyak SJ, Kimmey MB, Veenstra DL, Brentnall TA (2003) Cost-effectiveness of pancreatic cancer screening in familial pancreatic cancer kindreds. Gastrointest Endosc 57:23–29

177. Brentnall TA (2000) Cancer surveillance of patients from familial pancreatic cancer kindreds. Med Clin North Am 84:707–718

178. Barnhill RL, Hurwitz S, Duray PH, Arons MS (1988) The dysplastic nevus: recognition and management. Plast Reconstr Surg 81:280–289

179. Crutcher WA (1988) The dysplastic nevus and its clinical management. Adv Dermatol 3:187–203

180. Sober AJ, Burstein JM (1995) Precursors to skin cancer. Cancer 75:645–650

181. Bafounta ML, Beauchet A, Aegerter P, Saiag P (2001) Is dermoscopy (epiluminescence microscopy) useful for the diagnosis of melanoma? Results of a meta-analysis using techniques adapted to the evaluation of diagnostic tests. Arch Dermatol 137:1343–1350

182. Carli P, de Giorgi V, Chiarugi A, Nardini P, Weinstock MA, Crocetti E, Stante M, Giannotti B (2004) Addition of dermoscopy to conventional naked-eye examination in melanoma screening: a randomized study. J Am Acad Dermatol 50:683–689

183. Carli P, De Giorgi V, Crocetti E, Mannone F, Massi D, Chiarugi A, Giannotti B (2004) Improvement of malignant/benign ratio in excised melanocytic lesions in the 'dermoscopy era': a retrospective study 1997-2001. Br J Dermatol 150:687–692

184. Haenssle HA, Vente C, Bertsch HP, Rupprecht R, Abuzahra F, Junghans V, Ellinghaus B, Emmert S, Hallermann C, Rosenberger A et al (2004) Results of a surveillance programme for patients at high risk of malignant melanoma using digital and conventional dermoscopy. Eur J Cancer Prev 13:133–138

185. Kittler H, Pehamberger H, Wolff K, Binder M (2000) Follow-up of melanocytic skin lesions with digital epiluminescence microscopy: patterns of modifications observed in early melanoma, atypical nevi, and common nevi. J Am Acad Dermatol 43:467–476

186. Menzies SW, Gutenev A, Avramidis M, Batrac A, McCarthy WH (2001) Short-term digital surface microscopic monitoring of atypical or changing melanocytic lesions. Arch Dermatol 137:1583–1589

187. Berwick M, Begg CB, Fine JA, Roush GC, Barnhill RL (1996) Screening for cutaneous melanoma by skin self-examination. J Natl Cancer Inst 88:17–23

188. U.S. Preventative Services Task Force (2009) Screening for skin cancer: U.S. Preventative Services Task Force recommendation statement. Ann Intern Med 150:188–193

Chapter 11
Multiple Endocrine Neoplasia

Yariv J. Houvras and Gilbert H. Daniels

Keywords Multiple endocrine neoplasia • Medullary thyroid cancer • Pheochromocytoma • Hyperparathyroidism • RET • MENIN • Gastrinoma • Insulinoma • Pituitary adenoma

Introduction

Several genetic syndromes are associated with multiple endocrine tumors. In this chapter, we focus on Multiple Endocrine Neoplasia (MEN) types 2 and 1. Von Hippel Lindau and Neurofibromatosis will be discussed in other sections.

MEN 1 and MEN 2 are often taught and learned together, yet these are quite distinct genetic and clinical entities (see Tables 11.1 and 11.3). MEN 2 arises from activating mutations in RET, a receptor tyrosine kinase. Advances in genetic testing have improved the diagnosis and management of patients with MEN 2 and have had a dramatic impact on the outcome of this syndrome. This is, in part, due to the molecular understanding of RET function, and the strong correlation between RET mutation and MEN 2 phenotype. In contrast, MEN 1 arises from mutations in MENIN, a nuclear protein whose precise molecular function remains unclear. Genetic testing for MEN 1 has proven useful in identifying carriers, but has not been shown to improve clinical outcome. There is a strong consensus about management decisions in MEN 2, whereas the appropriate testing and therapeutic strategies for MEN 1 remain less well defined. Finally, targeted therapy for medullary thyroid carcinoma is an emerging area in which an understanding of RET biology has led to the development of new drugs for patients with advanced medullary thyroid carcinoma. Medullary thyroid carcinoma represents one of the first hereditary cancer syndromes susceptible to targeted molecular therapy.

Y.J. Houvras (✉)
Massachusetts General Hospital Cancer Center,
Boston, MA, USA
e-mail: yhouvras@partners.org

MEN 2 Overview

Multiple endocrine neoplasia type 2 (MEN 2) is a hereditary cancer syndrome caused by germline mutations in the RET proto-oncogene. Although descriptions of thyroid cancer and pheochromocytoma first appeared in the 1930s, Sipple was the first to confirm this association [1]. Over the next 7 years, medullary thyroid cancer (MTC) was described and shown to be part of this syndrome, calcitonin was shown to be a marker for and a product of the C-cells (parafollicular cells) which give rise to MTC, MEN 2 was shown to be dominantly inherited, and the term Multiple Endocrine Neoplasia was coined.

MEN 2 is a rare syndrome with an incidence of approximately 1 in 30,000 individuals. Almost 1,000 kindreds have been described; many others have never been reported. Three clinical syndromes of MEN 2 have been described and are summarized in Table 11.1. The unifying feature of MEN 2 syndromes is the presence of MTC. The association with pheochromocytomas is an important feature of MEN 2-related disease, since pheochromocytomas can result in life-threatening hypertensive crises. An interesting historical note is that the first described case of classical pheochromocytoma was in a patient recently tracked to an MEN 2 family [2].

Overall, up to 50% of MEN 2 patients develop pheochromocytomas, and approximately 30% develop hyperparathyroidism. However, these percentages vary considerably with different RET mutations.

MEN 2 Molecular Genetics

MEN 2 arises from activating mutations in the RET gene, a feature which distinguishes medullary thyroid carcinoma from other hereditary cancer syndromes which generally arise from loss of function mutations in tumor suppressor genes. Mutations in RET exhibit a strong correlation between genotype and phenotype, which has been the basis for establishing clinical risk levels based on the RET mutation (Fig. 11.1) [22]. The human *RET* gene encompasses 21 exons on chr 10q11.2

and encodes three splice variants – Ret 51, Ret 43, and Ret 9 – which differ by their C terminal amino acids [3]. RET is a receptor tyrosine kinase (RTK) which functions as a coreceptor for the glial derived neurotrophic factor (GDNF) family of ligands (GDNF, artemin, neurturin, and persephin) bound to GDNF receptor-alpha family of receptors. Binding of the GDNF ligand-GDNF receptors to RET triggers dimerization and activation of the intracellular tyrosine kinase (TK). Ret dimers exhibit trans-autophosphorylation of intracellular tyrosine residues and activation of downstream signaling pathways. Ret activation has been shown to stimulate Ras/ERK, phosphotidylinositol-3-kinase/AKT, beta-catenin/WNT, phospholipase C gamma, and Src pathways.

Table 11.1 Clinical features of MEN 2 syndromes (adapted from ref. [20])

MEN 2A (Sipple's syndrome)
Medullary thyroid carcinoma or C-cell hyperplasia
Pheochromocytoma or adreno-medullary hyperplasia
Hyperparathyroidism, usually involving all four parathyroid glands
Cutaneous lichen amyloidosis

MEN 2B
Medullary thyroid carcinoma or C cell hyperplasia
Pheochromocytoma or adrenomedullary hyperplasia
Intestinal and mucosal ganglioneuromatosis
Thickened corneal nerves
Thickened lips
Characteristic marfanoid body habitus
Hyperextensibility of upper extremities
Tearless crying in infancy
Constipation in infancy
Note: absence of hyperparathyroidism

FMTC (Familial Medullary Thyroid Carcinoma)
Medullary thyroid carcinoma without other endocrine gland involvement

The RET protein consists of an N terminal signal peptide, an extracellular region with 4 cadherin-like repeats, a calcium-binding site and a cysteine-rich domain, a transmembrane region, and an intracellular portion with two tyrosine kinase domains (Fig. 11.1) [4].

RET mutations in the cysteine-rich extracellular domain (exons 8, 10, 11) generally lead to ligand-independent homodimerization and cross-phosphorylation, causing receptor activation. Mutations in the intracellular domain (exons 13, 14, 15, 16) are rarer, and may lead to alteration in the substrate recognition pocket of the catalytic core with constitutive activation of the Ret kinase enzyme catalytic site leading to autophosphorylation [5]. The four major tissues affected by RET mutations in humans are: C cells in the thyroid, parathyroid cells, chromaffin cells of the adrenal medulla and enteric autonomic neurons. Gain of function RET mutations lead to ligand-independent activation, which results in C-cell hyperplasia or MTC, and, depending on the mutation, pheochromocytoma, parathyroid hyperplasia, and mucosal ganglioneuromas.

In contrast to MEN 1, a limited number of RET mutations explain the majority of MEN 2 diseases [6]. RET mutations in MEN 2 are typically missense mutations that lead to ligand-independent receptor activation [3]. Such gain-of-function mutations are well described in other RTKs associated with human cancer, but are uncommon for a hereditary cancer gene. MEN 2 is almost always inherited in an autosomal dominant pattern, so an affected individual has a 50% chance of passing a disease-causing RET gene on through his/her germline to the next generation. This underscores the importance of genetic testing to identify carriers, and provide appropriate counseling for disease detection and prevention. RET mutations have been identified in 98% of MEN 2A and 2B families and 95% of familial medullary thyroid carcinoma (FMTC) families.

The RET mutations with the worst clinical outcome (918 and 833) have the highest in vitro transforming activity [7, 8].

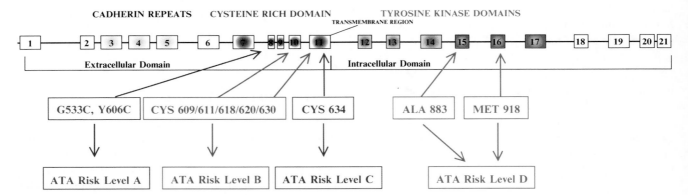

Fig. 11.1 RET gene structure and common MEN 2-associated mutations. A schematic diagram depicting the human RET gene exons and associated protein domains. Representative mutations of each of the ATA risk levels (A–D) are indicated. ATA risk level A mutations (see Table 11.2) are associated with the least aggressive clinical phenotypes. ATA risk level D mutations are associated with the most aggressive clinical behavior. ATA risk levels C and D mutations are associated with intermediate clinical phenotypes

Insertion of appropriate MEN 2A and 2B mutants in transgenic mice leads to overt C-cell hyperplasia at 3 weeks of age and subsequent multifocal MTC [9, 10].

There has been a report of a family in which two individuals homozygous for the A883T mutation (due to consanguinity) developed MTC, while other family members heterozygous for the A883T mutation did not, indicating the relative potency of specific RET mutations to transform C cells [11]. The more common mutation at codon 883, A883F (risk level D), is linked to MEN 2B and causes pheochromocytoma in addition to MTC.

Translocations involving RET are commonly seen in radiation-induced papillary thyroid carcinoma [12, 13]. RET amplification has also been described in radiation-induced papillary and anaplastic thyroid cancers [14].

Loss of function mutations in RET are strongly associated with Hirschsprung disease [15–17]. RET is required for the normal migration of enteric neurons during embryonic development, and targeted disruption of murine Ret leads to aganglionic megacolon in mouse [18]. Aberrant expression of RET in thyroid follicular cells, through translocation with PTC (RET/PTC) or NRTRK, leads to papillary thyroid carcinoma [6].

Increasing knowledge about RET mutations may lead to innovative and more successful therapy of MTC in the future.

Genotype–Phenotype Correlations in MEN 2

Different mutations in the RET oncogene lead to the distinct clinical syndromes of MEN 2A, MEN 2B, and FMTC. A strong correlation exists between particular RET gene mutations and clinical features and disease course of MEN 2-related medullary thyroid cancer [19]. Initially patients were stratified into least high (1), high (2), and highest risk (3) categories [20]. Based on this classification, the risk of Stage III or IV MTC disease increased 14-fold for incremental change from mutations in level 1 to level 3 [21]. Recent guidelines from the American Thyroid Association (ATA) propose a graded 4-tier category A–D, with level D mutations denoting the highest risk for early onset or aggressive medullary thyroid cancer, and level A mutations carrying the lowest risk [22]. Table 11.2 is based on the 2009 ATA classification scheme.

The MEN 2B-associated mutations at codons 883 and 918 are associated with the highest penetrance of MTC, the most aggressive disease course, and are categorized as level D. Prophylactic thyroidectomy is recommended as soon as the diagnosis is made and if possible within the first year of life for patients with risk level D mutations. Mutations at codon 634 are uniquely categorized as level C and are associated with

Table 11.2 RET mutations organized by ATA risk level (from ref. [22])

ATA risk level	Exon	Mutation
A	1	R321G
A	8	531/9 bp duplication
A	8	532 duplication
A	8	C515S
A	8	G533C
A	10	R600Q
A	10	K603E
A	10	Y606C
A	11	635/insertion ELCR; T636P
A	11	S649L
A	11	K666E
A	13	E768D
A	13	N777S
A	13	L790F
A	13	Y791F
A	14	V804L/M
A	14	G819K
A	14	R833C
A	14	R844Q
A	15	R866W
A	15	S891A
A	16	R912P
B	10	C609F/R/G/S/Y
B	10	C611R/G/F/S/W/Y
B	10	C618R/G/F/S/Y
B	10	C620R/G/F/S/W/Y
B	11	C630R/F/S/Y
B	11	D631Y
B	11	633/9 bp duplication
B	11	634/12 bp duplication
B	13/14	V804M + V778I
C	11	C634R
C	11	C634G/F/S/W/Y
D	14	V804M + E805K
D	14	V804M + Y806C
D	14/15	V804M + S904C
D	15	A883F
D	16	M918T

relatively early MTC and a strong association with pheochromocytoma and hyperparathyroidism. Prophylactic thyroidectomy is recommended for patients before age 5 for risk level C mutations. Some individuals with less penetrant mutations, (risk levels A and B) may delay prophylactic thyroidectomy after age 5 under special circumstances (see below). The most appropriate timing for thyroidectomy for these RET mutations continues to be debated.

Depending upon genotype at least 90% of RET mutation carriers will develop MTC. Some of the less aggressive mutations may take many decades to develop. For example, a recent patient with a V804M mutation presented with MTC at age 69. Three children who harbored the same mutation underwent surgery at ages 42, 45, and 47; one had C-cell hyperplasia and two had normal thyroid pathology [23]. Mutations in the 804 codon may be particularly vexing. Although these mutations are generally indolent, they become more serious when a second germline or somatic mutation occurs [24].

The families with FMTC are particularly enriched with mutations in exons 8, 10, 13, and 14 and are generally associated with lower ATA risk groups A and B. Some mutations (particularly codons 532, 533, 630, 769, V804M, 844, 912) are thought to be relatively specific for FMTC, but only time and observation in large numbers of families can confirm this specificity [4].

As specific RET mutations have been identified, heterogeneity of the genotype–phenotype correlation has been identified. The heterogeneity is greatest for mutations associated with ATA risk levels A and B. Marked heterogeneity may occur within families. The following family history may prove instructive. The proband in an MEN 2A family was diagnosed with MTC at age 18 (codon 618 mutation, ATA risk level B). His thyroid pathology revealed bilateral MTC and multiple positive lymph nodes, many with extra-nodal extension. Over the next several years, he developed diffuse hepatic and bony metastases and is currently enrolled in a clinical trial with a tyrosine kinase inhibitor. As a result of family screening, his mother was diagnosed at age 40 with MTC with 13 nodal metastases and a unilateral pheochromocytoma. Seven years after diagnosis, she is disease-free. The proband's maternal aunt was diagnosed with MTC at age 36 and is currently disease-free. The proband's maternal grandmother was diagnosed with MTC with lymph node involvement at age 64. Seven years after surgery, she has an isolated calcitonin elevation (16 pg/mL) but no radiographic evidence of measurable disease. A maternal great grandfather was diagnosed with a pheochromocytoma at postmortem examination (1954), but unfortunately there is no description of the thyroid. What additional germline or somatic mutations contributed to the more aggressive behavior in the proband in the family is unknown.

Clinical Features of Medullary Thyroid Carcinoma

Medullary thyroid carcinoma (MTC) arises from C cells (also called parafollicular cells) in the human thyroid, which are neural crest-derived cells specialized for secretion of calcitonin (CTN). C cell hyperplasia is a precursor for MTC in MEN 2 individuals.

Clinically MTC generally presents with a thyroid nodule. The diagnosis is generally not suspected unless suggested by a fine-needle aspiration biopsy. Common cytologic features of MTC are plasmacytoid or spindled cells with round nuclei and "salt and pepper" chromatin. In addition, a thyroid FNA which reveals unusual single cells or where the diagnosis of an anaplastic thyroid carcinoma is suggested in a younger patient should prompt consideration of MTC. If possible, the FNA specimen should be immunostained for calcitonin. However, the diagnosis of MTC should be confirmed by measuring serum calcitonin, which is almost invariably elevated in MTC. As a general rule, the serum calcitonin concentration is roughly proportional to the size of the MTC.

Although routine calcitonin screening in patients with thyroid nodules is common in Europe, it is not common practice in the US. The role of calcitonin screening continues to be debated [25]. Although elevated serum calcitonin is quite sensitive for the diagnosis of MTC, there are other benign conditions which are associated with a mildly elevated serum calcitonin (e.g., autoimmune thyroiditis, chronic renal failure, mastocytosis, achlorhydria) [25]. Elevated calcitonin in the appropriate clinical setting suggests MTC, but it is important to recognize that other tumors have occasionally been reported to secrete calcitonin [26]. In addition to calcitonin, patients with MTC may have elevated levels of other neuroendocrine markers including CEA, chromogranin A, serotonin, histamine, and tryptase [27]. With the advent of ultrasensitive calcitonin assays (sensitivity of 1–2 pg/mL) stimulated calcitonin testing using infusions of calcium or pentagastrin is no longer necessary.

Prior to surgery, all patients with MTC should be screened for pheochromocytoma either with plasma fractionated metanephrines or 24 h urine testing for fractionated metanephrines and/or catecholamines.

Surgery for medullary thyroid carcinoma generally includes a bilateral thyroidectomy with central lymph node dissection. When ultrasound or CT imaging suggests the presence of lateral lymph node involvement, appropriate neck compartment dissections should be performed. In MEN 2A patients without evidence of pathologically enlarged lymph nodes on neck ultrasound and a CTN < 40 pg/mL, a prophylactic lymph node dissection is not recommended [22].

Calcitonin is an extremely sensitive tumor marker for patients with MTC. CEA is also an important adjunctive tumor marker.

After thyroidectomy, an undetectable serum calcitonin (using modern ultra-sensitive assays) argues strongly against residual disease. Modest postoperative CTN elevations suggest residual nodal disease. Higher CTN concentrations and CEA concentrations suggest distant metastatic disease. Medullary thyroid carcinoma commonly metastasizes to liver, lungs, bones, and lymph nodes, but a variety of other sites are also seen. Patients with metastatic disease can survive for many years, but the prognosis is quite variable. Active surveillance and management are required. Calcitonin doubling time helps predict the outcome with the worst prognosis in patients with doubling times less than 6 months, intermediate course in those with 6–24 month doubling time, and excellent prognosis in those with >24 month doubling time [28].

When CTN exceeds 10,000 severe, often intractable diarrhea may result. Patients should undergo treatment with antimotility agents such as loperamide as first-line therapy. For patients whose diarrhea cannot be medically controlled, surgical resection, radiofrequency ablation, or alcohol ablation of specific lesions may prove helpful. Treatment with somatostatin analogs may be beneficial in some patients [29]. Some patients with advanced MTC develop Cushing's syndrome secondary to ectopic ACTH production.

The clinical behavior of medullary thyroid cancer may change dramatically in some patients. Patients with stable disease over the course of many years can occasionally experience a sudden increase in tumor growth, accompanied by increasing calcitonin and/or CEA, and symptoms related to the sites of disease. Unfortunately, dramatic changes in the growth of MTC generally herald a poor prognosis for the individual patient.

Conventional chemotherapy has a disappointing record in the treatment of patients with metastatic medullary thyroid carcinoma. Recently, several tyrosine kinase inhibitors with anti-RET activity have been developed for the treatment of patients with MTC [30, 31]. Zactima (AZ6474, Astra Zeneca) has completed a phase 2 and a randomized phase 3 trial in patients with MTC. At the time of this writing, the results from the phase 3 study were not yet available. XL184 (Exelixis) has completed a phase 1 study, in which an expansion cohort was enrolled for patients with MTC. A randomized, placebo-controlled, phase 3 study of XL184 is under way. Both agents have shown significant clinical activity in patients with medullary thyroid cancer across a range of RET mutations. In addition to these agents, sorafenib and sunitinib poses anti-RET activity and have demonstrated clinical efficacy in MTC [32, 33]. Sorafenib and sunitinib are FDA approved for other malignancies, but are available "off-label" for use in the appropriate clinical setting.

A young age at diagnosis of MTC or multifocal MTC should suggest hereditary disease. However, only genetic testing by RET gene sequencing from peripheral blood lymphocytes clearly distinguishes hereditary (MEN 2) from sporadic MTC. Although the majority of MTC is due to sporadic disease, all patients with newly diagnosed MTC should undergo RET genetic testing to exclude MEN 2 after appropriate counseling. Screening of individuals with apparently sporadic MTC may uncover germline RET mutations in approximately 7% of cases [34]. Complete *RET* gene sequencing should be considered for patients with confirmed MEN 2 clinical features but negative results on standard mutation testing (exons 10–14, 15, 16) or for patients presenting with apparently sporadic MTC at a young age. If no mutations are identified, haplotype or genetic linkage testing around the RET locus should be considered.

If an MEN 2 proband is identified, additional family screening almost invariably uncovers additional cases. Genetic testing should be performed in conjunction with formal genetic counseling and should include all available family members.

Genetic analysis of the medullary thyroid carcinoma in individuals with sporadic MTC reveals somatic (but not germline) RET mutations in about two thirds of individuals [35, 36]. The most common somatic mutations occur in codons 918 and 833 (exons 15 and 16). Less commonly somatic mutations in exons 10 and 11 are found. The prognosis is worse for those sporadic MTC with exon 15 and 16 mutations. Tumor genotyping of sporadic MTC is not currently part of usual clinical practice. However, if RET directed therapies prove successful, such tumor genotyping may become necessary in the future, and may help predict clinical course and response to treatment.

A single nucleotide polymorphism (SNP) of RET, G961S, has been shown to be more frequent in patients with sporadic MTC as compared with control subjects, associated with an earlier age of MTC, and with higher calcitonin levels [37–39].

Sporadic Medullary Thyroid Carcinoma

There are approximately 1,400 new cases of MTC each year in the USA. Approximately 80% of MTC is sporadic and 20% is hereditary. Sporadic MTC tends to present in the fifth to sixth decade, whereas hereditary MTC tends to present much earlier, depending on the penetrance of the specific RET mutation. Hyperplasia of C-cells is thought to be a constant precursor for hereditary medullary thyroid carcinoma. However, the relationship between C-cell hyperplasia (a relatively common "normal" finding with careful thyroid histological examination) and sporadic MTC is uncertain. Hereditary medullary thyroid carcinoma is generally bilateral and sporadic MTC is generally unilateral.

Familial Medullary Thyroid Carcinoma

The hallmark of FMTC is the presence of hereditary medullary thyroid cancer in a large kindred, without any other associated MEN 2 endocrine disorders. FMTC has been variously defined as a multigenerational kindred with isolated MTC, or four MTC affected family members without other manifestations of MEN 2A. Given the variable penetrance of pheochromocytoma, there are many families with MEN 2A who may initially appear to have FMTC, and subsequently develop another manifestation of MEN 2A. It is particularly important to focus on the older members of such kindreds, since the disease often has delayed penetrance.

FMTC is best thought of as a clinical subtype of MEN 2A with less penetrant pheochromocytoma and hyperparathyroidism rather than a distinct disorder. For this reason, we recommend screening for pheochromocytoma in families with isolated hereditary medullary thyroid cancer, since the consequence of missing a pheochromocytoma is so important.

In familial MTC without evident RET mutation, full RET gene sequencing may be necessary. For example, some laboratories do not routinely sequence exon 8 which may, rarely, harbor a causative mutation [40].

MEN 2A

Mutations in cysteine 634 are the most common mutations in MEN 2A and the most likely to be associated with pheochromocytomas and hyperparathyroidism. MTC is generally the first manifestation, with pheochromocytomas and hyperparathyroidism occurring at later dates. MTC is the leading cause of death in MEN 2A. In one study of 86 patients in 12 kindreds, the average age of diagnosis of MTC was 29, pheochromocytoma 37 and hyperparathyroidism 36. Overall 42% developed pheochromocytomas and 35% developed hyperparathyroidism in this study but dramatic inter-kindred differences were noted [41].

The timing of thyroidectomy in MEN is discussed in a subsequent section.

Pheochromocytoma in MEN 2A

In some studies, up to 25% of all pheochromocytomas are hereditary, particularly those occurring at younger ages and when bilateral or extra-adrenal. Genetic abnormalities associated with hereditary pheochromocytomas include RET (MEN 2), Von Hippel Lindau mutations, Neurofibromatosis 1 (NF1) mutations and mutations in succinate dehydrogenase (SDH) genes B, C, and D [42]. Approximately 1% of patients with MEN 1 will develop pheochromocytomas [43].

MEN 2 affected individuals are at risk for developing unilateral or bilateral pheochromocytoma, a malignant proliferation of adrenal chromaffin cells. Pheochromocytomas cause a spectrum of clinical features as a result of catecholamine secretion. The classic "P" signs and symptoms of pheochromocytoma include paroxysms, perspiration, pallor, pressure (hypertension), palpitations (tachycardia), and pounding headaches. The majority of pheos in MEN 2 are confined to the adrenal and benign [44]. Approximately 4% of pheos in MEN 2 are malignant. Currently, with aggressive surveillance, most patients with MEN 2 and pheochromocytoma

are asymptomatic at the time of diagnosis. However, sudden death associated with pheochromocytoma still occurs.

Screening for pheochromocytoma is best accomplished by either a 24-h urine collection and assay for fractionated catecholamines (epinephrine, norepinephrine, dopamine) and metanephrines (metanephrine and normetanephrine) or plasma fractionated metanephrines. These tests have excellent performance characteristics for the diagnosis of pheochromocytoma. In some MEN 2 patients with pheos, elevated urine epinephrine is the only abnormality noted. MEN 2 pheo patients are more likely to have normal biochemical screening tests than the general pheo population. MEN 2 patients with abnormal 24-h urine or plasma metanephrine testing should undergo adrenal protocol CT imaging. MEN 2 patients with signs or symptoms suggestive of pheochromocytoma should undergo biochemical testing and imaging. Due to the high risk associated with pheochromocytomas in pregnancy, women should be screened prior to conception or if not possible shortly after conception. Since these tumors are almost always confined to the adrenal, MIBG imaging is rarely necessary.

Most agree that even asymptomatic MEN 2 individuals should undergo annual biochemical screening for pheochromocytoma. The age to begin screening depends in part on the RET gene mutation. Individuals with MEN 2A associated mutations in codons 630 or 634, and MEN 2B individuals (codons 804, 883, 918) should undergo annual biochemical screening starting at age 8. Screening annually beginning at age 20 is appropriate for all other RET mutations. However, since pheos may occur as early as age 5, some experts recommend beginning screening at age 5 in all patients with MEN 2 particularly in those undergoing surgery [45]. Some recommend adrenal imaging studies every 3–5 years after age 15 even with negative testing. We agree with this approach in families with a high risk of pheochromocytoma.

In preparing patients for surgery to remove pheos, we generally use traditional preoperative preparation with alpha blockade (phenoxybenzamine) followed by beta blockers, when adequate alpha blockade has been achieved. Metyrosine, an inhibitor of catecholamine synthesis, is rarely used. Some centers do not use preoperative alpha blockade but use arterial and pulmonary artery catheters with intraoperative treatment with calcium channel blockers, magnesium or nitroprusside.

Pheochromocytomas are generally removed by endoscopic adrenalectomy. Many surgeons employ cortical sparing adrenalectomy on one side when bilateral adrenalectomy is necessary. This maintains adequate glucocorticoid function in about 65% of patients, however 10–25% require subsequent reoperation because of ipsilateral recurrence [4, 46]. Some groups use open adrenalectomy when cortical sparing procedures are done, but our adrenal surgeons are comfortable performing endoscopic cortical sparing surgery.

For MEN 2 patients diagnosed with unilateral pheochromocytoma, there is a risk of developing contralateral disease after surgery. We recommend continued surveillance, but we do not endorse prophylactic contralateral adrenalectomy in this setting.

When bilateral adrenalectomy is necessary in MEN 2 patients, adrenal insufficiency is a potentially important cause of morbidity. Patients require glucocorticoid and mineralocorticoid therapy and education about increased glucocorticoid dosing during illness. They should keep medical alert or other medical identifying information with them at all times.

Although MTC almost invariably precedes pheochromocytoma in MEN 2, there are families in which the initial presentation is pheochromocytoma with C-cell disease discovered at the time of thyroidectomy. In one family, patients had either C-cell hyperplasia or microscopic MTC after presentation with pheochromocytoma [47].

Hyperparathyroidism in MEN 2A

Overall, primary hyperparathyroidism (PHPT) occurs in 20–30% of patients with MEN 2A, generally manifested by the involvement of all four glands. The highest prevalence of PHPT occurs with the MEN 2A associated codon 634 mutation. Hyperparathyroidism is diagnosed by hypercalcemia with inappropriately normal or elevated parathyroid hormone concentrations. Hyperparathyroidism in MEN 2A is generally less severe than in MEN 1.

There is no consensus on the management of the parathyroid glands in MEN 2A and wide practice variations exist [46]. Some surgeons recommend removing the lower two parathyroid glands when performing thyroidectomy when the calcium is normal. Our surgeons recommend removing 3½ parathyroid glands as the treatment for hyperparathyroidism, leaving a silk suture to mark the remaining gland. Others, concerned with the risk of recurrent disease, advocate removing all four glands and autografting parathyroid tissue into the forearm; some surgeons do this only when total parathyroidectomy is required. Some centers perform autografting into the sternocleidomastoid muscle for patients with RET mutations conferring low risk of PHPT and MTC recurrence. Recurrent hyperparathyroidism is common.

Medical management of recurrent PHPT with cinacalcet may be considered in select cases where surgery is not feasible.

Other Manifestations of MEN 2A

Cutaneous lichen amyloidosis (CLA) is a rare skin lesion characterized by patches of pruritic, scaly, pigmented skin commonly in the interscapular region of the back or extensor surfaces of the extremities. Severe itching generally precedes the rash. There is a strong association between RET codon 634 mutations and CLA, with CLA occurring in up to 36% of patients [48, 49]. Biopsy of the affected lesions demonstrates amyloid, which contains calcitonin. The identification of CLA should prompt evaluation for other manifestations of MEN 2A and RET genetic testing. Topical capsaicin (0.025%) may ameliorate the itching to some extent [50].

Hirschsprung Disease (HD) is a developmental disorder in which enteric neurons fail to migrate correctly and innervate the distal colon. The result is aganglionic megacolon in which the distal bowel fails to relax appropriately and intestinal obstruction ensues. Loss of function of the RET gene is found in 50% of familial and 20% of sporadic Hirschprung disease [51]. This is supported by RET knockout studies in mice which display a similar phenotype [18]. Several exon 10 mutations in RET are associated with both MEN 2 features and Hirschsprung disease (codons 609, 611, 618, 620), so called Janus mutations [52, 53]. Individuals with Hirschsprung Disease should undergo RET genetic testing to exclude a mutation. It is also important to realize that individuals with the HD associated RET gene mutations may have mild symptoms of obstruction.

MEN 2B

MEN 2B is characterized by highly penetrant, early onset and aggressive MTC, in association with pheochromocytoma (50%) but not hyperparathyroidism. MEN 2B is often very aggressive with high stage MTC appearing at very young ages. About 90% of MEN 2B cases arise de novo making family screening very difficult. The M918T mutation in exon 16 accounts for >95% of patients with MEN 2B, the remainder are mutations at codons 883, and compound mutants involving codon 804. MEN 2B makes up approximately 5 % of MEN 2 cases with an annual incidence of approximately 1 per million.

The clinical phenotype of MEN 2B includes: ganglioneuromas on the tongue, lips (giving the appearance of swollen lips) and conjunctivae, intestinal ganglioneuromatosis, a marfanoid body habitus, hyperflexibility of the upper extremities, medullated corneal nerve fibers, and reduced tear production. MEN 2B patients may present with such gastrointestinal manifestations as nausea, vomiting, chronic constipation, and intestinal obstruction.

Metastatic disease has been demonstrated within the first 6 months of life in patients with hereditary MEN 2B [54]. Genetic testing should be done at birth if possible. If MEN 2B associated RET mutations are confirmed, total thyroidectomy should be performed as soon as the diagnosis is made (and certainly before 1 year of age). Unfortunately the diagnosis is often delayed. Given the rarity of a family history of MEN

2B and the fact that the typical habitus and manifestations above often appear between age 4 and 8, the majority of patients are diagnosed later in childhood and present with evidence of nodal or more distant metastases. MTC is a common cause of death in MEN 2B. It is therefore very important for pediatricians to be educated about two early signs of MEN 2B, namely constipation and tearless crying [55].

Impact of Screening on Clinical Outcomes in MEN 2

MEN 2 serves as a historical model for approaching the early diagnosis of hereditary tumors. Once calcitonin was demonstrated to be the product of C-cells (parafollicular cells), basal and stimulated calcitonin measurements served as a screening test in MEN 2 families and as a trigger for thyroidectomy. Initial calcitonin assays were too insensitive to diagnose C-cell hyperplasia or early MTC, so calcitonin stimulation by pentagastrin (no longer available in the US) was incorporated into the evaluation. Based on the families available for study at that time, abnormal pentagastrin stimulated calcitonin tests were found in 90–100% of presumed carriers by age 30.

Biochemical screening of family members in MEN 2A kindreds has been shown to alter the course of disease. In one large kindred followed for 14 years after prophylactic thyroidectomy, 19/22 patients who underwent thyroidectomy remained disease free [56]. This is in contrast to the historical cure rate of 50%. Unfortunately, false-positive and false-negative CTN screening tests occurred in 5–10% of patients.

Since 1997, initial screening with CTN measurements has been supplanted by RET genetic testing which facilitates carrier detection and effective clinical intervention [20]. With the more penetrant mutations, virtually 100% of patients will have C-cell hyperplasia or MTC by age 30–35. Several studies have demonstrated improved outcome and early disease detection with this approach. When genetic testing has been applied to patients who had previously undergone thyroidectomy based on CTN screening without C-cell disease, RET mutations were absent in all six patients [57]. In the same study, eight patients who screened positive for RET mutations with negative CTN screening tests had microscopic foci of MTC. These results illustrate the improved rates of false positives and false negatives by screening with a genetic test.

At the time genetic testing was introduced and applied to MEN families, some patients would have been necessarily older at the time of testing. The older the age of the patient undergoing thyroidectomy, the greater is the risk of finding Stage III or Stage IV disease.

Germline RET mutation testing should be offered for all patients with newly diagnosed medullary thyroid carcinoma, or an MEN 2-related malignancy. Individuals with intestinal ganglioneuromatosis, or lichen planus amyloidosis or pruritis in the central upper back, should also be considered for RET genetic testing and/or other evaluation for occult MEN 2-related malignancy [22]. Germline RET testing should also be considered for all family members in kindreds with confirmed MEN 2 or FMTC.

A European multicenter study (1993–2001) studied 207 patients from 145 families aged 20 years or younger [58]. All had total thyroidectomy after an RET mutation was identified. Patients with MTC larger than 1 cm or with distant metastases were not included. No nodal metastases were noted in patients under the age of 14. Twenty-nine families had FMTC, 112 had MEN 2A, and 4 had MEN 2 B. At the time of surgery, normal architecture was found in 5.3%, C cell hyperplasia in 31.9%, MTC without nodal involvement in 59.4% and MTC with nodal metastases in 3.4%. The most common mutation involved codon 634 (63%). Twelve of 16 codon 634 carriers younger than age 5 had node negative MTC. At age 20, the cumulative risk of nodal metastases with codon 634 mutations was 42%. Virtually, 100% of codon 634 carriers developed MTC by age 20. These data confirm the significant age related progression from C-cell hyperplasia to MTC and ultimately nodal metastases and emphasize the importance of early diagnosis and the timing of surgical intervention.

Genetic screening for RET carriers has the potential to eliminate MEN 2 associated MTC in families. Preimplantation genetic diagnosis can identify embryos without an RET mutation, and should be considered when clinically appropriate. Unfortunately, even intensive family genetic screening cannot eliminate all MEN 2, due to new mutations arising in the germline and the often delayed clinical manifestations. In European MEN 2 families, where geography facilitates genealogical studies, some RET mutations have been traced to the early twentieth or even late nineteenth century [59]. However, relatively new germline mutations (such as Y791F) have recently appeared, usually in men.

Timing and Extent of Surgery

The dilemma of surgery in young patients with MEN 2 involves the optimal time to prevent MTC or metastatic MTC ("window of opportunity" [60]) versus the optimal time to operate without complications. It is axiomatic that a skilled and experienced thyroid surgeon should perform these operations, and such surgeons are generally found at major referral centers specializing in thyroid disease. The ideal time to operate would be just before MTC appears or just before it metastasizes and that precise time cannot be determined. There is debate about whether central nodes (level VI) should be removed at the time of surgery. Removing these nodes increases the risk of hypoparathyroidism and recurrent laryngeal nerve injury. Unfortunately, reoperation to remove these nodes when the patient has not been cured, carries an even greater risk of injury. There is debate about whether surgery should be performed before the earliest reported age or the average age that metastatic disease appears in a given kindred or with a given mutation.

There is preliminary evidence that metastatic disease is rare when a primary tumor is less than 5 mm (by ultrasound examination), abnormal lymph nodes are absent on ultrasound examination, and the serum calcitonin is lower than 40 pg/mL. However, additional confirmation of these criteria is necessary.

There is a general agreement that surgery on MEN 2B should be carried out at the earliest age possible, despite the risks of surgery in very young infants. There is no consensus about whether the central nodes should be removed in those patients who do not meet the criteria for metastatic disease. Patients with ATA class C mutations should undergo surgery prior to age 5, usually between age 3 and 5. The same controversy about central node dissection exists in this group. Many groups would consider surgery before age 5 in patients with ATA Level B mutations. For patients with ATA Level A mutations, surgery may be delayed beyond age 5 if basal (and or stimulated) age adjusted calcitonin is normal, an annual neck ultrasound is normal, there is a less aggressive family history, and based on family preference.

If serum calcitonin is elevated, all would agree that a central neck dissection is needed and if nodes are noted on ultrasound, a lateral neck dissection is needed.

Some groups utilize the old carpenters adage of "measure twice, cut once" and repeat the RET genetic testing to be certain of the carrier status before operating on young patients [45].

MEN 1 Overview

Multiple endocrine neoplasia type 1 (MEN 1) is a hereditary cancer syndrome characterized by a spectrum of tumors involving the parathyroid, endocrine pancreas, and the pituitary (Table 11.3). MEN 1 was first described by Erdheim in 1903 as a constellation of multiple endocrine tumors. However, the autosomal dominant nature of the syndrome awaited the insights of Wermer in 1954 [61]. The prevalence of the syndrome is thought to be two to three cases per 100,000. The clinical manifestations of MEN 1 extend beyond the traditional three P's (parathyroid, pancreas, pituitary), and may include carcinoid and adrenal lesions. The age of onset of MEN 1 tumors of the parathyroid and pancreas is about 20 years earlier than sporadic tumors; the age of onset of pituitary tumors in MEN 1 is roughly comparable to sporadic tumors.

Recognition of germline loss of heterozygosity (LOH) at 11q13 [62] in MEN 1 kindreds led to the discovery of the tumor suppressor MENIN. Advances in medical and surgical therapy have dramatically decreased the morbidity related to

Table 11.3 Clinical features of MEN 1 (adapted from ref. [20])

Lesion	Malignant potential	Estimated incidence
Parathyroid adenomas	Uncommon	90%
Functional entero-pancreatic		
Gastrinoma	Yes	40%
Insulinoma	Yes	10%
Glucagonoma	Yes	1%
VIPoma	Yes	1%
Somatostatinoma	Yes	1%
Non-functional tumors (PP-omas)	Yes	20–34%
Carcinoid (thymic, bronchial)	Yes	2–4%
Anterior pituitary tumors		
Prolactinoma	Uncommon	20%
GH, PRL, NF	Uncommon	5%
ACTH	Uncommon	1–2%
TSH	Uncommon	<1%
Adrenal cortex (non-functional)	Uncommon	25%
Pheochromocytoma	Uncommon	1%
Non-endocrine lesions		
Angiofibromas	Uncommon	85%
Lipomas	Uncommon	30%
Collagenomas	Uncommon	30%
Ependymoma	Uncommon	1%

hormonal overproduction in MEN 1. However, death from MEN 1 malignancies remains a significant clinical problem.

MEN 1 Molecular Genetics

The MEN 1 gene encodes a 610 amino acid protein, menin. The MEN 1 gene is a tumor suppressor gene which exhibits LOH in most MEN 1 tumors [5]. Menin is a nuclear protein which has been shown to interact with a number of transcription factors and regulators of gene transcription including JunD, Smad3, mSin3a, HDAC1, and MLL1. It has no known recognizable protein domain, and its precise biochemical function remains unclear. Menin has been shown to interact with Cdx4 to regulate Hox genes in acute myeloid leukemia, and it has been implicated in a complex with the histone methyltransferase MLL1 [63, 64]. Menin has also been implicated in the epigenetic regulation of p27 and p18 by methylating histone H3, lysine 4 (H3K4) in the promoter regions of these tumor suppressor genes [65].

Murine MEN 1 exhibits striking sequence conservation (98% amino acid identity), gene structure, and protein subcellular localization compared to the human gene. Targeted disruption of mouse MEN 1 is embryonic lethal in its homozygous form, indicating a role for MEN 1 in early embryonic development [66]. Heterozygous MEN 1 mice exhibit multiple parathyroid tumors, pancreatic islet tumors, and hyperplastic growth of adenomas in the anterior pituitary [67,

68], but hypercalcemia is not found. A range of other mouse tumors including adrenal cortical carcinoma, thyroid tumors, and gonadal tumors have been observed in these models. Mouse models of MEN 1 reveal important conservation of the tumor suppressor functions of MEN 1 gene and recapitulate some of the key features of the MEN 1 syndrome.

In humans, over 1,000 mutations in MEN 1 have been described, including missense, nonsense, deletions, insertions, and splice mutations [69]. There are four mutations which account for approximately 10% of mutations in families. The majority of mutations are predicted to lead to a truncated protein. There is no apparent correlation between a particular mutant MEN 1 genotype and clinical disease manifestations (phenotype).

There may be differences between MEN 1 kindreds. For example, some families with pituitary tumors have primarily prolactinomas, whereas others have somatotroph adenomas. Some are enriched with thymic carcinoids. Thymic carcinoids are restricted to men; most MEN 1 bronchial carcinoids are found in women. Dramatic differences between individuals in the same family and even between identical twins have been described. One of our families is illustrative. The proband presented in her 40s with metastatic adrenal cortical carcinoma, which led to her demise. At autopsy, she was found to have a pituitary tumor, four abnormal parathyroid glands, and multiple pancreatic neuroendocrine tumors. Over the last three decades, four of her seven children have been found to have hyperparathyroidism (one also had a prolactinoma), and none have demonstrated pancreatic or adrenal tumors despite extensive testing.

Somatic mutations in MEN 1 have been detected in sporadic endocrine tumors including parathyroid hyperplasia, and parathyroid carcinoma [70, 71] but are not common.

Clinical Definition and Penetrance

MEN 1 is suspected in an individual who has biochemical or other evidence, of at least two characteristic tumor types [20]. Familial MEN 1 is suspected when an individual with these tumors has a first degree relative with at least one tumor in these tissues.

However, more stringent definitions have been applied by some investigators, requiring three or more tumors.

An extensive study of multiple kindreds from six referral centers in Germany found the following penetrance of tumors by birth cohort analysis: parathyroid (90%); enteropancreatic (60%); pituitary (40%); adrenal cortical (26%); carcinoids (17%) [72]. Tumors may appear as early as age 5 and into the late eighth decade of life, so these figures may represent an underestimation.

There are rare examples of clinical syndromes resembling MEN 1 due to other mutations. Individuals with MEN 1 syndrome who test negative for germline mutations in the MEN 1 gene may harbor mutations in a cyclin-dependent kinase inhibitor [73].

Primary Hyperparathyroidism in MEN 1

Primary hyperparathyroidism is the most common and often the first clinical manifestation of MEN 1. Almost all cases appear by age 50 in MEN 1 kindreds. Hyperparathyroidism is diagnosed by hypercalcemia with inappropriately normal or elevated parathyroid hormone concentrations. Hyperparathyroidism in MEN 1 involves all four parathyroid glands usually with independent clonal neoplasms. In sporadic hyperparathyroidism, at most 15% of cases are due to involvement of all four parathyroid glands. It is common to see marked heterogeneity in these MEN 1 tumors; the volume of the largest parathyroid tumor may be 10 or 20 times the volume of the smallest within the same patient [74]. Although the consequences of hyperparathyroidism and hypercalcemia can be life threatening, the parathyroid gland generally exhibits hyperplasia without malignant transformation. Parathyroid carcinoma is not generally associated with MEN 1, but it has been described in several case reports of individuals with clinical features consistent with MEN 1 [75].

Guidelines for therapy of sporadic hyperparathyroidism generally recommend surgery for all individuals under the age of 50. However, the surgical indications for hyperparathyroidism in MEN 1 are less clear, since permanent cure remains an elusive goal. Many academic centers remove 3½ parathyroid glands leaving a silk suture to mark the location of the remaining gland. A cervical thymectomy is often performed in case a fifth parathyroid gland is present [76]. However, recurrent hyperparathyroidism occurs in about half of patients within 8–10 years of surgery [77, 78]. Other centers perform total parathyroidectomy with autotransplantion of a small amount of parathyroid tissue into the forearm. This facilitates removal of additional parathyroid tissue when hyperparathyroidism recurs. In some centers, parathyroid tissue is cryopreserved, but the utility of this is uncertain. Rarely, total parathyroidectomy with conventional hypoparathyroidism therapy (calcitriol and calcium supplementation) is intentionally performed. Recombinant human parathyroid hormone (rPTH) is being tested for replacement therapy of hypoparathyroidism. It is uncertain if improved therapy of hypoparathyroidism with rPTH would permit different treatment strategies in MEN 1 hyperparathyroidism.

Cinacalcet is a calcimimetic which stimulates the parathyroid gland's calcium sensor to inhibit the release of parathyroid hormone. Cinacalcet is FDA approved for treatment of secondary hyperparathyroidism in patients with chronic kidney disease undergoing dialysis, and for patients with parathyroid carcinoma. In primary hyperparathyroidism, it has been shown to lower the calcium and parathyroid hormone concentration, but not to improve bone density [79].

Cinacalcet has been reported to restore normal PTH and serum calcium levels in an MEN 1 patient with recurrent hyperparathyroidism who refused surgery [80]. The role of this and future generations of calcimimetics in recurrent hyperparathyroidism in MEN 1 and in sporadic hyperparathyroidism requires additional study.

Familial isolated hyperparathyroidism has many etiologies including calcium sensor mutations (Familial Hypocalciuric Hypercalcemia) [81], cyclin-dependent kinase inhibitor mutations [73], and rarely MEN 1 mutations [82].

Entero-Pancreatic Neuroendocrine Tumors

Neuroendocrine tumors involving the pancreatic islet cells or the duodenal sub-mucosa are the second most common manifestation of MEN 1. Multiple tumors may be found in the pancreas with multiple different hormones being produced. Pancreatic endocrine microadenomas and mono-hormonal endocrine cell clusters (MECCs) display high rates of MEN 1 LOH, whereas islet cell hyperplasia does not [83]. These results suggest that islet hyperplasia may not be a requisite step in tumorigenesis.

Functional (and some nonfunctional) pancreatic tumors may be suspected by measuring basal and stimulated hormone and pancreatic polypeptide levels [84].

Other tumors are discovered with cross sectional imagining (CT scans and MRIs), somatostatin receptor scintigraphy (e.g., pentreotide scanning) [85], and endoscopic ultrasonography. The relative value and role of each test continues to be explored.

The extent and timing of surgical intervention for these tumors varies by institution and tumor type. Some authors recommend a conservative approach of surveillance for patients with smaller (<1–2 cm) tumors. Others consider all macroscopic tumors potentially malignant and recommend a more aggressive surgical approach including resection of isolated hepatic metastases [86, 87]. In some instances a Whipple procedure may be performed. Surgical morbidity may be significant and surgical deaths have occurred. Some institutions perform blind distal pancreatectomy in all MEN 1 patients with macroscopic tumors and use intraoperative ultrasound guidance for enucleation of tumors in the head of the pancreas.

Gastrinomas

Gastrinomas occur in nearly 40% of patients with MEN 1 and are among the most vexing MEN 1 tumors. Up to 25% of Zollinger–Ellison syndrome (ZES) patients are thought to have MEN 1. ZES due to excess gastrin may cause solitary or multiple peptic ulcers, recurrent ulcers, ulcers distal to the duodenum, and diarrhea. Proton pump inhibitors, often in high doses, effectively prevent gastric acid hypersecretion, essentially eradicating the previously devastating clinical consequences of ZES related to acid secretion. Individuals with ZES may experience a decrease in acid hypersecretion after surgery for hyperparathyroidism, since elevated calcium exacerbates acid secretion.

The diagnosis of a gastrinoma is confirmed by either an elevated fasting gastrin level or the secretin stimulation test. An elevated gastrin greater than 1,000 pg/mL, in the setting of a measured gastric pH below 5.0 is diagnostic. Elevated values that are lower than 1,000 pg/mL pose a diagnostic challenge that can be addressed with the secretin stimulation test. A rise in serum gastrin of 120 pg/mL or greater, after intravenous secretin has a sensitivity of 93% and a specificity of 100% in diagnosing gastrinomas in a prospective series of 293 ZES patients composed of both sporadic ZES (71%) and MEN 1 patients (29%) [88]. A calcium infusion study is a less effective alternative to the secretin stimulation test. Serum chromogranin A may be elevated in ZES but has poor specificity. Even in normal individuals, proton pump inhibitors, cause marked hypergastrinemia and elevation of chromogranin A. Other causes of elevated gastrin and chromogranin A include atrophic gastritis, and Helicobacter pylori infections [89].

Gastrinomas in MEN 1 patients are commonly multifocal, and localization is often the biggest challenge. They are often found in the duodenal submucosa, where they escape detection. A majority of gastrinomas will be found in the "gastrinoma triangle," a region bounded by the cystic and common bile duct, the junction of the second and third portions of the duodenum, and the junction of the neck and body of the pancreas. They may be malignant with metastatic disease present at the time of diagnosis. [90]. Whereas surgery for sporadic ZES results in a cure rate in about one third of patients, there are virtually no long term biochemical cures after surgery for ZES in MEN 1. Malignant gastrinomas may metastasize and are the most common cause of death from MEN 1. However, as in sporadic ZES, metastatic gastrinomas may have a relatively indolent course or progress more virulently [91]. Unfortunately, there is no prospective method of distinguishing between these entities. The role of surgery in preventing mortality with gastrinomas is actively debated. Some recommend early surgery on the pancreas with duodenal exploration/resection, whereas others rarely recommend surgery for MEN 1 ZES [92, 93]. The optimal surgical strategy for MEN 1 patients with ZES remains to be defined.

The therapy of metastatic gastrinomas is beyond the scope of this chapter, and is well reviewed elsewhere [94]. Liver metastases may be amenable to embolization or surgical resection in selected cases [95]. For patients with metastatic disease, streptozocin/5-FU based chemotherapy has been associated with variable response rates between 20 and 40% [96, 97] but with significant treatment related toxicity.

Newer agents, such as the multi-targeted tyrosine kinase inhibitor sunitinib, have shown efficacy in a phase II study of patients with neuroendocrine cancers [98].

Gastric pathology is almost universal in MEN 1 ZES. Advanced enterochromaffin cell proliferation (53%), gastric carcinoids (23%) and gastric nodules (44%) have been described. The malignant potential of the gastric carcinoids is unknown [99].

Insulinomas

Insulinomas are generally benign tumors which arise from pancreatic islet cells. Due to the clinical presentation of recurrent hypoglycemia, they are among the oldest recognized manifestations of MEN 1. Hypoglycemia generally appears in the second or third decade of life but has been diagnosed as early as age 5. Fasting hypoglycemia is most common, but postprandial symptoms may occur [100]. The diagnosis is confirmed by an inappropriately normal or elevated insulin concentration in the face of fasting hypoglycemia. The evaluation of hypoglycemic disorders may require specialized laboratory testing [23].

Insulinomas in MEN 1 may be multicentric as was found in 89% (16/18) of patients with MEN 1 associated insulinomas treated at the Mayo Clinic between 1970 and 1991 [101]. Surgery is the treatment of choice including local tumor excision plus distal subtotal pancreatectomy for most MEN 1 patients [91]. Recurrence is more common in patients with MEN 1 and has been reported to be as high as 21% at 10 years [102]. Repeat surgery is generally recommended for MEN 1 patients with recurrent disease. The therapy of metastatic insulinomas or untreatable hypoglycemia is far from satisfactory. Therapy for hypoglycemia includes diazoxide [103], verapamil and somatostatin analogs, such as octreotide [104]. Recently, four patients with refractory insulinomas were treated with everolimus, a rapamycin analog and inhibitor of mTOR. All patients had normalization of blood glucose and two had a partial response by RECIST criteria [105].

Rare Functional Tumors in MEN 1: VIPomas, Glucagonomas, Somatostatinomas, GRH-omas [106]

These tumors are very rare in MEN 1 patients and affect 1–2% of patients. About 80% of VIP-omas occur in the pancreas. They are usually solitary, greater than 3 cm at the time of diagnosis, most commonly found in the pancreatic tail and are malignant in 60% of cases. Metastatic disease occurs in 50% of patients at the time of diagnosis. Vasoactive intestinal peptide (VIP) is elevated and causes profuse watery diarrhea

(700–8,000 cc per day), hypokalemia, and hypochlorhydria. Glucagonomas oversecrete glucagon and may present with a clinical syndrome which includes the typical rash of necrolytic migratory erythema, cheilitis, diabetes mellitus, anemia, weight loss, venous thrombosis with pulmonary emboli, and neuropsychiatric symptoms. These tumors are often large (5–10 cm) and are commonly malignant. Somatostatinomas hypersecrete somatostatin and may present with abdominal pain, weight loss, diabetes, cholelithiasis, and diarrhea with steatorrhea. They occur in the pancreas or small bowel. Most are solitary and large (>5 cm) and present with metastases to lymph nodes and the liver; they are often incidental findings. GRH-omas secrete growth hormone releasing hormone which stimulates growth hormone release and may cause acromegaly. These tumors may be found in the pancreas, lung, or small intestine. The tumor is often multifocal, large, and metastatic. Surgery is the treatment of choice for these tumors [107]. Metastatic disease carries a poor prognosis [108].

Non-functional Tumors in MEN 1

Nonfunctional pancreatic neuroendocrine tumors (NFPNET) are common in MEN 1. The prevalence of these lesions was 34% in a cohort of 579 MEN 1 patients, making NFPNET among the most prevalent tumor types. These tumors typically stain positive for chromogranin A but not for a specific hormone. Many of these tumors secrete pancreatic polypeptide (up to 75% in some series), and some authors refer to those tumors as PP-omas. Elevated PP levels do occur in nontumor situations as well.

NFPNET patients may be symptomatic from the size or location of the tumor. These tumors are associated with a relatively high rate of metastasis at presentation (up to 60% in some series) [109]. Tumor size correlates with metastatic disease and shortened survival.

Pituitary Adenomas in MEN 1

The diagnosis and treatment of pituitary adenomas in MEN 1 is similar to that in sporadic pituitary tumors [110]. However, tumors in MEN 1 may be larger and more likely to recur after surgery, are more likely to express multiple hormones, and may be multifocal. Pituitary tumors may present in the first decade of life in MEN 1 affected individuals [111–113]. Prolactinomas are most common and are diagnosed by hyperprolactinemia, once pregnancy and drugs which elevate prolactin are excluded. In prolactinomas, the prolactin concentration is proportional to the size of the tumor. Prolactinomas are treated medically, generally with long-acting dopamine agonists such as cabergoline. A pituitary macroadenoma (greater than 1 cm) with modest prolactin elevation (e.g., 50–200 ng/mL) is not a prolactinoma and should be considered a nonfunctioning tumor. Somatotroph adenomas are the next most frequent tumor and are generally treated surgically. Corticotroph adenomas, gonadotropin secreting adenomas and nonfunctioning macroadenomas are treated surgically. Cushing's syndrome may result from pituitary corticotroph adenomas, ectopic ACTH production from gastrinomas or adrenal autonomy.

Carcinoid Tumors in MEN 1

MEN 1 patients may also develop carcinoid tumors in the thymus, lung, small intestine, and stomach. [114–116]. Carcinoids are composed of neuroendocrine cells which stain for immunohistochemical markers such as chromogranin A and neuron specific enolase, and exhibit neurosecretory granules by electron microscopy. Thymic carcinoids are almost always found in men, are found in conjunction with hyperparathyroidism and smoking, and are highly lethal [117]. Although rare, a high index of clinical suspicion is therefore justified. Unfortunately, cervical thymectomy (often performed during surgery for hyperparathyroidism) may not prevent this aggressive malignancy. Patients with apparently sporadic thymic carcinoids should be screened for MEN 1 [118]. Although no apparent genotype–phenotype correlation exists for MEN 1 thymic carcinoids, some MEN 1 families exhibit strong tropism for this malignancy. Bronchial carcinoids in MEN 1 are much more frequent in women.

Adrenal Abnormalities

Adrenal lesions, including adrenal enlargement, functional and nonfunctional cortical adenomas and adrenal cortical carcinomas are more common in MEN 1 individuals compared with normal subjects. The prevalence of adrenal abnormalities ranges from 30 to 70% depending upon the screening studies used. The prevalence of adrenal adenomas was 35% in a cohort of 20 patients with MEN 1 [119]. Another series evaluated the adrenal in 33 patients with MEN 1. Thirty-seven percent ($n = 12$) had bilateral adrenal enlargement. Histopathology revealed diffuse and nodular cortical hyperplasia, adenomas and one case of adrenocortical adenomas [120]. Another study found mean adrenal size in MEN 1 significantly larger than in normal. Nodules were demonstrated in 60% of patients (versus 0.4–2% in the normal population) [121].

MEN 1 mutations in adrenal adenomas are generally heterozygous and without LOH. Therefore, the mechanism by which germline mutations in MEN 1 contribute to an increased incidence in adrenal adenomas is uncertain. The majority of adrenal adenomas are nonfunctional and therefore observation is often reasonable [122].

Although generally associated with MEN 2, pheochromocytomas may occur in 1% of MEN 1 individuals. Hence, testing for pheochromocytomas in MEN 1 patients with adrenal abnormalities is important. Most patients with pancreatic neuroendocrine tumors and pheochromocytomas will prove to have VHL rather than MEN 1.

Skin Changes in MEN 1

Several cutaneous lesions have been associated with MEN 1 including multiple angiofibromas, collagenomas, café au lait macules, lipomas, confetti like hypopigmentation, and multiple gingival papules [123]. The angiofibromas are identical to those seen in tuberous sclerosis complex. In one series, 88% of MEN 1 patients not selected for skin lesions had angiofibromas; half had five or more [42]. More than three angiofibromas plus collagenomas (single or multiple) had 75% sensitivity for MEN 1 and 95% specificity. In individuals with ZES, angiofibromas and collagenomas were more frequent in MEN 1 patients than sporadic (64% vs. 8% and 62% vs. 5%; $P < 0.00001$) and were multiple in 77–81% of the MEN 1 patients [124]. These skin findings may suggest MEN 1 in a patient with primary hyperparathyroidism or ZES. MEN 1 loss of heterozygosity has been described in angiofibromas, suggesting a causal role for MEN 1 in the development of these lesions [125].

Miscellaneous Findings in MEN 1

Several CNS tumors including meningiomas, ependymomas, astrocytomas, and schwannomas have been reported as associated with MEN 1 [126–128]. In one study, meningiomas were found in six of 74 MEN 1 individuals (8%) [129]. One patient with a meningioma was found to have LOH at the MEN 1 locus on 11q13 indicating a possible role for MEN 1 in the pathogenesis of meningioma. Leiomyomas of the esophagus and uterus have been found in MEN 1. In one study, ten of 12 (83%) were found to have LOH at the MEN 1 locus. However, LOH was not found in three lung smooth muscle tumors from a single patient with MEN 1 [130].

Genetic Screening in MEN 1

MEN 1 is transmitted as an autosomal dominant trait, as is the case with other tumor suppressor genes. Once the mutation or syndrome has been detected in an individual family screening is indicated. The primary purpose of identifying family members as gene carriers is to ensure that appropriate biochemical and imaging surveillance is performed. Carrier detection can similarly avoid unnecessary testing in individuals who have not inherited an MEN 1 mutation. It is generally not appropriate to pursue prophylactic surgery based on MEN 1 mutation status alone. Although one study suggested that clinical outcome was better in individuals diagnosed by genetic testing, lead-time bias could not be excluded [131].

Direct DNA sequencing of the entire MEN 1 gene from peripheral blood lymphocytes can detect germline mutations in 70–80% of cases from MEN 1 kindreds [132] The remaining 20–30% of families with MEN 1 clinical features likely have regulatory or epigenetic alterations, or represent phenocopies of the disease. In some series which required more stringent criteria for diagnosis, MEN 1 mutations were found in up to 94% of familial cases. Sporadic cases with apparent MEN 1 syndrome are much less likely to demonstrate MEN 1 gene mutations [133, 134].

Individuals with a family history suggestive of MEN 1 in first degree relatives should be screened for this disorder. In addition to family history, various criteria have been proposed for initiating genetic testing. These include:

Multiple parathyroid tumors before age 30
Recurrent hyperparathyroidism after successful surgery
Gastrinomas or multiple islet cell tumors at any age
Familial isolated hyperparathyroidism when FHH has been
    excluded.
Age less than age 35 with one of the five principal tumors
More than one MEN 1 associated lesion in one organ
Two or more MEN 1-related tumors
All cases of thymic carcinoid

In one series, haplotype analysis of chromosome 11q13 or microrarray-based detection of small deletions was employed in families where DNA sequencing failed to identify a causative mutation. Genetic counseling and detailed family history is a critical component in the evaluation of a new kindred suspected of harboring an MEN 1 mutation. When a mutation is not found or when patients refuse genetic testing, biochemical and hormonal testing may be appropriate screening modalities.

Surveillance of MEN 1 Affected Individuals

Biochemical screening may identify manifestations of MEN 1-related tumors early in the disease course. Since disease morbidity is often caused by hormonal excess in MEN 1, biochemical screening of known carriers is important. Although, there is no evidence that an aggressive screening program results in decreased morbidity, establishing a program of biochemical screening for mutation carriers is recommended [20]. As a general rule, the penetrance of MEN 1 manifestations is near 0 before age 5, around 50% at age 20 and around 95% by age 40. Lifelong surveillance for MEN 1 disease manifestations is necessary.

Establishing a program of biochemical and radiographic screening is recommended for patients with a confirmed MEN 1 mutation. A minimal biochemical battery would include annual measurement of serum calcium, parathyroid hormone, gastrin, and prolactin to exclude hyperparathyroidism, ZES and prolactinoma. Others would recommend adding IGF-1 (to exclude growth hormone excess) and pancreatic polypeptide (as a marker for neuroendocrine pancreatic tumors). Consensus guidelines recommend yearly biochemical screening and imaging studies every 3–5 years (Table 11.4) [20]. Clinical symptoms suggestive of less common MEN 1 manifestations (hypoglycemia) should prompt further biochemical evaluation. We have generally performed imaging studies every 1–2 years in MEN 1 individuals. Periodic screening for gastrinomas by upper endoscopy may be reasonable.

Periodic CT or MRI-based cross-sectional images are necessary in MEN 1 mutation carriers [135]. MRI of the pituitary (with gadolinium) is most appropriate for diagnosing pituitary adenomas. The relative role of abdominal CT or MRI, somatostatin receptor imaging and endoscopic ultrasonography for the diagnosis of pancreatic neuroendocrine tumors requires continued study. Chest imaging is particularly important in kindreds where thymic carcinoids are common. It is appropriate to tailor the screening program to the MEN 1-related tumors which are present in a particular family.

Table 11.4 Recommended screening guidelines for MEN 1 patients (from ref. [131])	Modality	Starting age	Frequency	Tests
	Clinic visit	5	Twice yearly	History and physical exam
	Laboratory studies	5	Twice yearly	Ionized calcium, chloride, phosphate, PTH, fasting glucose, fasting insulin, fasting c-peptide, glucagon, fasting gastrin, pancreatic polypeptide, PRL, IGF-1, platelet serotonin, chromogranin A
	Imaging studies	15	Every 2 years	MRI upper abdomen MRI with gadolinium of pituitary MRI of mediastinum in males

Carney Complex and McCune Albright Syndrome

Although quite rare, Carney Complex and McCune Albright Syndrome are worthy of brief commentary since both are associated with multiple endocrinopathies. The Carney complex is an autosomal dominant disorder which includes benign tumors autonomously producing cortisol (with multiple small cortical pigmented nodules), thyroid hormone, growth hormone, prolactin, androgens and/or estrogens in conjunction with myxomas, lentigines, and schwannomas. The majority are caused by inactivating mutations in a tumor suppressor gene, protein kinase type 1 A regulatory subunit (PRKAR1A) [136, 137].

The McCune Albright syndrome is characterized by autonomous overproduction of androgen, estrogen, growth hormone, prolactin, cortisol, or thyroid hormone, café au lait spots, fibrous dysplasia and rarely sarcomas [138]. It is due to somatic mutations in the gene that codes for the alpha subunit of the stimulatory G protein (GNAS1). These gain of function mutations are mosaic in affected individuals and likely arise somatically in early development. It is not hereditary.

References

1. Sipple JH (1961) The association of pheochromocytoma with carcinomas of the thyroid gland. Am J Med 31:163–166
2. Neumann HP et al (2007) Evidence of MEN-2 in the original description of classic pheochromocytoma. N Engl J Med 357(13):1311–1315
3. Arighi E, Borrello MG, Sariola H (2005) RET tyrosine kinase signaling in development and cancer. Cytokine Growth Factor Rev 16(4–5):441–467
4. Kouvaraki MA et al (2005) RET proto-oncogene: a review and update of genotype-phenotype correlations in hereditary medullary thyroid cancer and associated endocrine tumors. Thyroid 15(6):531–544
5. Marx SJ (2005) Molecular genetics of multiple endocrine neoplasia types 1 and 2. Nat Rev Cancer 5(5):367–375
6. Santoro M et al (2002) Molecular mechanisms of RET activation in human cancer. Ann N Y Acad Sci 963:116–121
7. Santoro M et al (1995) Activation of RET as a dominant transforming gene by germline mutations of MEN2A and MEN2B. Science 267(5196):381–383
8. Borrello MG et al (1995) RET activation by germline MEN2A and MEN2B mutations. Oncogene 11(11):2419–2427
9. Michiels FM et al (1997) Development of medullary thyroid carcinoma in transgenic mice expressing the RET protooncogene altered by a multiple endocrine neoplasia type 2A mutation. Proc Natl Acad Sci USA 94(7):3330–3335
10. Smith-Hicks CL et al (2000) C-cell hyperplasia, pheochromocytoma and sympathoadrenal malformation in a mouse model of multiple endocrine neoplasia type 2B. EMBO J 19(4):612–622
11. Elisei R et al (2004) Identification of a novel point mutation in the RET gene (Ala883Thr), which is associated with medullary thyroid carcinoma phenotype only in homozygous condition. J Clin Endocrinol Metab 89(11):5823–5827
12. Ito T et al (1994) Activated RET oncogene in thyroid cancers of children from areas contaminated by Chernobyl accident. Lancet 344(8917):259
13. Nikiforov YE et al (1997) Distinct pattern of ret oncogene rearrangements in morphological variants of radiation-induced and sporadic thyroid papillary carcinomas in children. Cancer Res 57(9):1690–1694
14. Nakashima M et al (2007) RET oncogene amplification in thyroid cancer: correlations with radiation-associated and high-grade malignancy. Hum Pathol 38(4):621–628
15. Angrist M et al (1995) Mutation analysis of the RET receptor tyrosine kinase in Hirschsprung disease. Hum Mol Genet 4(5):821–830
16. Edery P et al (1994) Mutations of the RET proto-oncogene in Hirschsprung's disease. Nature 367(6461):378–380
17. Romeo G et al (1994) Point mutations affecting the tyrosine kinase domain of the RET proto-oncogene in Hirschsprung's disease. Nature 367(6461):377–378
18. Schuchardt A et al (1994) Defects in the kidney and enteric nervous system of mice lacking the tyrosine kinase receptor Ret. Nature 367(6461):380–383
19. Machens A et al (2003) Early malignant progression of hereditary medullary thyroid cancer. N Engl J Med 349(16):1517–1525
20. Brandi ML et al (2001) Guidelines for diagnosis and therapy of MEN type 1 and type 2. J Clin Endocrinol Metab 86(12): 5658–5671
21. Yip L et al (2003) Multiple endocrine neoplasia type 2: evaluation of the genotype-phenotype relationship. Arch Surg 138((4):409–416, discussion 416
22. Kloos RT et al (2009) Medullary thyroid cancer: management guidelines of the American Thyroid Association. Thyroid 19(6):565–612
23. Shaha AR et al (2006) Late-onset medullary carcinoma of the thyroid: need for genetic testing and prophylactic thyroidectomy in adult family members. Laryngoscope 116(9):1704–1707
24. Lesueur F et al (2005) Germline homozygous mutations at codon 804 in the RET protooncogene in medullary thyroid carcinoma/multiple endocrine neoplasia type 2A patients. J Clin Endocrinol Metab 90(6):3454–3457
25. Costante G et al (2009) Determination of calcitonin levels in C-cell disease: clinical interest and potential pitfalls. Nat Clin Pract Endocrinol Metab 5(1):35–44
26. Schwartz KE et al (1979) Calcitonin in nonthyroidal cancer. J Clin Endocrinol Metab 49(3):438–444
27. de Groot JW et al (2006) Biochemical markers in the follow-up of medullary thyroid cancer. Thyroid 16(11):1163–1170
28. Laure Giraudet A et al (2008) Progression of medullary thyroid carcinoma: assessment with calcitonin and carcinoembryonic antigen doubling times. Eur J Endocrinol 158(2):239–246
29. Mahler C et al (1990) Long-term treatment of metastatic medullary thyroid carcinoma with the somatostatin analogue octreotide. Clin Endocrinol (Oxf) 33(2):261–269
30. Ye L, Santarpia L, Gagel RF (2009) Targeted therapy for endocrine cancer: the medullary thyroid carcinoma paradigm. Endocr Pract 1–24
31. Carlomagno F et al (2002) ZD6474, an orally available inhibitor of KDR tyrosine kinase activity, efficiently blocks oncogenic RET kinases. Cancer Res 62(24):7284–7290
32. Hong D et al (2008) Medullary thyroid cancer: targeting the RET kinase pathway with sorafenib/tipifarnib. Mol Cancer Ther 7(5):1001–1006
33. Kelleher FC, McDermott R (2008) Response to sunitinib in medullary thyroid cancer. Ann Intern Med 148(7):567
34. Elisei R et al (2007) RET genetic screening in patients with medullary thyroid cancer and their relatives: experience with 807 individuals at one center. J Clin Endocrinol Metab 92(12):4725–4729

35. Moura MM et al (2009) Correlation of RET somatic mutations with clinicopathological features in sporadic medullary thyroid carcinomas. Br J Cancer 100(11):1777–1783

36. Elisei R et al (2008) Prognostic significance of somatic RET oncogene mutations in sporadic medullary thyroid cancer: a 10-year follow-up study. J Clin Endocrinol Metab 93(3):682–687

37. Cardot-Bauters C et al (2008) Does the RET variant G691S influence the features of sporadic medullary thyroid carcinoma? Clin Endocrinol (Oxf) 69(3):506–510

38. Robledo M et al (2003) Polymorphisms G691S/S904S of RET as genetic modifiers of MEN 2A. Cancer Res 63(8):1814–1817

39. Elisei R et al (2004) RET exon 11 (G691S) polymorphism is significantly more frequent in sporadic medullary thyroid carcinoma than in the general population. J Clin Endocrinol Metab 89(7): 3579–3584

40. Da Silva AM et al (2003) A novel germ-line point mutation in RET exon 8 (Gly(533)Cys) in a large kindred with familial medullary thyroid carcinoma. J Clin Endocrinol Metab 88(11): 5438–5443

41. Howe JR, Norton JA, Wells SA Jr (1993) Prevalence of pheochromocytoma and hyperparathyroidism in multiple endocrine neoplasia type 2A: results of long-term follow-up. Surgery 114(6):1070–1077

42. Nakamura E, Kaelin WG Jr (2006) Recent insights into the molecular pathogenesis of pheochromocytoma and paraganglioma. Endocr Pathol 17(2):97–106

43. Erlic Z, Neumann HP (2009) Familial pheochromocytoma. Hormones (Athens) 8(1):29–38

44. Machens A et al (2005) Codon-specific development of pheochromocytoma in multiple endocrine neoplasia type 2. J Clin Endocrinol Metab 90(7):3999–4003

45. Waguespack SG (2009) A perspective from pediatric endocrinology on the hereditary medullary thyroid carcinoma syndromes. Thyroid 19(6):543–546

46. Brauckhoff M, Gimm O (2009) Extrathyroidal manifestations of multiple endocrine neoplasia type 2. Thyroid 19(6):555–557

47. Kinlaw WB et al (2005) Multiple endocrine neoplasia 2A due to a unique C609S RET mutation presents with pheochromocytoma and reduced penetrance of medullary thyroid carcinoma. Clin Endocrinol (Oxf) 63(6):676–682

48. Nunziata V et al (1989) Cutaneous lichen amyloidosis associated with multiple endocrine neoplasia type 2A. Henry Ford Hosp Med J 37(3–4):144–146

49. Verga U et al (2003) Frequent association between MEN 2A and cutaneous lichen amyloidosis. Clin Endocrinol (Oxf) 59(2):156–161

50. Verga U, Beck-Peccoz P, Cambiaghi S (2002) Cutaneous lichen amyloidosis in multiple endocrine neoplasia type 2A. Thyroid 12(12):1149

51. Amiel J et al (2008) Hirschsprung disease, associated syndromes and genetics: a review. J Med Genet 45(1):1–14

52. Mulligan LM, Ponder BA (1995) Genetic basis of endocrine disease: multiple endocrine neoplasia type 2. J Clin Endocrinol Metab 80(7):1989–1995

53. Arighi E et al (2004) Biological effects of the dual phenotypic Janus mutation of ret cosegregating with both multiple endocrine neoplasia type 2 and Hirschsprung's disease. Mol Endocrinol 18(4):1004–1017

54. O'Riordain DS et al (1994) Medullary thyroid carcinoma in multiple endocrine neoplasia types 2A and 2B. Surgery 116(6):1017–1023

55. Wray CJ et al (2008) Failure to recognize multiple endocrine neoplasia 2B: more common than we think? Ann Surg Oncol 15(1):293–301

56. Gagel RF et al (1988) The clinical outcome of prospective screening for multiple endocrine neoplasia type 2a. An 18-year experience. N Engl J Med 318(8):478–484

57. Lips CJ et al (1994) Clinical screening as compared with DNA analysis in families with multiple endocrine neoplasia type 2A. N Engl J Med 331(13):828–835

58. Machens A (2004) Early malignant progression of hereditary medullary thyroid cancer. N Engl J Med 350(9):943

59. Machens A, Dralle H (2008) Familial prevalence and age of RET germline mutations: implications for screening. Clin Endocrinol (Oxf) 69(1):81–87

60. Machens A, Dralle H (2009) Prophylactic thyroidectomy in RET carriers at risk for hereditary medullary thyroid cancer. Thyroid 19(6):551–554

61. Wermer P (1954) Genetic aspects of adenomatosis of endocrine glands. Am J Med 16(3):363–371

62. Chandrasekharappa SC et al (1997) Positional cloning of the gene for multiple endocrine neoplasia-type 1. Science 276(5311):404–407

63. Yokoyama A et al (2004) Leukemia proto-oncoprotein MLL forms a SET1-like histone methyltransferase complex with menin to regulate Hox gene expression. Mol Cell Biol 24(13):5639–5649

64. Yan J et al (2006) Cdx4 and menin co-regulate Hoxa9 expression in hematopoietic cells. PLoS ONE 1:e47

65. Karnik SK et al (2005) Menin regulates pancreatic islet growth by promoting histone methylation and expression of genes encoding p27Kip1 and p18INK4c. Proc Natl Acad Sci USA 102(41): 14659–14664

66. Bertolino P et al (2003) Genetic ablation of the tumor suppressor menin causes lethality at mid-gestation with defects in multiple organs. Mech Dev 120(5):549–560

67. Crabtree JS et al (2001) A mouse model of multiple endocrine neoplasia, type 1, develops multiple endocrine tumors. Proc Natl Acad Sci USA 98(3):1118–1123

68. Loffler KA et al (2007) Broad tumor spectrum in a mouse model of multiple endocrine neoplasia type 1. Int J Cancer 120(2): 259–267

69. Lemos MC, Thakker RV (2008) Multiple endocrine neoplasia type 1 (MEN1): analysis of 1336 mutations reported in the first decade following identification of the gene. Hum Mutat 29(1):22–32

70. Sato K et al (2000) Somatic mutations of the multiple endocrine neoplasia type 1 (MEN1) gene in patients with sporadic, nonfamilial primary hyperparathyroidism. Surgery 127(3):337–341

71. Haven CJ et al (2007) Identification of MEN1 and HRPT2 somatic mutations in paraffin-embedded (sporadic) parathyroid carcinomas. Clin Endocrinol (Oxf) 67(3):370–376, 67

72. Machens A et al (2007) Age-related penetrance of endocrine tumours in multiple endocrine neoplasia type 1 (MEN1): a multi-centre study of 258 gene carriers. Clin Endocrinol (Oxf) 67(4): 613–622

73. Agarwal SK, Mateo CM, Marx SJ (2009) Rare germline mutations in cyclin-dependent kinase inhibitor genes in MEN1 and related states. J Clin Endocrinol Metab 94(5):1826–1834

74. Marx SJ et al (1991) Heterogeneous size of the parathyroid glands in familial multiple endocrine neoplasia type 1. Clin Endocrinol (Oxf) 35(6):521–526

75. Agha A et al (2007) Parathyroid carcinoma in multiple endocrine neoplasia type 1 (MEN1) syndrome: two case reports of an unrecognised entity. J Endocrinol Invest 30(2):145–149

76. Akerstrom G, Malmaeus J, Bergstrom R (1984) Surgical anatomy of human parathyroid glands. Surgery 95(1):14–21

77. Rizzoli R, Green J 3rd, Marx SJ (1985) Primary hyperparathyroidism in familial multiple endocrine neoplasia type I. Long-term follow-up of serum calcium levels after parathyroidectomy. Am J Med 78(3):467–474

78. Burgess JR et al (1998) The outcome of subtotal parathyroidectomy for the treatment of hyperparathyroidism in multiple endocrine neoplasia type 1. Arch Surg 133(2):126–129

79. Peacock M et al (2005) Cinacalcet hydrochloride maintains long-term normocalcemia in patients with primary hyperparathyroidism. J Clin Endocrinol Metab 90(1):135–141

80. Falchetti A et al (2008) A patient with MEN1-associated hyperparathyroidism, responsive to cinacalcet. Nat Clin Pract Endocrinol Metab 4(6):351–357

81. D'Souza-Li L et al (2002) Identification and functional characterization of novel calcium-sensing receptor mutations in familial hypocalciuric hypercalcemia and autosomal dominant hypocalcemia. J Clin Endocrinol Metab 87(3):1309–1318

82. Hannan FM et al (2008) Familial isolated primary hyperparathyroidism caused by mutations of the MEN1 gene. Nat Clin Pract Endocrinol Metab 4(1):53–58

83. Perren A et al (2007) Multiple endocrine neoplasia type 1 (MEN1): loss of one MEN1 allele in tumors and monohormonal endocrine cell clusters but not in islet hyperplasia of the pancreas. J Clin Endocrinol Metab 92(3):1118–1128

84. Skogseid B et al (1987) A standardized meal stimulation test of the endocrine pancreas for early detection of pancreatic endocrine tumors in multiple endocrine neoplasia type 1 syndrome: five years experience. J Clin Endocrinol Metab 64(6):1233–1240

85. Yim JH et al (1998) Prospective study of the utility of somatostatin-receptor scintigraphy in the evaluation of patients with multiple endocrine neoplasia type 1. Surgery 124(6):1037–1042

86. Triponez F et al (2006) Is surgery beneficial for MEN1 patients with small (< or = 2 cm), nonfunctioning pancreaticoduodenal endocrine tumor? An analysis of 65 patients from the GTE. World J Surg 30(5):654–662, discussion 663–664

87. Fendrich V et al (2006) An aggressive surgical approach leads to long-term survival in patients with pancreatic endocrine tumors. Ann Surg 244(6):845–851, discussion 852–853

88. Berna MJ et al (2006) Serum gastrin in Zollinger-Ellison syndrome: II. Prospective study of gastrin provocative testing in 293 patients from the National Institutes of Health and comparison with 537 cases from the literature. evaluation of diagnostic criteria, proposal of new criteria, and correlations with clinical and tumoral features. Medicine (Baltimore) 85(6):331–364

89. Murugesan SV, Varro A, Pritchard DM (2009) Review article: Strategies to determine whether hypergastrinaemia is due to Zollinger-Ellison syndrome rather than a more common benign cause. Aliment Pharmacol Ther 29(10):1055–1068

90. Pipeleers-Marichal M et al (1990) Gastrinomas in the duodenums of patients with multiple endocrine neoplasia type 1 and the Zollinger-Ellison syndrome. N Engl J Med 322(11):723–727

91. Gibril F et al (2001) Prospective study of the natural history of gastrinoma in patients with MEN1: definition of an aggressive and a nonaggressive form. J Clin Endocrinol Metab 86(11):5282–5293

92. Doherty GM, Thompson NW (2003) Multiple endocrine neoplasia type 1: duodenopancreatic tumours. J Intern Med 253(6):590–598

93. Cisco RM, Norton JA (2007) Surgery for gastrinoma. Adv Surg 41:165–176

94. Jensen RT et al (2006) Gastrinoma (duodenal and pancreatic). Neuroendocrinology 84(3):173–182

95. Ruszniewski P et al (1993) Hepatic arterial chemoembolization in patients with liver metastases of endocrine tumors. A prospective phase II study in 24 patients. Cancer 71(8):2624–2630

96. von Schrenck T et al (1988) Prospective study of chemotherapy in patients with metastatic gastrinoma. Gastroenterology 94(6):1326–1334

97. Ruszniewski P et al (1991) [Intravenous chemotherapy with streptozotocin and 5 fluorouracil for hepatic metastases of Zollinger-Ellison syndrome. A prospective multicenter study in 21 patients]. Gastroenterol Clin Biol 15(5):393–398

98. Kulke MH et al (2008) Activity of sunitinib in patients with advanced neuroendocrine tumors. J Clin Oncol 26(20):3403–3410

99. Berna MJ et al (2008) A prospective study of gastric carcinoids and enterochromaffin-like cell changes in multiple endocrine neoplasia type 1 and Zollinger-Ellison syndrome: identification of risk factors. J Clin Endocrinol Metab 93(5):1582–1591

100. Placzkowski KA et al (2009) Secular trends in the presentation and management of functioning insulinoma at the Mayo Clinic, 1987-2007. J Clin Endocrinol Metab 94(4):1069–1073

101. Grant CS (2005) Insulinoma. Best Pract Res Clin Gastroenterol 19(5):783–798

102. Service FJ et al (1991) Functioning insulinoma – incidence, recurrence, and long-term survival of patients: a 60-year study. Mayo Clin Proc 66(7):711–719

103. Gill GV, Rauf O, MacFarlane IA (1997) Diazoxide treatment for insulinoma: a national UK survey. Postgrad Med J 73(864):640–641

104. Vezzosi D et al (2005) Octreotide in insulinoma patients: efficacy on hypoglycemia, relationships with Octreoscan scintigraphy and immunostaining with anti-sst2A and anti-sst5 antibodies. Eur J Endocrinol 152(5):757–767

105. Kulke MH, Bergsland EK, Yao JC (2009) Glycemic control in patients with insulinoma treated with everolimus. N Engl J Med 360(2):195–197

106. Levy-Bohbot N et al (2004) Prevalence, characteristics and prognosis of MEN 1-associated glucagonomas, VIPomas, and somatostatinomas: study from the GTE (Groupe des Tumeurs Endocrines) registry. Gastroenterol Clin Biol 28(11):1075–1081

107. Dralle H et al (2004) Surgery of resectable nonfunctioning neuroendocrine pancreatic tumors. World J Surg 28(12):1248–1260

108. O'Toole D et al (2006) Rare functioning pancreatic endocrine tumors. Neuroendocrinology 84(3):189–195

109. Triponez F et al (2006) Epidemiology data on 108 MEN 1 patients from the GTE with isolated nonfunctioning tumors of the pancreas. Ann Surg 243(2):265–272

110. Chanson P, Salenave S (2004) Diagnosis and treatment of pituitary adenomas. Minerva Endocrinol 29(4):241–275

111. Verges B et al (2002) Pituitary disease in MEN type 1 (MEN1): data from the France-Belgium MEN1 multicenter study. J Clin Endocrinol Metab 87(2):457–465

112. Padberg B et al (1995) Multiple endocrine neoplasia type 1 (MEN 1) revisited. Virchows Arch 426(6):541–548

113. Trouillas J et al (2008) Pituitary tumors and hyperplasia in multiple endocrine neoplasia type 1 syndrome (MEN1): a case-control study in a series of 77 patients versus 2509 non-MEN1 patients. Am J Surg Pathol 32(4):534–543

114. Rosai J, Higa E, Davie J (1972) Mediastinal endocrine neoplasm in patients with multiple endocrine adenomatosis. A previously unrecognized association. Cancer 29(4):1075–1083

115. Lee CH et al (1986) Carcinoid tumor of the pancreas causing the diarrheogenic syndrome: report of a case combined with multiple endocrine neoplasia, type I. Surgery 99(1):123–129

116. Debelenko LV et al (1997) Identification of MEN1 gene mutations in sporadic carcinoid tumors of the lung. Hum Mol Genet 6(13):2285–2290

117. Ferolla P et al (2005) Thymic neuroendocrine carcinoma (carcinoid) in multiple endocrine neoplasia type 1 syndrome: the Italian series. J Clin Endocrinol Metab 90(5):2603–2609

118. Teh BT et al (1998) Thymic carcinoids in multiple endocrine neoplasia type 1. Ann Surg 228(1):99–105

119. Barzon L et al (2001) Multiple endocrine neoplasia type 1 and adrenal lesions. J Urol 166(1):24–27

120. Skogseid B et al (1992) Clinical and genetic features of adrenocortical lesions in multiple endocrine neoplasia type 1. J Clin Endocrinol Metab 75(1):76–81

121. Whitley SA et al (2008) The appearance of the adrenal glands on computed tomography in multiple endocrine neoplasia type 1. Eur J Endocrinol 159(6):819–824

122. Waldmann J et al (2007) Adrenal involvement in multiple endocrine neoplasia type 1: results of 7 years prospective screening. Langenbecks Arch Surg 392(4):437–443

123. Darling TN et al (1997) Multiple facial angiofibromas and collagenomas in patients with multiple endocrine neoplasia type 1. Arch Dermatol 133(7):853–857

124. Asgharian B et al (2004) Cutaneous tumors in patients with multiple endocrine neoplasm type 1 (MEN1) and gastrinomas: prospective study of frequency and development of criteria with high

sensitivity and specificity for MEN1. J Clin Endocrinol Metab 89(11):5328–5336

125. Pack S et al (1998) Cutaneous tumors in patients with multiple endocrine neoplasia type 1 show allelic deletion of the MEN1 gene. J Invest Dermatol 110(4):438–440

126. Kato H et al (1996) Multiple endocrine neoplasia type 1 associated with spinal ependymoma. Intern Med 35(4):285–289

127. Doumith R et al (1982) Pituitary prolactinoma, adrenal aldosterone-producing adenomas, gastric schwannoma and colonic polyadenomas: a possible variant of multiple endocrine neoplasia (MEN) type I. Acta Endocrinol (Copenh) 100(2):189–195

128. Karges W et al (2003) Bi-allelic inactivation of the MEN1 tumor suppressor gene in human grade II astrocytoma. Cancer Lett 196(1):23–27

129. Asgharian B et al (2004) Meningiomas may be a component tumor of multiple endocrine neoplasia type 1. Clin Cancer Res 10(3):869–880

130. McKeeby JL et al (2001) Multiple leiomyomas of the esophagus, lung, and uterus in multiple endocrine neoplasia type 1. Am J Pathol 159(3):1121–1127

131. Pieterman CR et al (2009) Multiple endocrine neoplasia type 1 (MEN1): its manifestations and effect of genetic screening on clinical outcome. Clin Endocrinol (Oxf) 70(4):575–581

132. Agarwal SK et al (2004) Molecular pathology of the MEN1 gene. Ann N Y Acad Sci 1014:189–198

133. Tham E et al (2007) Clinical testing for mutations in the MEN1 gene in Sweden: a report on 200 unrelated cases. J Clin Endocrinol Metab 92(9):3389–3395

134. Ellard S et al (2005) Detection of an MEN1 gene mutation depends on clinical features and supports current referral criteria for diagnostic molecular genetic testing. Clin Endocrinol (Oxf) 62(2):169–175

135. Geerdink EA, Van der Luijt RB, Lips CJ (2003) Do patients with multiple endocrine neoplasia syndrome type 1 benefit from periodical screening? Eur J Endocrinol 149(6):577–582

136. Bertherat J et al (2009) Mutations in regulatory subunit type 1A of cyclic adenosine 5′-monophosphate-dependent protein kinase (PRKAR1A): phenotype analysis in 353 patients and 80 different genotypes. J Clin Endocrinol Metab 94(6):2085–2091

137. Horvath A, Stratakis CA (2008) Clinical and molecular genetics of acromegaly: MEN1, Carney complex, McCune-Albright syndrome, familial acromegaly and genetic defects in sporadic tumors. Rev Endocr Metab Disord 9(1):1–11

138. Lietman SA, Schwindinger WF, Levine MA (2007) Genetic and molecular aspects of McCune-Albright syndrome. Pediatr Endocrinol Rev 4 Suppl 4:380–385

Chapter 12
Pediatric Malignancies: Retinoblastoma and Wilms' Tumor

David A. Sweetser and Eric F. Grabowski

Keywords Retinoblastoma • Wilms tumor • WT1 gene • RB1 gene • Cell cycle • Beckwith Wiedemann syndrome • WTX gene • Knudsen hypothesis

The retinoblastoma section of this chapter was written by Eric Grabowski, and the Wilms' tumor section was written by David Sweetser

Introduction

Retinoblastoma and Wilms' tumor represent two childhood tumors with both sporadic and familial forms. Delineation of the molecular etiology of these cancers identified the retinoblastoma gene Rb as the first example of a tumor suppressor gene and provided the first example of imprinting and cancer predisposition in Wilms' tumor. In this chapter, we review the clinical features and genetics of these two disorders and the implications for management, early detection and potential prevention of these disorders.

Retinoblastoma

Clinical Features

Epidemiology

Retinoblastoma is the most common primary ocular malignancy of childhood, affecting approximately one in every 20,000 live births [1–4]. This fact makes the disease as common as severe hemophilia. Of an estimated 200–300

new cases each year in the United States, 30% prove to be bilateral. The tumor is a generally slow-growing one that may remain contained in the eye for months or even years. Yet it is responsible for 5% of all childhood blindness, and it rapidly leads to death when the tumor extends beyond the globe [5]. In fact, death remains the likely outcome in poorly developed countries where access to timely surgery, chemotherapy, and/or radiation therapy is limited. Furthermore, the tumor confers lifelong risk of second (or even third, fourth, and fifth) nonocular malignancies on the 40% of patients who harbor a germinal mutation as origin of the disease [6].

Clinical Presentation

Most children with retinoblastoma are first identified by parents, who generally consult an ophthalmologist for one or more of several presenting complaints. In order of frequency, these are leukokoria (56%), strabismus (20%), painful eye with glaucoma (7%), and decreased visual acuity (5%). Less common presenting signs are orbital cellulitis, unilaterally dilated pupil, heterochromia, hyphema, nystagmus, and even failure to thrive [7]. Figure 12.1 shows leukokoria in a child with bilateral retinoblastoma.

About 5% of children with germinal retinoblastoma have cognitive and somatic abnormalities, including mental retardation and failure to thrive, which are part of a syndrome known as the chromosome 13 deletion syndrome (see Sect. 12.2.4.1).

Signs of extraocular tumor are, fortunately, uncommon in developed countries. Nonetheless, children with orbital tumor may present with proptosis, or with forward displacement of a prosthesis in the case of an already enucleated eye, while those with central nervous system tumor may show lethargy or irritability. Children with bone and bone marrow metastases almost always have bony masses arising from skull bones, but long bones can also be affected [7]. A presentation common in third world countries, but rare elsewhere, is a mass protruding forward from one or both orbits with regional spread of tumor into the oral cavity and, by means of lymphatics, the neck. One of us (EFG) has taken care of an infant with small bilateral retinoblastomas but a large suprasellar tumor who presented

D.A. Sweetser (✉) and E.F. Grabowski (✉)
Department of Pediatric Hematology/Oncology,
Harvard Medical School, Massachusetts General Hospital,
Boston, MA, USA
e-mail: dsweetser@partners.org; EGrabowski@partners.org

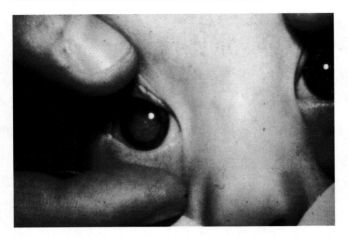

Fig. 12.1 Germinal retinoblastoma: Leukokoria in an infant with bilateral retinoblastoma, with tumor in the right globe extending anteriorly to the lens

with wandering eye movements and a head circumference at the 95th percentile. The presence of a tumor in the pineal gland or suprasellar space in a child with bilateral retinoblastoma constitutes "trilateral" retinoblastoma [6, 8], since tumors in these locations contain photoreceptor elements.

Diagnosis

Diagnosis of intraocular retinoblastoma is made visually by an ophthalmologist, ideally a retina specialist. In contrast to the situation for most other tumors, biopsy is contraindicated insofar as such a procedure carries with it an unacceptable risk of introducing tumor cells to the globe exterior (extraocular tumor). The differential diagnosis includes persistent fetal vasculature (formerly known as persistent hyperplastic primary vitreous), Coat's disease (an inflammatory condition giving rise to subretinal fluid), ocular toxicariasis, astrocytic hamartoma, and retinopathy of prematurity.

Evaluation for Extraocular Tumor

The workup for extraocular tumor includes a careful review of the globe and optic nerve pathology for any enucleated eye. Although not employed for primary diagnosis, the pathology for any enucleated globe and optic nerve segment yields important information as to the (a) presence of extraocular tumor and/or (b) the risk of micrometastatic disease. Tumor cells at the margin of nerve resection or on the episcleral surface are considered as part of an extraocular tumor. The presence of a tumor beyond the lamina cribosa (that structure of the sclerae through which optic nerve fibers exit the globe), massive choroidal tumor, and tumor involving the uvea are considered high-risk features for micrometastatic

disease. Both situations warrant prophylactic combination chemotherapy [9].

The evaluation also includes a baseline MR of the brain and orbits to exclude occult orbital tumor or optic nerve extension of disease, as well, for germinal cases, to exclude the presence of trilateral tumor in the pineal or suprasellar region. In the presence of optic nerve tumor or trilateral tumor, one should also perform a lumbar puncture for cerebrospinal fluid cytology. In the presence of bone lesions and/or bone pain, one should also perform bilateral bone marrow aspirates and biopsies, along with a bone scan. Retinoblastoma in the bone marrow, like neuroblastoma in the bone marrow, need not be disseminated.

Management of Retinoblastoma

The management of retinoblastoma has seen striking advances over the past 20 years. These include the use of chemotherapy, with or without radiation therapy, for intraocular tumors >3 mm in diameter; the identification of children who, based on globe and optic nerve pathology, may be at high risk for micrometastases; the successful use of chemotherapy for localized bulky tumor (orbital recurrence, optic nerve tumor at the margin of surgical section) or cerebrospinal fluid (CSF) tumor only; and the successful application of combination chemotherapy followed by autologous stem cell rescue for bone and bone marrow disease. For intraocular tumor, a new "ABC" staging system is gaining widespread acceptance and has been adopted internationally by the Children's Oncology Group (COG). For an excellent review of the ABC staging system and current stage-related chemotherapy, see Grabowski [9].

Intraocular tumors confined to the retina and <3 mm in diameter are treated with local opthalmologic measures: photocoagulation, cryotherapy, and diathermy. Enucleation is reserved for cases of unilateral tumor that are so extensive as to pose a risk for extraocular dissemination and/or unilateral cases for which the affected eye has no chance of useful vision. Enucleation is also employed in bilateral tumors when one eye satisfies one or both of the above criteria, while the other has a lower stage of disease and is amenable to treatment with combination chemotherapy and/or radiation therapy.

Molecular Biology, The RB1 Gene, Specific Mutations, and Tumor Penetrance

Molecular Biology

Children with the germinal mutation for retinoblastoma include all those with bilateral disease (30% of cases) and 15% of those with unilateral disease (70% of cases). Although a close association between genetics and cancer has been obvious for years from studies of families and children with retinoblastoma, only 12% of affected children have a positive family history. The other 88% represent the first mutation within the kindred. From a genetics standpoint, germinal retinoblastoma behaves like an autosomal-dominant syndrome with a very high degree of penetrance, yet the abnormal tumor-predisposing mutant allele is recessive [10, 11]; see below.

In 1971 Knudsen proposed a two-hit hypothesis for retinoblastoma [12]. In both germinal and nongerminal types of this cancer, a mutation is required in both alleles of what is now considered to be a tumor suppressor gene located in the q14 band of chromosome 13. In the germinal (and inherited) form, one allele is affected in all the cells of the body, a first mutation occurring as a prezygotic event. A second, postzygotic mutation occurs in the second allele, generally in the first year of life, leading to bilateral and multiple tumors in a given eye. The mean number of tumor foci in a given eye follows the Poisson distribution about an observed mean of 5.3, lending support to the Knudsen hypothesis that at least two chromosomal events are required for the development of cancer. In practice, approximately 90% of those heterozygous for an inactivation mutation (RB+RB−) develop retinoblastoma owing to the high probability of a second mutation (RB+RB+), and this high probability is what give rise to the multifocal nature of tumors as well as a near-certainty of a second mutation. The heterozygous state consequently behaves as an autosomal dominant one even though it is recessive at the gene level [13, 14]. Conversely, nongerminal and nonhereditary retinoblastoma nearly universally is associated with unilateral, unifocal tumors, with both mutation events being postzygotic [15–17]. The joint probability of two postzygotic mutation events is so low that tumors are virtually always solitary.

The RB1 Gene

The RB1 gene is located at human chromosome 13q14 and possesses 27 introns [18, 19]. Importantly, it encodes the RB polypeptide (pRB), a 110 kDa phosphoprotein that shares homology with two related other proteins, p130 and p107. Together, these proteins comprise the RB family of proteins, each containing an N-terminal, a C-terminal, and intervening A/B domains. The A/B region mediates binding to most RB-associated proteins and codes for a polypeptide-pocket domain that is necessary for protein–protein interactions with endogenous protein mediators of cell growth and differentiation, and with exogenous viral proteins [20–22]. The latter (viral proteins) include adenovirus E1A, SV40 T antigen, and HPV E7. The polypeptide-pocket domain is capable of binding several polypeptides at the same time, as indicated from the existence of multiple protein-binding interface regions via crystallographic analysis [23]. The C-terminal region, while

not well characterized, is involved in suppressing cell growth. It has a nuclear-localization signal, which regulates the transport of pRB from the cytoplasm to the nucleus, and the concurrent transport of pRB-associated polypeptides, which lacks nuclear-localization capability, as inferred from sequence analysis [18]. A mutation in this region has been described which yields lower penetrance of retinoblastoma [24]. The N-terminal region binds the A/B pocket [18]. Mutations in this region lead to loss of phosphorylation sites that mediate pRB function [25].

The Protein Product pRB

The protein product of the RB1 gene, known as pRB, is considered to be the master regulator of proteins mediating cell growth in this tumor. pRB binds the E2F family of transcription factors, which assist cell entry into the S phase of the cell cycle [26, 27]. pRB binds a number of polypeptides in the E2F family, which functionally blocks the cell from entering the S phase. In particular, the hypophosphorylated form of pRB, the form predominant in differentiated cells, binds to the transactivation domain of E2F, which in turn determines the binding of E2F to DNA within promoters of genes responsible for regulation of the cell cycle. In contrast, hyperphosphorylation inactivates the tumor-suppressor function of pRB by releasing the bound E2F and permitting subsequent DNA synthesis [28, 29]. A higher-order suppression also occurs: E2F places pRB near other transcription factors important to gene expression, thereby allowing E2F to block these factors also from interacting with the basal transcription complex [30, 31]. As a result, the pRB-E2F complex blocks the function of additional enhancers, suppressing the transcription of genes proximal to the E2F sites.

pRB also inhibits transcription of genes involved in cell proliferation by means of its interaction with histone deacetylases (HDACs) [32]. HDACs work by removing acetyl groups from certain histones, which enhances the stability of the histone-DNA complex and reduces the ability of chromatin to access transcription machinery. pRB localizes HDACs to DNA-bound E2F, stabilizing the histone-DNA interaction and thereby suppressing gene transcription [33–35].

Gene Mutations in Retinoblastoma

Heterozygous carriers of an RB1 mutation can demonstrate variable phenotypic expression [36]. For example, the child in Fig. 12.2 had the chromosome 13q14 deletion syndrome (including bilateral retinoblastoma), while her mother, the daughter of a man with bilateral tumor, had unilateral retinoblastoma and no nonocular somatic abnormalities. Moreover, there are kindred in which no tumor at all has developed in

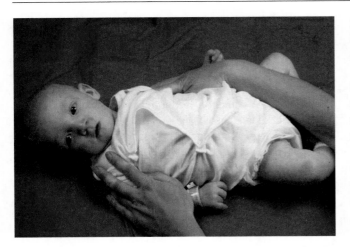

Fig. 12.2 Chromosome 13q14 deletion syndrome: Microcephaly and failure-to-thrive in a 5-month-old infant with bilateral retinoblastoma

obligate carriers. Such variability in phenotypic expression might be expected in a small number of cases insofar as a chance second and inactivating mutation is required for tumor formation, and this second mutation might lead to a partially functional pRB. In reality, the situation is more complex; specific mutations are now known to confer variation in phenotypic expression. Of more than 1,000 families for whom mutations have been characterized, the majority of mutations are nonsense or frameshift mutations [37]. These are located within exons 2–25 and almost always cause bilateral tumor. The exact location of a stop codon within RB1, interestingly, does not appear to affect phenotype [36]. This is believed to be due to a process known as nonsense-mediated decay, a process in which transcripts of RB1 alleles containing internal stop codons are detected by posttranscriptional surveillance mechanisms, causing the mutant transcripts to degrade with total loss of functional pRB [36, 38]. Therefore, there is no intermediate state reached for which there is a partially functional pRB and consequently variable penetrance. Nonetheless, cases have been reported in which there is a nonsense mutation in patients with unilateral tumor or even no tumor [16, 39]. This phenotype has been shown to be due to somatic mosaicism, present in less than 10% of families with hereditary retinoblastoma.

Point mutations in introns or exons that lead to splice-site mutations comprise another major group of RB1 mutations. Commonly these give rise to a premature stop codon. Because of nonsense-mediated decay, these mutations, too, are usually associated with high penetrance and expressivity (bilateral tumors) [36]. However, similar mutations can also occur at less well-conserved splice sites, as within introns, resulting in leaky mutations. In such mutations, a portion of the total transcript is normal RNA, with a consequent reduction in

functional protein [40]. Such germ-line carriers can thus have unilateral disease [36, 40]. A similar situation exists for mutations in the RB1 promoter.

In-frame and missense mutations occur less commonly in RB1 and lead to normal quantities of stable transcript. These mutations, associated with amino acid insertion, deletion, or substitution within the A/B pocket, cause decreased penetrance and expressivity [24, 36, 41].

Finally, there are rare cases in which two isolated instances of unilateral retinoblastoma, or bilateral and unilateral retinoblastoma, are separated by several generations. One explanation for these cases is the presence of two independent genetic events in a single kindred, provided the kindred is large enough [42].

Penetrance and Mutation Detection Rates

Regarding penetrance in germinal retinoblastoma, one can state that penetrance is mutation-dependent. Approximately 95% of mutations have virtually 100% penetrance, while 5% have 30–50% penetrance. The former are generally frame shift, nonsense, and gene deletion mutations. The latter tend to be hypomorphic in-frame and missense mutations, which give rise to a reduced amount of the protein product pRB, not the absence of pRB.

With regard to mutation detection rates in germinal cases, one can presently identify mutations in 80–90% of tumor specimens, while the detection rate with peripheral blood is only 15–70%, owing to the heterozygous nature of mutations found in nontumor tissue (Dr. Theodore Dryga, personal communication, June 2009). In nongerminal cases, mutation detection rates with tumor tissue are similar, but peripheral blood is by definition noninformative.

The Role of p53

Early mouse models of retinoblastoma from the 1970s demonstrated the development of retinoblastoma in response to either injection of adenovirus 12 E1A into wild type mice [22], or, in response to the breeding of a transgenic mouse expressing SV 40T antigen in the retina [43]. We now know that adenovirus 12 E1A in the first model bound and inactivated pRB, and also bound p53. The T antigen in the second model inactivated not only pRB, but also p130, p107, and p53. In a third model, transgenic mice expressing HPV E7, pRB but not p53 was inhibited and retinoblastoma did not develop [44]. In fact, in mice, but not in humans, p107 must be inactivated to compensate for upregulation of p107 when pRB is inactivated; this leads to the formation of retinoblastomas of low penetrance [45].

Finally, in a fourth model, mice in which p53 is also inactivated yield retinoblastomas of high penetrance [44]. While p53 is not inactivated in human retinoblastoma, the p53 pathway is suppressed by other means: amplification of the MDMX and MDM2 genes [46].

The role of p53 in human retinoblastoma becomes clearer when one considers that most human cancers are known to escape apoptosis by acquiring mutations which block the p53 pathway. In fact, they have mutations which inactivate both pRB and the p53 pathway [47–49]. Loss of pRB, for example, might similarly be thought to lead to apoptosis and abrogation of clonal expansion of a retinoblastoma cell. Yet p53 in human retinoblastoma remains functional [50, 51]. One possible explanation for this state of affairs is that retinoblastoma cells are inherently resistant to apoptosis and do not depend upon p53 inactivation to proliferate [52]. This explanation has been disproved. An alternative one is the above-mentioned amplification of the MDMX and MDM2 genes [46, 52].

Genetic Diagnosis

Since 45–50% of the offspring of patients who have a germinal mutation will be affected, prenatal diagnosis (from choriovillus sampling or amniocentesis), presymptomatic diagnosis, preimplantation testing of embryos for in vitro fertilization, and cord-blood testing are all of great importance. Before the cloning of the RB1 gene and the availability of molecular genetic techniques for genetic diagnosis, the risk that a given person is a carrier of a retinoblastoma-inducting mutation was estimated from clinical findings and family history. Factors were the number of tumors in the affected relative, the relationship of the person to the affected relative, the number of affected relatives, and the number of unaffected siblings of the relative [53]. Moreover, direct detection of mutations was limited to a small number of cases in which high-resolution chromosome analyses permitting detection of relatively large deletions involving chromosome 13q14.2. However, an indirect approach was reported which is based upon the recognition of mutations at the retinoblastoma locus. Recognition of these mutations is made by means of genetic linkage analysis with the neighboring esterase D locus and chromosome 13-specific DNA polymorphisms as genetic markers [54–56]. (Esterase D is an enzyme marker, which is linked to RB1.) This indirect approach is applied to family members with at least two affected members and to those with affected members whose chromosomes show the genetic markers. Confidence in the risk assessment is further limited by the possibility of meiotic recombination between the retinoblastoma gene and the marker loci.

The first form of molecular diagnosis of retinoblastoma started with the isolation in the 1980s of DNA probes on chromosome 13 that detected restriction fragment length polymorphisms [57–59]. These probes were used in two ways. First, they were employed in indirect detection of disease-causing mutations by haplotype analyses. Second, they were used in direct detection of large deletions (20–25% of germinal cases) and reduction to homozygosity. The accuracy of these analyses, however, depended upon the distance between the marker and the gene mutation. With the cloning of RB1 in 1986 [10, 13, 14], it became possible to isolate intragenic polymorphic markers for linkage and haplotype analyses, and to directly detect tumor-producing mutations by means of sequencing [60–65]. If today a mutation cannot be found, haplotype analysis of the individual, family members, and any available tumor tissue can still be important in genetic counseling of the family, for it can exclude risk of tumor in some cases.

To detect mutations directly, today we sequence the 25 exons, the flanking introns, and the promoter region of RB1 [60–62, 64, 65]. There remains some difficulty in that the RB1 gene is large and no "hot spots" for mutations have been found. Therefore, a variety of screening techniques have been introduced to screen for the area of the mutation prior to direct sequencing of the PCR-amplified DNA. These techniques include single-strand conformation polymorphism, ribonuclease protection, and denaturing gel electrophoresis.

Genetic Counseling

All children with germinal retinoblastoma (bilateral disease, or unilateral disease with a positive family history) or suspected germinal tumor (unilateral disease with multiple tumors and age <18 months) should be referred for genetic counseling. As germinal retinoblastoma is a genetic disease, it is most important that the family as well as the comprehensive care team (generally, ophthalmologist and retina specialist, pediatric hematologist/oncologist, radiation oncologist, and social worker), understand the implications of the germinal state. First and foremost is confirmation of the germinal state via mutation analysis of peripheral blood leukocytes and/or tumor tissue. Children with germinal retinoblastoma have a lifelong risk of second (or higher order) nonocular malignancies, a risk which is about 1% per year following a latency period of about 4 years from diagnosis of intraocular tumor [6, 66]. These nonocular tumors include pineal and suprasellar tumors ("trilateral retinoblastoma," Fig. 12.3) in the first decade of life, osteogenic sarcoma and other sarcomas in the second decade, and melanomas in the third and fourth. In developed countries, such nonocular tumors pose a greater

Fig. 12.3 "Trilateral retinoblastoma": Suprasellar tumor in a
5-month-old with bilateral
retinoblastoma

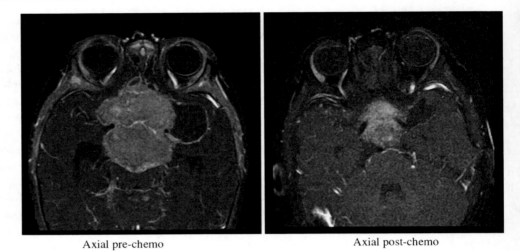

Axial pre-chemo   Axial post-chemo

risk to life than does the primary retinoblastoma itself
[6, 67]. Such children require aggressive diagnostic workup
of any change in mental status, or any persistent localized
pain, swelling, or limp.

Next in importance is assessment of risk of tumor development in siblings and other family members. The professional providing counseling, which preferably should be a
geneticist but may in special situations also be an ophthalmologist or pediatric oncologist with special experience in
retinoblastoma, should be able to (a) explain the genetic
nature of retinoblastoma, (b) evaluate individual risk based
on clinical features of the index case as well as family history, (c) present the availability and limitations of molecular testing, (d) assist the family in interpreting the test
results, and (e) discuss with the family other options for
having children, including adoption [53]. It must be kept in
mind, on the other hand, that the existence of genetic mosaicism [39, 68], low-penetrance retinoblastoma [69–71], and
variable expressivity in retinoblastoma [71] can complicate
risk assessments.

Finally, there are syndromes that include retinoblastoma
such as the 13q14 deletion syndrome (approximately 5% of
germinal retinoblastoma) in which mental retardation is
common, as are somatic abnormalities [72]. These somatic
abnormalities include microcephaly and failure-to-thrive
(Fig. 12.2), broad prominent nasal bridge, hypertelorism,
microophthalmos, epicanthal folds, ptosis, protruding
upper incisors, micrognathia, short neck with lateral folds,
low set ears, imperforate anus or perineal fistula, hypoplas-
tic or absent thumbs, cleft palate, and supernumary digits
or toes (Fig. 12.4). Rarely, identification of dysmorphic
features and the presence of psychomotor retardation in a
young child has preceded recognition of concomitant retinoblastoma [73].

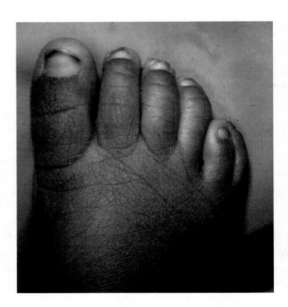

Fig. 12.4 Chromosome 13q14 deletion syndrome: Polydactyly

Summary of Retinoblastoma

The Knudson hypothesis has become today a widely
accepted, useful, and elegant conceptual model for tumor
development that has been applied to other tumors, including
Wilms tumor. Subsequent cloning and sequencing of the
RB1 gene has led to a remarkable understanding of the
structure and function of the RB1 gene and its protein
product, pRB. This understanding extends to the complex
regulation of transcription, translation, and post-translational
tumor-suppressor function. Today, we are able to detect specific
pathogenic mutations in RB1 and use knowledge of these

mutations in genetic diagnosis of retinoblastoma. As we become more skillful in correlating the results of mutation analyses with retinoblastoma phenotypes, we should be able better to predict risk of tumor development, offer more reliable genetic counseling, and even one day develop mutation-specific approaches to treatment.

Wilms' Tumor

Introduction

Wilms' tumor is a relatively common childhood tumor whose complex genetics have fascinated geneticists and oncologists for many decades [74]. Few other cancers have given as many insights into cancer genetics and epigenetics as well as the relationship between development and tumorigenesis. In this section, we review what is known about the causes and origins of Wilms' tumor and how the study of the genetics of this tumor has shed light on the pathogenesis of this disease and how genetic testing can predict the risk of disease development in certain subgroups of individuals.

Clinical Features

Epidemiology

Wilms' tumor, also known as nephroblastoma, is the most common malignant renal tumor in children. It affects 1 in 10,000 children and accounts for 6% of all childhood tumors with about 460 new cases diagnosed each year in the United States. Among ethnic groups, rates of Wilms' tumor are highest among blacks and lowest in East Asian populations including Asian-Americans [75, 76]. There is a peak incidence between 2 and 5 years of age and 95% of cases are diagnosed by 10 years of age [77]. Rates are slightly higher in females (male to female ratio 0.89:1) [78], and patients with bilateral tumors are twice as likely to be female [79]. High birth weight has been associated with an increased risk of Wilms' tumor [80, 81]. Advanced paternal age has been inconsistently associated with an increased risk of Wilms' tumor [81, 82]. Several environmental factors have been linked to Wilms' tumor including household pesticides, paternal exposures to pesticides and metals, and maternal hormone exposures. Inconsistencies in exposure assessment and lack of reproducibility have prevented firm conclusions [81, 83–85], but environmental exposures are thought not to play a major role in the etiology of Wilms' tumor [79].

Clinical Presentation

Wilms' tumor most commonly presents as an asymptomatic abdominal mass in an otherwise well appearing child. However, up to one third of patients can present with abdominal pain, vomiting, anorexia, or malaise. Those with abdominal pain are more likely to have unfavorable histology, a higher stage and subcapsular hemorrhage or tumor rupture [86]. Uncommonly, Wilms' tumor can present with features of an acute abdomen [86]. Hematuria, fever or hypertension can also be seen, the latter in up to 55% of patients and associated with elevated plasma rennin concentrations [87]. In most cases, routine blood tests including a complete blood count and differential, serum chemistries, liver function tests, and renal function tests are normal. Wilms' tumor is associated with a number of clinical anomalies including hemihypertrophy, genitourinary tract malformations, and aniridia [88]. One detailed study in the UK found congenital anomalies in 45% of patients with Wilms' tumor who underwent a detailed clinical evaluation [89]. These anomalies may be isolated, but a variety of clinical syndromes as described later in this chapter are associated with Wilms' tumor.

Diagnosis

An abdominal ultrasound is often the first radiographic study performed to evaluate an abdominal mass. This study can often determine the origin and extent of the tumor, invasion of associated structures, and importantly in the case of Wilms' tumor, whether the tumor has invaded the renal vein or extended into the inferior vena cava. A contrast computed tomography (CT) scan of the abdomen is usually performed to better evaluate the tumor (Fig. 12.5) and the opposite kidney and either a CXR or more commonly a CT scan of the chest is

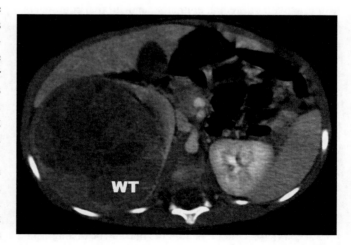

Fig. 12.5 Wilms' tumor (WT) as visualized by computerized tomography

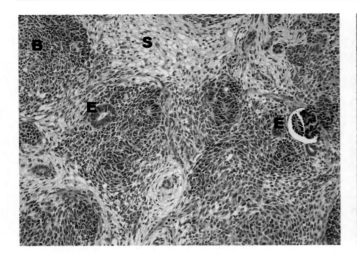

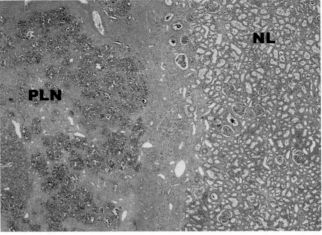

Fig. 12.6 Favorable Histology Wilms' tumor. This tumor displays a classic triphasic histology with blastemal (B), stromal (S), and epithelial (E) features. Epithelial components include tubule (*left*) and pseudoglomerular (*right*) elements. Photomicrograph provided by Dr. Kamran Badizadegan, James Homer Wright Pathology Laboratories, Massachusetts General Hospital, Boston, MA, 20×

Fig. 12.7 Perilobar Nephroblastomatosis. This section was taken from a child with extensive bilateral perilobar nephrogenic rests (PLN) and shows normal kidney (NL) on the right. Photomicrograph provided by Dr. Kamran Badizadegan, James Homer Wright Pathology Laboratories, Massachusetts General Hospital, Boston, MA, 4×

also performed, since the lung and liver are the most common sites of distant metastatic disease. Neuroblastoma, may invade the kidney and appear radiographically similar to Wilms' tumor but can usually be distinguished from Wilms' tumor by the presence of calcifications, encasement of major vessels, and often invasion of neural foramina [90]. Most Wilms' tumors present as solitary lesions, but 12% have multifocal disease in a single kidney and 6% have bilateral disease [91].

Histology

Most Wilms' tumor exhibits typical triphasic ("favorable") histology with blastemal, epithelial, and stromal components (Fig. 12.6). Undifferentiated blastemal cells are small basophilic cells with little cytoplasm. Epithelial components tend to form rosettes, tubules, or pseudo-glomeruli; while stromal components include primarily collagenous fibrous tissue, or striated and smooth muscle but can also include bone, cartilage, and fat cells. The presence of anaplasia (large hyperchromatic nuclei and irregular mitotic figures), is associated with adverse outcome, although focal anaplasia has a better prognosis when compared with diffuse anaplasia [92]. Mutations in tumor protein 53 (TP53) are rarely found in favorable histology Wilms' tumor, but are found in 75% of Wilms' tumor with anaplasia [93]. In Wilms' tumor with focal anaplasia, TP53 mutations are confined to foci of anaplastic cells [94]. Other renal tumors that can be distinguished histologically from Wilms' tumor include congenital mesoblastic nephroma, rhabdoid tumors, and clear cell sarcoma of the kidney [95]. Similar to neuroblastoma, Wilms' tumor is

thought to arise from persistent clusters of relatively undifferentiated embryonic mesenchymal cells, termed nephrogenic rests (NR) in the case of Wilms' tumor (Fig. 12.7), which may persist for variable periods after birth. These NRs have been incidentally found on autopsy in about 1% of neonates [96], but most undergo sclerosis and involution, and are normally rarely seen after 3 months of age [96]. When diffuse throughout the kidney or in multiple sites this condition is termed nephroblastomatosis and can be confused with Wilms' tumor [97]. The limited persistence of these primitive mesenchymal rests may explain why neuroblastoma and Wilms' tumors are almost exclusively malignancies of childhood.

Sporadic Versus Hereditary Wilms' Tumor

Hereditary Wilms' tumor is rare. The National Wilms' Tumor Study (NWTS) documented a positive family history in only 1.5% of 6,209 patients [98]. Those with a family history were more likely to present with bilateral disease (16.1% as compared with 7.1% of sporadic cases) and at an earlier age. The mean age at diagnosis of bilateral disease with familial Wilms' tumor was 15.8 as compared to 32 months for sporadic bilateral disease. Similarly, unilateral disease in familial cases occurred earlier as compared with unilateral sporadic cases (35.2 vs. 44.7 months). Familial cases were slightly more likely to present with higher stage disease, but after adjusting for stage, there was no difference in the relapse rate or overall survival as compared with sporadic cases. Familial cases of Wilms' tumor can appear in the context of syndromes such as Beckwith-Wiedemann and aniridia.

Such patients accounted for 17.2% of the familial case as compared with 7.8% of sporadic Wilms' tumor patients. Most familial cases involved multiple affected siblings with very few instances of direct parent-to-child transmission. This could reflect gonadal mosaicism in one of the parents [98, 99]. Alternatively, this could reflect noninherited epigenetic processes, or even decreased fertility from germline mutations in Wilms' tumor genes affecting genitourinary development [74]. The relative lack of parent-to-child transmission has been postulated to reflect the poor survivability of Wilms' tumor up until recently [98, 99]. However, one study of 179 offspring of 96 long-term survivors of Wilms' tumor found no instance of Wilms' tumor [100]. Thus, the risk to offspring of sporadic unilateral Wilms' tumor patients is extremely low.

The earlier occurrence of bilateral disease was encompassed in Knudson "two-hit" hypothesis originally proposed for retinoblastoma and extended to Wilms' tumor [12, 101]. In this hypothesis, all individuals with bilateral disease carry one germline mutation and require a single postnatal hit for cancer to develop, as compared with unilateral cases in which two hits must develop in somatic cells with cancer developing at a later age [101]. This hypothesis has served as a framework for understanding the pathogenesis of childhood malignancies and presaged the discovery of tumor suppressor genes. However, Wilms' tumor has turned out to be quite a bit more complex than predicted by this model with the discovery of multiple predisposing genes as well as epigenetic forms of gene regulation. The Knudson hypothesis does not explain why only a minority (16.1%) of familial cases are bilateral or why familial bilateral cases occur at such a younger age as compared with familial unilateral cases or bilateral cases without a family history [98]. The epidemiologic features suggest that somatic mosaicism, rather than a germline mutation, may be responsible for some of the bilateral and multicentric cases [79].

Genetics, Genotype/Phenotype Correlations

The pathogenesis of Wilms' tumor involves a complex interaction of genetic mutations and epigenetic alterations that are slowly beginning to be understood.

The *WT1* Gene

The *WT1* tumor suppressor gene on chromosome 11p13 was the first Wilms' tumor gene to be identified. The WT1 gene is a zinc finger transcription factor essential for renal development [102]. Ten to fifteen percent of sporadic Wilms' tumor possess a variety of inactivating point mutations and deletions of the *WT1* gene [103, 104] that often affect both alleles [104, 105]. *WT1* was identified from studies of patients with dele-

tions of the 11p14-p12 chromosomal region who manifest an association of Wilms' tumor, Aniridia, Genitourinary malformations, and mental Retardation, now known as WAGR syndrome [106, 107]. The genitourinary abnormalities include cryptorchidism, hypospadius, and ambiguous genitalia, renal hypoplasia, ureteral hypoplasia, streak ovaries or a bicornate uterus [107]. The deletion interval is varied in size but includes the *PAX6* gene, responsible for aniridia, and the *WT1* gene, whose loss contributes both to Wilms' tumor as well as genitourinary abnormalities. About 30–57% of individuals with WAGR syndrome develop Wilms' tumor [88, 107]. The risk of developing chronic renal failure at 20 years from diagnosis may be as high as 53% [108]. The etiology of the mental retardation seen in 70% is unclear, but a variety of other nonclassical abnormalities seen in patients with this syndrome may be caused by deletions of a variable number of flanking genes in this contiguous gene deletion syndrome [109]. While deletion of a single allele of *WT1* is responsible for the genitourinary abnormalities in the WAGR syndrome, heterozygous germline missense mutations in the zinc finger region of WT1 disrupting DNA binding and creating a potential dominant negative WT1 protein are associated with more severe phenotype seen in the Deny-Drash syndrome characterized by severe genitourinary abnormalities including intersex disorders such as gonadal dysgenesis with male pseudohermaphroditism (normal female external genitalia, streak gonads and XY karyotype), renal mesangial sclerosis with early kidney failure, and a very high rate (90%) of Wilms' tumor [110]. A third syndrome associated with *WT1* mutations is Frasier syndrome. Frasier syndrome is caused by intronic point mutations that disrupt alternative splicing of exon 9 and reduce synthesis of the usually more abundant +KTS isoform of *WT1* [111]. This syndrome is similarly characterized by male pseudo-hermaphroditism and progressive glomerulopathy leading to end-stage renal failure in adolescence of early childhood, but does not carry an increased risk of Wilms' tumor [111, 112].

About 75% of Wilms' tumors with *WT1* mutations also harbor activating mutations in the *CTNNB1* gene encoding β-catenin [113]. Such *CTNNB1* mutations are largely confined to Wilms' tumors with *WT1* mutations indicating a cooperative relationship between loss of *WT1* and activation of Wnt signaling.

Chromosome 11p15

A second distinct Wilms' tumor locus has been identified at 11p15. Characterization of this region has uncovered a complex locus containing several imprinted genes whose expression depends on the parent of origin. Altered imprinting of 11p15 can cause a somatic overgrowth syndrome known as Beckwith Wiedemann syndrome (BWS). This syndrome was localized to 11p15 from linkage of rare familial cases [114,

115] as well as rare individuals with cytogenetic abnormalities [116, 117]. Loss of heterozygosity (LOH) of 11p has been reported in 30% of Wilms' tumor but does not carry any prognostic significance [118]. BWS can include features of an enlarged tongue, hemihypertrophy, enlarged abdominal organs, namely liver and spleen, in some cases resulting in an umbilical hernia or more severe midline abdominal wall defects. In addition, these individuals may have islet cell hyperplasia at birth leading to severe hypoglycemia, and 7–10% develop malignancies, most commonly, Wilms' tumor but also hepatoblastoma, hemangiomas, or adrenocortical carcinoma [119, 120]. Analysis of this region provided the first evidence of imprinting in cancer. The predisposition to Wilms' tumor, as well as some of the overgrowth features of BWS, are felt to be caused by the upregulation of the *IGF2*

gene at 11p15. This gene, along with the nontranslated antisense RNA *LIT1/KCNQ1OT1* located within the *KCNQ1* gene, is normally expressed exclusively from the paternal allele. The *H19* gene, which encodes an untranslated RNA transcript with tumor suppressor-like activities [121], along with the *CDKN1C/p57^{KIP2}* gene, is normally expressed from the maternal allele. In BWS, several imprinting abnormalities can be seen including unipaternal disomy, as well as loss of imprinting of *IGF2* or *LIT1* (Fig. 12.8). The imprinting pattern appears to be controlled by two distinct differentially methylated regions (DMRs) [122]. Loss of imprinting of these loci can be caused by abnormal methylation or microdeletions of one of these imprinting control elements [123]. Unipaternal disomy has been found in 10% of individuals with Beckwith-Wiedemann [124]. Molecular abnormalities

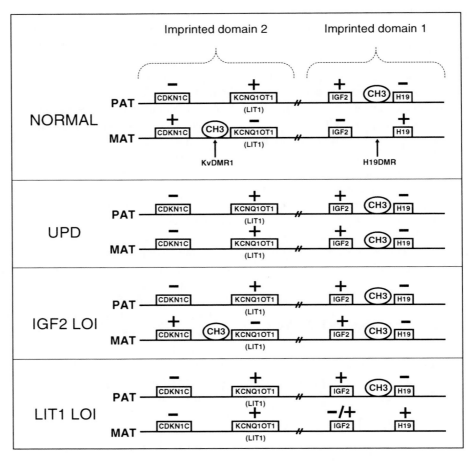

Fig. 12.8 Diagram of the imprinted 11p15 locus and examples of different patterns of expression and imprinting defects seen in BWS adapted from Weksberg et al. [127]. There are two imprinted domains in this region each controlled by a distinct differentially methylated region (DMR). On the normal paternal allele the KvDMR1 is unmethylated with expression of KCNQ1OT1/LIT1 and repression of the CDKN1/p57^{KIP2}, while the H19DMR is methylated (CH3) with repression of H19 expression and permitting IGF2 expression. These patterns are reversed on the maternal allele. In the case of unipaternal disomy (UPD) the maternal allele is replaced by a second paternal allele with biallelic expression of IGF2 and repression of H19. This pattern of expression is also seen with loss of imprinting of IGF2 (IGF2 LOI), although in this case there is normal expression of CDKN1C/p57^{KIP2} and LIT1. In the case of loss of imprinting of LIT1 (LIT1 LOI), there is hypomethylation and increased expression of LIT1 with repression of CDKN1C/p57^{KIP2}, and variable IGF2 LOI but normal methylation and repression of H19

of 11p15 have been demonstrated in 70% of individuals with BWS [125]. Of these mutations 8% had mutations in *CDKN1C*, 58% hypomethylation of KvDMR1, 7% hypermethylation of H19DMR, and 27% had uniparental disomy (UPD) [126]. Hypomethylation of LIT1 in the KvDMR1 imprinting center is a common diagnostic test for BWS [127, 128]. Molecular abnormalities of 11p15 have been found in 3% of sporadic Wilms' tumors and 12% of bilateral cases [122]. Mutations in *CDKN1C/p57(KIP2)* gene found in a minority of individuals with BWS [129], have not been found in sporadic Wilms' tumors. About 15% of BWS cases are familial, and over 40% of these families have been found to carry germline *CDKN1C* mutations as compared to 4–5% of sporadic cases [129, 130]. There is an association of isolated hemihypertrophy and UPD [131]. The highest risk of developing Wilms' tumor risk is in the presence of hypermethylation of the H19DMR imprinting center and UPD, both of which are characterized by biallelic expression of *IGF2*. In contrast, those with hypomethylation of KvDMR1 appear to have a quite low risk of Wilms' tumor development [122, 123, 126, 132], but a higher risk of hepatoblastomas, rhabdomyosarcomas, and gonadoblastoma [133].

There is accruing evidence that assisted reproductive technologies may be associated with a slight increase in imprinting disorders such as BWS, although the absolute risk is still extremely small [134]. So far, there have been no studies showing an increase in the risk of Wilms' tumor with assisted reproductive technology, although this is currently being studied through the Children's Oncology Group.

Chromosomes 1p and 16q

A third Wilms' tumor locus has been mapped by LOH studies to 16q [135]. Fluorescence in situ hybridization combined with allelic analyses has detected both hemizygous deletions of 16q as well as apparent UPD [136]. In contrast to 11p15, there is no evidence of paternal or maternal bias for the lost 16q chromosome [135]. Unbalanced translocations involving 16q and resulting in partial monosomy of 16q are also recurring cytogenetic abnormalities seen in Wilms' tumor. A common translocation partner in these cases is the long arm of chromosome 1, 1q with the generation of der(16)t(1q;16q) [137, 138]. A similar translocation is seen in numerous other tumor types. Chromosome 1q is also involved in unbalanced translocations with 9q, 17p and 21p resulting in partial 1q trisomy in Wilms' tumor [139]. LOH of 16q has been found in 14.6–20% of Wilms' tumor [140, 141]. It has a higher incidence in anaplastic histology Wilms' (32.4%) as compared to favorable histology (17.4%) [141]. LOH of 1p has been reported in 10–15% of Wilms' tumor [140, 141], with a similar incidence in anaplastic and favorable histology Wilms' tumor. The simultaneous LOH

of both 16q and 1p has been found in 2.6–4.6% of Wilms' tumor [140, 141], and this has been shown to have adverse prognostic significance in favorable histology but not anaplastic Wilms' tumor [141]. The presence of allelic loss of both 1p and 16q reduced the 4 year event free survival rate of patients with Stage IV (primarily patients with lung metastases) favorable histology Wilms' tumor from 83 to 66%. The unbalanced der(16q)t(1q:16q) observed in Wilms' tumor could potentially account for 16q and 1p LOH if there was isodisomy for 1p (scored as LOH) from a duplication and subsequent nondisjunction of the normal chromosome 1, along with trisomy 1q and monosomy 16q [141].

Chromosome 7p

LOH of 7p14 was identified in 12 of 73 Wilms' tumors, and mapping studies narrowed the commonly deleted region to 390 kb [142, 143]. A putative tumor suppressor gene, *POU6F2*, was the only expressed gene identified in this region and two germline nucleotide substitutions, not detected in controls were identified in this gene in two Wilms' tumor patients whose tumor DNA exhibited loss of the constitutionally wild-type allele. Based on these findings and the detected expression in fetal and adult kidney, it was suggested that this gene was a tumor suppressor gene involved in hereditary predisposition to Wilms' tumor [142].

The WTX Gene

A genome-wide search for somatic deletions in Wilms' tumor using array comparative genomic hybridization led to the identification of a third Wilms' tumor gene, *WTX*, or "Wilms' Tumor Gene on the X chromosome." This study identified inactivation mutations, either small deletions or point mutations, in 30% (15 of 51) of examined tumors [144]. Several addition studies verified functional inactivation of the *WTX* gene in Wilms' tumor, albeit at a lower frequency (7–18%) [145, 146]. The *WTX* gene has a similar temporal pattern of expression in the developing kidney, as the *WT1* gene. They are both expressed in the pluripotent condensing metanephric mesenchyme, the presumed precursors of Wilms' tumor [144]. WTX has been shown to complex with beta-catenin, AXIN, beta-TrCP2, and APC to promote beta-catenin ubiquitination and degradation. Thus, the loss of *WTX* can result in activation of WNT/beta-catenin signaling [147]. *CTNNB1* mutations frequently accompany *WT1* mutations but are not seen in conjunction with *WTX* mutations [144]. Apparently *WTX* loss can cause a similar activation of the Wnt pathway by itself. This indicates a major involvement of activation of the Wnt/beta-catenin pathway in the pathogenesis of Wilms' tumor.

Despite the potential involvement of this pathway in other tumors, mutations in *WTX* were not seen in leukemia, gastric, colorectal, and hepatocellular carcinomas [148–151]. Identification of the *WTX* gene as a putative tumor suppressor gene on the X chromosome provided the first potential example of a single hit inactivation of a tumor suppressor gene, in contrast to the biallelic Knudson model [101]. Mutations in females preferentially involved the active X-chromosome in this study, although this was apparently not the case in a second study [145]. The lower than expected tumor development from a gene requiring a single hit in males was presumed due to the limited developmental period of competency for tumorigenesis of the target cell population [144]. Interestingly, germline mutations of *WTX* can cause an X-linked sclerosing bone dysplasia known as osteopathia striate congenital with cranial sclerosis. These individuals do not have any tumor predisposition [152].

Familial Wilms' Tumor Loci

About 2% of individuals with Wilms' tumor have a family history of Wilms' tumor. None of these rare cases of nonsyndromic familial Wilms' tumor map to the *WT1* gene on 11p13, the 11p15 BWS locus, or to *WTX*. One such familial Wilms' tumor predisposition gene, FWT1, was mapped to 17q21-q21 in two unrelated families, each with 7 cases of Wilms' tumor [153, 154]. FWT1 does not appear to be a tumor suppressor gene as the average onset is about 1 year later compared with sporadic Wilms' tumor and these tumors are predominately unilateral [153, 155]. A second familial Wilms' tumor locus, FWT2, has been mapped to 19q13.4 in five families [156]. There are other familial Wilms' tumor predisposition genes to be identified as several families do not map to either of these two loci [157]. Biallelic mutations in the *BRCA2* gene at 13q12.3 are responsible for Fanconi Anemia subgroup D1. While heterozygote mutations are associated with a risk of ovarian and breast cancer, biallelic mutations predispose to a high risk of solid tumors including brain tumors, leukemia, and perhaps as high as a 20% chance of developing Wilms' tumor [158–160].

Other Syndromes Associated with Wilms' Tumor

Wilms' tumor is also seen with increased frequency in several other overgrowth syndromes besides BWS [120]. Simpson-Golabi-Behmel syndrome is associated with pre and postnatal overgrowth, coarse facial features, cardiac defects, renal dysplasia, skeletal abnormalities, and in some families mental retardation and has been mapped to chromosome Xq26 [161, 162]. Mutations in the glypican 3 (*GPC3*) gene have been described in the majority of individuals with this syndrome [163] who have higher incidence (at least 10%), of not only Wilms' tumor, but also hepatoblastoma and other intra-abdominal tumors [120, 164]. The *GPC3* gene is apparently not involved in sporadic Wilms' [165]. Perlman syndrome, a presumed autosomal recessive condition whose molecular basis is not known, is characterized by macrosomia, polyhydramnios, visceromegaly, generalized hypotonia, cryptorchidism as well as an approximate 30% risk of developing Wilms' tumor [166]. Perlman syndrome is associated with a high infant mortality, for those surviving beyond the neonatal period the incidence of Wilms' tumor in one study was 64% [167]. Sotos syndrome is also considered among the overgrowth syndromes with features of macrocephaly, tall stature, typical facial features, and developmental delay [168]. This syndrome, caused by mutations and deletions of the *NSD1* histone methyltransferase, is associated with an approximate 2–3% risk of various malignancies, rarely Wilms' tumor, but more commonly acute leukemias and lymphomas [120, 169].

Wilms' tumor has also been reported in relatively high frequency among individuals with mosaic variegated aneuploidy syndrome. This syndrome presents with severe intrauterine growth retardation, macrocephaly, variable developmental delay, and a high risk of malignancies including Wilms' tumor, rhabdomyosarcoma, and leukemia. This appears to be caused by premature sister chromatid separation resulting in constitutional mosaic aneuploidy which, in many cases, is due to biallelic mutations in the BUB1B mitotic spindle checkpoint gene [170]. A low risk of Wilms' tumor has been reported in association with other tumor predisposition syndromes including Bloom syndrome and Li Fraumeni syndrome, as well as Trisomies 13 and 18 and constitutional deletions of chromosome 2q37 [159].

Management of Wilms' Tumor

Treatment for Wilms' tumor in the United States has evolved over sequential clinical trials of the National Wilms' Tumor Study Group (NWTSG), the first pediatric intergroup clinical research unit in North America. These trials transformed what was once a highly lethal disease, with cure rates of 10–40% in the mid 1960s, to one of the most curable types of cancer, with current survival rates for most patients with favorable histology of greater than 90% [171]. Treatment generally entails nephrectomy and chemotherapy with abdominal and pulmonary radiation added for more advance disease. The NWTSG incorporated into the Children's Oncology Group (COG) has focused their efforts on further reducing the toxicity of treatment for favorable histology Wilms' tumor, using genetic features such as 1p and 16q LOH to stratify treatments, and finding new strategies for the treatment of unfavorable histology or anaplastic Wilms' tumor.

Management Implications

Role for Genetic Testing

In the presence of specific syndromal features directed germline genetic testing may be performed to help verify the diagnosis, but is not otherwise generally indicated for routine management of Wilms' tumor. An exception might be considered in children who have a close family member with young onset breast or ovarian cancer or those with a known family history of *BRCA2* gene mutations. As mentioned above, evaluation of the tumor for 1p and 16q LOH does appear to have prognostic significance and is currently being used in the U.S. for treatment stratification of subgroups of patients enrolled in clinical trials.

Wilms' Tumor Screening

Routine radiographic screening to improve outcome has been recommended for groups at high risk for the development of Wilms' tumor. Patients registered on National Wilms' Tumor Studies who had undergone such screening were more likely to have low stage disease [172]. Although prospective studies showing such screenings improve survival are lacking, these screenings can allow the detection of smaller tumors avoiding toxicities of treating advanced stage disease and permitting partial nephrectomy in individuals at risk for metachronous and bilateral disease [173–175]. Screenings may potentially avoid the removal of an entire kidney in BWS patients at risk for reflux nephropathy or medullary sponge kidney, conditions that might eventually affect their renal function [176].

Groups with a risk for Wilms' tumor of >5% have been recommended to undergo these screenings. This includes individuals with Beckwith Wiedemann syndrome, idiopathic hemihypertrophy (IHH), WAGR, aniridia, Denys-Drash, Perlman Syndrome, and Simpson-Golabi-Behmel as well as members of some familial Wilms' tumor pedigrees. Routine screening has been recommended for these individuals with serial abdominal ultrasounds every 3 months until 7–8 years of age. These ultrasounds are best evaluated by radiologists experienced in the evaluation of children with referral to pediatric oncologists for further evaluation. In addition, serial serum alpha fetoprotein monitoring every 6 weeks for the first 4 years of life has also been recommended in BWS and IHH to detect early hepatoblastoma [176]. This period of monitoring covers the periods of highest risk as 90% of Wilms' tumor have been diagnosed by age 7 [174] and 90% of hepatoblastomas by age

4 [177]. Genetic testing can modify the risks of individuals within these groups. For example, in Beckwith-Wiedemann Syndrome hypomethylation of KvDMR1 appears to confer a lower risk of Wilms' tumor development in contrast to the higher rate seen with hypermethylation of the H19DMR imprinting center [122, 123, 126, 132]. It has been proposed to limit screening for this latter group; however, Wilms' tumor has been seen, albeit with a much lower frequency, in those with hypomethylation of KvDMR1 and these individuals appear to have a relatively higher risk of other tumors, including hepatoblastomas, rhabdomyosarcomas, and gonadoblastoma [133]. Similarly, there is evidence to suggest only those individuals with isolated aniridia that have deletions of the WT1 gene are at risk for the development of Wilms' tumor [178], and it appears that only individuals with Simpson-Golabi-Behmel with mutations in the GPC3 gene are at risk for Wilms' tumor [120].

Screening of all individuals with IHH for Wilms' tumor has been criticized because there is no consensus on diagnostic criteria and the distinction from normal variation in limb length and wide is not clear [159]. Indeed, hemihypertrophy was only diagnosed before Wilms' tumor diagnosis less than 50% of the time [172, 179], thus, the overall risk of Wilms' tumor in IHH is less than 5%. Screening of only those individuals with isolated hemihypertrophy who have abnormalities of 11p15 has been suggested [180]; however, these changes are often not present in IHH individuals with Wilms' tumor [181].

These screenings are not without cost, including discomfort and inconvenience, as well as the likelihood of finding nonmalignant lesions requiring further evaluations and the potential for unnecessary surgery. Individuals with BWS are more likely to have nephrogenic rests; however, with careful image interpretation these may be distinguishable from Wilms' tumor by distinctive characteristics on MRI [182]. Individuals with BWS also have a higher risk of nonmalignant renal abnormalities including complicated renal cysts, caliceal diverticula, hydronephrosis, nephroblastomatosis, and nephrolithiasis that have in rare cases resulted in unnecessary nephrectomies [176, 183]. The risks and benefits of screening an individual at risk and the length of screening must be weighed by each parent and physician after appropriate counseling.

Long-Term Side Effects

The relatively high cure rates for Wilms' tumor in the last two decades have allowed assessment of complications into adulthood. Wilms' tumor survivors in general appear to have fewer and less severe late effects compared to most other childhood cancer survivors [184]. However, survivors of Wilms' tumor are at increased risk for complications from secondary malignancies, cardiomyopathy, pulmonary fibrosis, reproductive problems, and renal failure that can compromise the quality of life and can lead to increased mortality [185]. The long-term side effects are related to the type and amount of therapy given. The late effects of treating low stage disease with vincristine and dactinomycin are quite low. However, individuals receiving whole lung irradiation experience demonstrable decrease in total lung capacity and vital capacity although clinically significant long-term pulmonary complications, including pulmonary fibrosis, are rare [186]. Female survivors of Wilms' tumor are at increased risk of reproductive problems including decreased fertility, prematurity, decreased birth weight, and congenital malformations in their offspring [187, 188]. Some of these problems including fetal malformations appear due to uterine constraints perhaps due to radiation fibrosis, while some birth defects are within the spectrum of defects associated with Wilms' tumor and might represent inheritance of Wilms' tumor associated mutations or imprinting [188]. Interestingly, there does not seem to be an increase in the risk of birth defects in the children of male Wilms' tumor survivors [188]. A major aim of current protocols is to reduce the toxicities wherever possible.

Summary of Wilms' Tumor

The study of Wilms' tumor has yielded remarkable insights into the links between development and cancer. Wilms' tumor, together with retinoblastoma, and neuroblastoma, was used by Knudsen over 35 years ago in one of the first models for understanding the epidemiology of childhood cancer. His work helped explain the relationship between hereditary and sporadic cancers and a mechanism for penetrance in hereditary cancer. The role of abnormal imprinting in cancer was first described in Wilms' tumor. Advancements in our treatment of Wilms' tumor represent one of the major successes in oncology with cure rates for most individual in excess of 85%. However, much still remains to be done to stratify patients requiring less toxic therapies to reduce the risk of long-term complications while still maintaining high cure rates. In addition, new treatment schemes are needed for those patients with high-risk disease. The recent discovery of the WTX gene and further understanding of the genetic pathways leading to the development of Wilms' tumor will hopefully lead to additional targets for drug development.

References

1. Devesa SS (1975) The incidence of retinoblastoma. Am J Ophthalmol 80(2):263–265
2. Francois J, Matton MT, De Bie S, Tanaka Y, Vandenbulcke D (1975) Genesis and genetics of retinoblastoma. Ophthalmologica 170(5):405–425
3. Mahoney MC, Burnett WS, Majerovics A, Tanenbaum H (1990) The epidemiology of ophthalmic malignancies in New York State. Ophthalmology 97(9):1143–1147
4. Vogel F (1979) Genetics of retinoblastoma. Hum Genet 52(1):1–54
5. Abramson DH, Ellsworth RM, Grumbach N, Kitchin FD (1985) Retinoblastoma: survival, age at detection and comparison 1914–1958, 1958–1983. J Pediatr Ophthalmol Strabismus 22(6):246–250
6. Abramson DH (1999) Second nonocular cancers in retinoblastoma: a unified hypothesis. The Franceschetti Lecture. Ophthalmic Genet 20(3):193–204
7. Grabowski EF, Abramson DH (1987) Intraocular and extraocular retinoblastoma. Hematol Oncol Clin North Am 1(4):721–735
8. Zimmerman LE, Burns RP, Wankum G, Tully R, Esterly JA (1982) Trilateral retinoblastoma: ectopic intracranial retinoblastoma associated with bilateral retinoblastoma. J Pediatr Ophthalmol Strabismus 19(6):320–325
9. Grabowski EF (2006) Intraocular and extraocular retinoblastoma. In: Burg FD, Polin RA, Ingelfinger JR, Wald ER (eds) Current pediatric therapy, 18th edn. WB Saunders Co, Philadelphia, pp 1101–1105
10. Friend SH, Bernards R, Rogelj S et al (1986) A human DNA segment with properties of the gene that predisposes to retinoblastoma and osteosarcoma. Nature 323(6089):643–646
11. Mukai S (1993) Molecular genetic diagnosis of retinoblastoma. Informa Healthcare 8:292–299
12. Knudson AG Jr (1971) Mutation and cancer: statistical study of retinoblastoma. Proc Natl Acad Sci USA 68(4):820–823
13. Fung YK, Murphree AL, T'Ang A, Qian J, Hinrichs SH, Benedict WF (1987) Structural evidence for the authenticity of the human retinoblastoma gene. Science 236(4809):1657–1661
14. Lee WH, Bookstein R, Hong F, Young LJ, Shew JY, Lee EY (1987) Human retinoblastoma susceptibility gene: cloning, identification, and sequence. Science 235(4794):1394–1399
15. Klutz M, Horsthemke B, Lohmann DR (1999) RB1 gene mutations in peripheral blood DNA of patients with isolated unilateral retinoblastoma. Am J Hum Genet 64(2):667–668
16. Lohmann DR, Gerick M, Brandt B et al (1997) Constitutional RB1-gene mutations in patients with isolated unilateral retinoblastoma. Am J Hum Genet 61(2):282–294
17. Shimizu T, Toguchida J, Kato MV, Kaneko A, Ishizaki K, Sasaki MS (1994) Detection of mutations of the RB1 gene in retinoblastoma patients by using exon-by-exon PCR-SSCP analysis. Am J Hum Genet 54(5):793–800
18. De Falco G, Giordano A (2006) pRb2/p130: a new candidate for retinoblastoma tumor formation. Oncogene 25(38):5333–5340
19. Toguchida J, McGee TL, Paterson JC et al (1993) Complete genomic sequence of the human retinoblastoma susceptibility gene. Genomics 17(3):535–543
20. DeCaprio JA, Ludlow JW, Figge J et al (1988) SV40 large tumor antigen forms a specific complex with the product of the retinoblastoma susceptibility gene. Cell 54(2):275–283
21. Dyson N, Howley PM, Munger K, Harlow E (1989) The human papilloma virus-16 E7 oncoprotein is able to bind to the retinoblastoma gene product. Science 243(4893):934–937
22. Whyte P, Buchkovich KJ, Horowitz JM et al (1988) Association between an oncogene and an anti-oncogene: the adenovirus E1A proteins bind to the retinoblastoma gene product. Nature 334(6178):124–129
23. Lee JO, Russo AA, Pavletich NP (1998) Structure of the retinoblastoma tumour-suppressor pocket domain bound to a peptide from HPV E7. Nature 391(6670):859–865
24. Bremner R, Du DC, Connolly-Wilson MJ et al (1997) Deletion of RB exons 24 and 25 causes low-penetrance retinoblastoma. Am J Hum Genet 61(3):556–570

25. Shen WJ, Kim HS, Tsai SY (1995) Stimulation of human insulin receptor gene expression by retinoblastoma gene product. J Biol Chem 270(35):20525–20529

26. Dyson N (1998) The regulation of E2F by pRB-family proteins. Genes Dev 12(15):2245–2262

27. Harbour JW, Dean DC (2000) Rb function in cell-cycle regulation and apoptosis. Nat Cell Biol 2(4):E65–E67

28. Chen PL, Scully P, Shew JY, Wang JY, Lee WH (1989) Phosphorylation of the retinoblastoma gene product is modulated during the cell cycle and cellular differentiation. Cell 58(6):1193–1198

29. Stein GH, Beeson M, Gordon L (1990) Failure to phosphorylate the retinoblastoma gene product in senescent human fibroblasts. Science 249(4969):666–669

30. Chow KN, Dean DC (1996) Domains A and B in the Rb pocket interact to form a transcriptional repressor motif. Mol Cell Biol 16(9):4862–4868

31. Weintraub SJ, Chow KN, Luo RX, Zhang SH, He S, Dean DC (1995) Mechanism of active transcriptional repression by the retinoblastoma protein. Nature 375(6534):812–815

32. Nielsen SJ, Schneider R, Bauer UM et al (2001) Rb targets histone H3 methylation and HP1 to promoters. Nature 412(6846):561–565

33. Brehm A, Miska EA, McCance DJ, Reid JL, Bannister AJ, Kouzarides T (1998) Retinoblastoma protein recruits histone deacetylase to repress transcription. Nature 391(6667):597–601

34. Luo RX, Postigo AA, Dean DC (1998) Rb interacts with histone deacetylase to repress transcription. Cell 92(4):463–473

35. Magnaghi-Jaulin L, Groisman R, Naguibneva I et al (1998) Retinoblastoma protein represses transcription by recruiting a histone deacetylase. Nature 391(6667):601–605

36. Lohmann DR, Gallie BL (2004) Retinoblastoma: revisiting the model prototype of inherited cancer. Am J Med Genet C Semin Med Genet 129C(1):23–28

37. Lohmann DR (1999) RB1 gene mutations in retinoblastoma. Hum Mutat 14(4):283–288

38. Frischmeyer PA, Dietz HC (1999) Nonsense-mediated mRNA decay in health and disease. Hum Mol Genet 8(10):1893–1900

39. Sippel KC, Fraioli RE, Smith GD et al (1998) Frequency of somatic and germ-line mosaicism in retinoblastoma: implications for genetic counseling. Am J Hum Genet 62(3):610–619

40. Boerkoel CF, Exelbert R, Nicastri C et al (1995) Leaky splicing mutation in the acid maltase gene is associated with delayed onset of glycogenosis type II. Am J Hum Genet 56(4):887–897

41. Otterson GA, Chen W, Coxon AB, Khleif SN, Kaye FJ (1997) Incomplete penetrance of familial retinoblastoma linked to germ-line mutations that result in partial loss of RB function. Proc Natl Acad Sci USA 94(22):12036–12040

42. Dryja TP, Rapaport J, McGee TL, Nork TM, Schwartz TL (1993) Molecular etiology of low-penetrance retinoblastoma in two pedigrees. Am J Hum Genet 52(6):1122–1128

43. Windle JJ, Albert DM, O'Brien JM et al (1990) Retinoblastoma in transgenic mice. Nature 343(6259):665–669

44. Howes KA, Ransom N, Papermaster DS, Lasudry JG, Albert DM, Windle JJ (1994) Apoptosis or retinoblastoma: alternative fates of photoreceptors expressing the HPV-16 E7 gene in the presence or absence of p53. Genes Dev 8(11):1300–1310

45. Robanus-Maandag E, Dekker M, van der Valk M et al (1998) p107 is a suppressor of retinoblastoma development in pRb-deficient mice. Genes Dev 12(11):1599–1609

46. Laurie NA, Donovan SL, Shih CS et al (2006) Inactivation of the p53 pathway in retinoblastoma. Nature 444(7115):61–66

47. Hahn WC, Weinberg RA (2002) Modelling the molecular circuitry of cancer. Nat Rev Cancer 2(5):331–341

48. Sherr CJ, McCormick F (2002) The RB and p53 pathways in cancer. Cancer Cell 2(2):103–112

49. Vogelstein B, Kinzler KW (2004) Cancer genes and the pathways they control. Nat Med 10(8):789–799

50. Kato MV, Shimizu T, Ishizaki K et al (1996) Loss of heterozygosity on chromosome 17 and mutation of the p53 gene in retinoblastoma. Cancer Lett 106(1):75–82

51. Nork TM, Poulsen GL, Millecchia LL, Jantz RG, Nickells RW (1997) p53 regulates apoptosis in human retinoblastoma. Arch Ophthalmol 115(2):213–219

52. Chen D, Livne-bar I, Vanderluit JL, Slack RS, Agochiya M, Bremner R (2004) Cell-specific effects of RB or RB/p107 loss on retinal development implicate an intrinsically death-resistant cell-of-origin in retinoblastoma. Cancer Cell 5(6):539–551

53. Mukai S (2009) Retinoblastoma. In: Orkin SH, Fisher DE, Look AT, Lux S, Ginsburg D, Nathan DG (eds) Oncology of infancy and childhood, WB Saunders Co, Philadelphia

54. Halloran SL, Boughman JA, Dryja TP et al (1985) Accuracy of detection of the retinoblastoma gene by esterase D linkage. Arch Ophthalmol 103(9):1329–1331

55. Mukai S, Rapaport JM, Shields JA, Augsburger JJ, Dryja TP (1984) Linkage of genes for human esterase D and hereditary retinoblastoma. Am J Ophthalmol 97(6):681–685

56. Sparkes RS, Murphree AL, Lingua RW et al (1983) Gene for hereditary retinoblastoma assigned to human chromosome 13 by linkage to esterase D. Science 219(4587):971–973

57. Botstein D, White RL, Skolnick M, Davis RW (1980) Construction of a genetic linkage map in man using restriction fragment length polymorphisms. Am J Hum Genet 32(3):314–331

58. Cavenee WK, Dryja TP, Phillips RA et al (1983) Expression of recessive alleles by chromosomal mechanisms in retinoblastoma. Nature 305(5937):779–784

59. Dryja TP, Cavenee W, White R et al (1984) Homozygosity of chromosome 13 in retinoblastoma. N Engl J Med 310(9):550–553

60. Bookstein R, Lee EY, To H et al (1988) Human retinoblastoma susceptibility gene: genomic organization and analysis of heterozygous intragenic deletion mutants. Proc Natl Acad Sci USA 85(7):2210–2214

61. Dunn JM, Phillips RA, Becker AJ, Gallie BL (1988) Identification of germline and somatic mutations affecting the retinoblastoma gene. Science 241(4874):1797–1800

62. Horsthemke B, Barnert HJ, Greger V, Passarge E, Hopping W (1987) Early diagnosis in hereditary retinoblastoma by detection of molecular deletions at gene locus. Lancet 1(8531):511–512

63. Wiggs J, Nordenskjold M, Yandell D et al (1988) Prediction of the risk of hereditary retinoblastoma, using DNA polymorphisms within the retinoblastoma gene. N Engl J Med 318(3):151–157

64. Yandell DW, Campbell TA, Dayton SH et al (1989) Oncogenic point mutations in the human retinoblastoma gene: their application to genetic counseling. N Engl J Med 321(25):1689–1695

65. Yandell DW, Dryja TP (1989) Detection of DNA sequence polymorphisms by enzymatic amplification and direct genomic sequencing. Am J Hum Genet 45(4):547–555

66. Kleinerman RA, Tucker MA, Tarone RE et al (2005) Risk of new cancers after radiotherapy in long-term survivors of retinoblastoma: an extended follow-up. J Clin Oncol 23(10):2272–2279

67. Abramson DH (1985) Treatment of retinoblastoma. In: Blodi FC (ed) Contemporary issues in ophthalmology, vol. 2, retinoblastoma. Churchill Livingston, New York, pp 88–93

68. Munier FL, Thonney F, Girardet A et al (1998) Evidence of somatic and germinal mosaicism in pseudo-low-penetrant hereditary retinoblastoma, by constitutional and single-sperm mutation analysis. Am J Hum Genet 63(6):1903–1908

69. Connolly MJ, Payne RH, Johnson G et al (1983) Familial, EsD-linked, retinoblastoma with reduced penetrance and variable expressivity. Hum Genet 65(2):122–124

70. Macklin MT (1960) A study of retinoblastoma in Ohio. Am J Hum Genet 12:1–43

71. Strong LC, Riccardi VM, Ferrell RE, Sparkes RS (1981) Familial retinoblastoma and chromosome 13 deletion transmitted via an insertional translocation. Science 213(4515):1501–1503

72. Alldderdice PW, Davis JG, Miller OJ et al (1969) The 13q-deletion syndrome. Am J Hum Genet 21(5):499–512

73. Seidman DJ, Shields JA, Augsburger JJ, Nelson LB, Lee ML, Sciorra LJ (1987) Early diagnosis of retinoblastoma based on dysmorphic features and karyotype analysis. Ophthalmology 94(6): 663–666

74. Rivera MN, Haber DA (2005) Wilms' tumour: connecting tumorigenesis and organ development in the kidney. Nat Rev Cancer 5(9):699–712

75. Breslow N, Olshan A, Beckwith JB, Moksness J, Feigl P, Green D (1994) Ethnic variation in the incidence, diagnosis, prognosis, and follow-up of children with Wilms' tumor. J Natl Cancer Inst 86(1):49–51

76. Stiller CA, Parkin DM (1990) International variations in the incidence of childhood renal tumours. Br J Cancer 62(6):1026–1030

77. National Cancer Institute (2004) Surveillance epidemiology and end results (SEER) pediatric monograph, National Cancer Institute, Bethesda, MD

78. Pastore G, Carli M, Lemerle J et al (1988) Epidemiological features of Wilms' tumor: results of studies by the International Society of Paediatric Oncology (SIOP). Med Pediatr Oncol 16(1):7–11

79. Breslow N, Olshan A, Beckwith JB, Green DM (1993) Epidemiology of Wilms tumor. Med Pediatr Oncol 21(3):172–181

80. Daniels JL, Pan IJ, Olshan AF, Breslow NE, Bunin GR, Ross JA (2008) Obstetric history and birth characteristics and Wilms tumor: a report from the Children's Oncology Group. Cancer Causes Control 19(10):1103–1110

81. Schuz J, Kaletsch U, Meinert R, Kaatsch P, Michaelis J (2001) High-birth weight and other risk factors for Wilms tumour: results of a population-based case-control study. Eur J Pediatr 160(6): 333–338

82. Olson JM, Breslow NE, Beckwith JB (1993) Wilms' tumour and parental age: a report from the National Wilms' Tumour Study. Br J Cancer 67(4):813–818

83. Cooney MA, Daniels JL, Ross JA, Breslow NE, Pollock BH, Olshan AF (2007) Household pesticides and the risk of Wilms tumor. Environ Health Perspect 115(1):134–137

84. Goel R, Olshan AF, Ross JA, Breslow NE, Pollock BH (2009) Maternal exposure to medical radiation and Wilms tumor in the offspring: a report from the Children's Oncology Group. Cancer Causes Control 20(6):957–963

85. Jurewicz J, Hanke W (2006) Exposure to pesticides and childhood cancer risk: has there been any progress in epidemiological studies? Int J Occup Med Environ Health 19(3):152–169

86. Davidoff AM, Soutter AD, Shochat SJ (1998) Wilms tumor presenting with abdominal pain: a special subgroup of patients. Ann Surg Oncol 5(3):213–215

87. Maas MH, Cransberg K, van Grotel M, Pieters R, van den Heuvel-Eibrink MM (2007) Renin-induced hypertension in Wilms tumor patients. Pediatr Blood Cancer 48(5):500–503

88. Miller RW, Fraumeni JF Jr, Manning MD (1964) Association of Wilms's tumor with aniridia, hemihypertrophy and other congenital malformations. N Engl J Med 270:922–927

89. Ng A, Griffiths A, Cole T et al (2007) Congenital abnormalities and clinical features associated with Wilms' tumour: a comprehensive study from a centre serving a large population. Eur J Cancer 43(9):1422–1429

90. Dickson PV, Sims TL, Streck CJ et al (2008) Avoiding misdiagnosing neuroblastoma as Wilms tumor. J Pediatr Surg 43(6):1159–1163

91. Breslow N, Beckwith JB, Ciol M, Sharples K (1988) Age distribution of Wilms' tumor: report from the National Wilms' Tumor Study. Cancer Res 48(6):1653–1657

92. Dome JS, Cotton CA, Perlman EJ et al (2006) Treatment of anaplastic histology Wilms' tumor: results from the fifth National Wilms' Tumor Study. J Clin Oncol 24(15):2352–2358

93. Bardeesy N, Falkoff D, Petruzzi MJ et al (1994) Anaplastic Wilms' tumour, a subtype displaying poor prognosis, harbours p53 gene mutations. Nat Genet 7(1):91–97

94. Bardeesy N, Beckwith JB, Pelletier J (1995) Clonal expansion and attenuated apoptosis in Wilms' tumors are associated with p53 gene mutations. Cancer Res 55(2):215–219

95. Isaacs H Jr (2008) Fetal and neonatal renal tumors. J Pediatr Surg 43(9):1587–1595

96. Beckwith JB, Kiviat NB, Bonadio JF (1990) Nephrogenic rests, nephroblastomatosis, and the pathogenesis of Wilms' tumor. Pediatr Pathol 10(1–2):1–36

97. Beckwith JB (1993) Precursor lesions of Wilms tumor: clinical and biological implications. Med Pediatr Oncol 21(3):158–168

98. Breslow NE, Olson J, Moksness J, Beckwith JB, Grundy P (1996) Familial Wilms' tumor: a descriptive study. Med Pediatr Oncol 27(5):398–403

99. Knudson AG Jr, Strong LC (1975) Letter: Familial Wilms's tumor. Am J Hum Genet 27(6):809–810

100. Li FP, Williams WR, Gimbrere K, Flamant F, Green DM, Meadows AT (1988) Heritable fraction of unilateral Wilms tumor. Pediatrics 81(1):147–149

101. Knudson AG Jr, Strong LC (1972) Mutation and cancer: a model for Wilms' tumor of the kidney. J Natl Cancer Inst 48(2):313–324

102. Kreidberg JA, Sariola H, Loring JM et al (1993) WT-1 is required for early kidney development. Cell 74(4):679–691

103. Gessler M, Konig A, Arden K et al (1994) Infrequent mutation of the WT1 gene in 77 Wilms' Tumors. Hum Mutat 3(3):212–222

104. Varanasi R, Bardeesy N, Ghahremani M et al (1994) Fine structure analysis of the WT1 gene in sporadic Wilms tumors. Proc Natl Acad Sci USA 91(9):3554–3558

105. Ton CC, Huff V, Call KM et al (1991) Smallest region of overlap in Wilms tumor deletions uniquely implicates an 11p13 zinc finger gene as the disease locus. Genomics 10(1):293–297

106. Riccardi VM, Sujansky E, Smith AC, Francke U (1978) Chromosomal imbalance in the Aniridia-Wilms' tumor association: 11p interstitial deletion. Pediatrics 61(4):604–610

107. Fischbach BV, Trout KL, Lewis J, Luis CA, Sika M (2005) WAGR syndrome: a clinical review of 54 cases. Pediatrics 116(4): 984–988

108. Breslow NE, Norris R, Norkool PA et al (2003) Characteristics and outcomes of children with the Wilms tumor-Aniridia syndrome: a report from the National Wilms Tumor Study Group. J Clin Oncol 21(24):4579–4585

109. Xu S, Han JC, Morales A, Menzie CM, Williams K, Fan YS (2008) Characterization of 11p14-p12 deletion in WAGR syndrome by array CGH for identifying genes contributing to mental retardation and autism. Cytogenet Genome Res 122(2):181–187

110. Pelletier J, Bruening W, Kashtan CE et al (1991) Germline mutations in the Wilms' tumor suppressor gene are associated with abnormal urogenital development in Denys-Drash syndrome. Cell 67(2):437–447

111. Klamt B, Koziell A, Poulat F et al (1998) Frasier syndrome is caused by defective alternative splicing of WT1 leading to an altered ratio of WT1 +/−KTS splice isoforms. Hum Mol Genet 7(4):709–714

112. Barbaux S, Niaudet P, Gubler MC et al (1997) Donor splice-site mutations in WT1 are responsible for Frasier syndrome. Nat Genet 17(4):467–470

113. Li CM, Kim CE, Margolin AA et al (2004) CTNNB1 mutations and overexpression of Wnt/beta-catenin target genes in WT1-mutant Wilms' tumors. Am J Pathol 165(6):1943–1953

114. Koufos A, Grundy P, Morgan K et al (1989) Familial Wiedemann-Beckwith syndrome and a second Wilms tumor locus both map to 11p15.5. Am J Hum Genet 44(5):711–719

115. Ping AJ, Reeve AE, Law DJ, Young MR, Boehnke M, Feinberg AP (1989) Genetic linkage of Beckwith-Wiedemann syndrome to 11p15. Am J Hum Genet 44(5):720–723

116. Waziri M, Patil SR, Hanson JW, Bartley JA (1983) Abnormality of chromosome 11 in patients with features of Beckwith-Wiedemann syndrome. J Pediatr 102(6):873–876

117. Pueschel SM, Padre-Mendoza T (1984) Chromosome 11 and Beckwith-Wiedemann syndrome. J Pediatr 104(3):484–485

118. Grundy PE, Telzerow PE, Breslow N, Moksness J, Huff V, Paterson MC (1994) Loss of heterozygosity for chromosomes 16q and 1p in Wilms' tumors predicts an adverse outcome. Cancer Res 54(9):2331–2333

119. Wiedemann H-R (1983) Tumours and hemihypertrophy associated with Wiedemann-Beckwith syndrome (letter). Eur J Pediatr 141:129

120. Lapunzina P (2005) Risk of tumorigenesis in overgrowth syndromes: a comprehensive review. Am J Med Genet C Semin Med Genet 137C(1):53–71

121. Hao Y, Crenshaw T, Moulton T, Newcomb E, Tycko B (1993) Tumour-suppressor activity of H19 RNA. Nature 365(6448): 764–767

122. Scott RH, Douglas J, Baskcomb L et al (2008) Constitutional 11p15 abnormalities, including heritable imprinting center mutations, cause nonsyndromic Wilms tumor. Nat Genet 40(11): 1329–1334

123. Sparago A, Russo S, Cerrato F et al (2007) Mechanisms causing imprinting defects in familial Beckwith-Wiedemann syndrome with Wilms' tumour. Hum Mol Genet 16(3):254–264

124. Feinberg AP, Williams BR (2003) Wilms' tumor as a model for cancer biology. Methods Mol Biol 222:239–248

125. Cooper WN, Luharia A, Evans GA et al (2005) Molecular subtypes and phenotypic expression of Beckwith-Wiedemann syndrome. Eur J Hum Genet 13(9):1025–1032

126. Bliek J, Gicquel C, Maas S, Gaston V, Le Bouc Y, Mannens M (2004) Epigenotyping as a tool for the prediction of tumor risk and tumor type in patients with Beckwith-Wiedemann syndrome (BWS). J Pediatr 145(6):796–799

127. Weksberg R, Shuman C, Smith AC (2005) Beckwith-Wiedemann syndrome. Am J Med Genet C Semin Med Genet 137C(1):12–23

128. DeBaun MR, Niemitz EL, McNeil DE, Brandenburg SA, Lee MP, Feinberg AP (2002) Epigenetic alterations of H19 and LIT1 distinguish patients with Beckwith-Wiedemann syndrome with cancer and birth defects. Am J Hum Genet 70(3):604–611

129. Lam WW, Hatada I, Ohishi S et al (1999) Analysis of germline CDKN1C (p57KIP2) mutations in familial and sporadic Beckwith-Wiedemann syndrome (BWS) provides a novel genotype-phenotype correlation. J Med Genet 36(7):518–523

130. Lee MP, DeBaun M, Randhawa G, Reichard BA, Elledge SJ, Feinberg AP (1997) Low frequency of p57KIP2 mutation in Beckwith-Wiedemann syndrome. Am J Hum Genet 61(2):304–309

131. Shuman C, Smith AC, Steele L et al (2006) Constitutional UPD for chromosome 11p15 in individuals with isolated hemihyperplasia is associated with high tumor risk and occurs following assisted reproductive technologies. Am J Med Genet A 140(14): 1497–1503

132. Rump P, Zeegers MP, van Essen AJ (2005) Tumor risk in Beckwith-Wiedemann syndrome: a review and meta-analysis. Am J Med Genet A 136(1):95–104

133. Weksberg R, Nishikawa J, Caluseriu O et al (2001) Tumor development in the Beckwith-Wiedemann syndrome is associated with a variety of constitutional molecular 11p15 alterations including imprinting defects of KCNQ1OT1. Hum Mol Genet 10(26): 2989–3000

134. Manipalviratn S, DeCherney A, Segars J (2009) Imprinting disorders and assisted reproductive technology. Fertil Steril 91(2): 305–315

135. Maw MA, Grundy PE, Millow LJ et al (1992) A third Wilms' tumor locus on chromosome 16q. Cancer Res 52(11):3094–3098

136. Shearer PD, Valentine MB, Grundy P et al (1999) Hemizygous deletions of chromosome band 16q24 in Wilms tumor: detection by fluorescence in situ hybridization. Cancer Genet Cytogenet 115(2):100–105

137. Sheng WW, Soukup S, Bove K, Gotwals B, Lampkin B (1990) Chromosome analysis of 31 Wilms' tumors. Cancer Res 50(9):2786–2793

138. Kondo K, Chilcote RR, Maurer HS, Rowley JD (1984) Chromosome abnormalities in tumor cells from patients with sporadic Wilms' tumor. Cancer Res 44(11):5376–5381

139. Betts DR, Ilg EC, Oezahin H, von der Weid N, Niggli FK (1999) Trisomy 1q generating translocations in Wilms tumor. Cancer Genet Cytogenet 112(2):138–143

140. Messahel B, Williams R, Ridolfi A et al (2009) Allele loss at 16q defines poorer prognosis Wilms tumour irrespective of treatment approach in the UKW1-3 clinical trials: a Children's Cancer and Leukaemia Group (CCLG) Study. Eur J Cancer 45(5):819–826

141. Grundy PE, Breslow NE, Li S et al (2005) Loss of heterozygosity for chromosomes 1p and 16q is an adverse prognostic factor in favorable-histology Wilms tumor: a report from the National Wilms Tumor Study Group. J Clin Oncol 23(29):7312–7321

142. Perotti D, De Vecchi G, Testi MA et al (2004) Germline mutations of the POU6F2 gene in Wilms tumors with loss of heterozygosity on chromosome 7p14. Hum Mutat 24(5):400–407

143. Perotti D, Testi MA, Mondini P et al (2001) Refinement within single yeast artificial chromosome clones of a minimal region commonly deleted on the short arm of chromosome 7 in Wilms tumours. Genes Chromosomes Cancer 31(1):42–47

144. Rivera MN, Kim WJ, Wells J et al (2007) An X chromosome gene, WTX, is commonly inactivated in Wilms tumor. Science 315(5812):642–645

145. Perotti D, Gamba B, Sardella M et al (2008) Functional inactivation of the WTX gene is not a frequent event in Wilms' tumors. Oncogene 27(33):4625–4632

146. Ruteshouser EC, Robinson SM, Huff V (2008) Wilms tumor genetics: mutations in WT1, WTX, and CTNNB1 account for only about one-third of tumors. Genes Chromosomes Cancer 47(6):461–470

147. Major MB, Camp ND, Berndt JD et al (2007) Wilms tumor suppressor WTX negatively regulates WNT/beta-catenin signaling. Science 316(5827):1043–1046

148. Chung NG, Kim MS, Chung YJ, Yoo NJ, Lee SH (2008) Tumor suppressor WTX gene mutation is rare in acute leukemias. Leuk Lymphoma 49(8):1616–1617

149. Yoo NJ, Kim S, Lee SH (2009) Mutational analysis of WTX gene in Wnt/ beta-catenin pathway in gastric, colorectal, and hepatocellular carcinomas. Dig Dis Sci 54(5):1011–1014

150. Owen C, Virappane P, Alikian M et al (2008) WTX is rarely mutated in acute myeloid leukemia. Haematologica 93(6):947–948

151. Virappane P, Gale R, Hills R et al (2008) Mutation of the Wilms' tumor 1 gene is a poor prognostic factor associated with chemotherapy resistance in normal karyotype acute myeloid leukemia: the United Kingdom Medical Research Council Adult Leukaemia Working Party. J Clin Oncol 26(33):5429–5435

152. Jenkins ZA, van Kogelenberg M, Morgan T et al (2009) Germline mutations in WTX cause a sclerosing skeletal dysplasia but do not predispose to tumorigenesis. Nat Genet 41(1):95–100

153. Rahman N, Arbour L, Tonin P et al (1996) Evidence for a familial Wilms' tumour gene (FWT1) on chromosome 17q12-q21. Nat Genet 13(4):461–463

154. Rahman N, Abidi F, Ford D et al (1998) Confirmation of FWT1 as a Wilms' tumour susceptibility gene and phenotypic characteristics of Wilms' tumour attributable to FWT1. Hum Genet 103(5):547–556

155. Rahman N, Arbour L, Tonin P et al (1997) The familial Wilms' tumour susceptibility gene, FWT1, may not be a tumour suppressor gene. Oncogene 14(25):3099–3102

156. McDonald JM, Douglass EC, Fisher R et al (1998) Linkage of familial Wilms' tumor predisposition to chromosome 19 and a two-locus model for the etiology of familial tumors. Cancer Res 58(7):1387–1390

157. Huff V, Amos CI, Douglass EC et al (1997) Evidence for genetic heterogeneity in familial Wilms' tumor. Cancer Res 57(10): 1859–1862

158. Hirsch B, Shimamura A, Moreau L et al (2004) Association of biallelic BRCA2/FANCD1 mutations with spontaneous chromosomal instability and solid tumors of childhood. Blood 103(7):2554–2559

159. Scott RH, Stiller CA, Walker L, Rahman N (2006) Syndromes and constitutional chromosomal abnormalities associated with Wilms tumour. J Med Genet 43(9):705–715

160. Reid S, Renwick A, Seal S et al (2005) Biallelic BRCA2 mutations are associated with multiple malignancies in childhood including familial Wilms tumour. J Med Genet 42(2):147–151

161. Xuan JY, Besner A, Ireland M, Hughes-Benzie RM, MacKenzie AE (1994) Mapping of Simpson-Golabi-Behmel syndrome to Xq25-q27. Hum Mol Genet 3(1):133–137

162. Neri G, Gurrieri F, Zanni G, Lin A (1998) Clinical and molecular aspects of the Simpson-Golabi-Behmel syndrome. Am J Med Genet 79(4):279–283

163. Pilia G, Hughes-Benzie RM, MacKenzie A et al (1996) Mutations in GPC3, a glypican gene, cause the Simpson-Golabi-Behmel overgrowth syndrome. Nat Genet 12(3):241–247

164. Lapunzina P, Badia I, Galoppo C et al (1998) A patient with Simpson-Golabi-Behmel syndrome and hepatocellular carcinoma. J Med Genet 35(2):153–156

165. Gillan TL, Hughes R, Godbout R, Grundy PE (2003) The Simpson-Golabi-Behmel gene, GPC3, is not involved in sporadic Wilms tumorigenesis. Am J Med Genet A 122A(1):30–36

166. Henneveld HT, van Lingen RA, Hamel BC, Stolte-Dijkstra I, van Essen AJ (1999) Perlman syndrome: four additional cases and review. Am J Med Genet 86(5):439–446

167. Alessandri JL, Cuillier F, Ramful D et al (2008) Perlman syndrome: report, prenatal findings and review. Am J Med Genet A 146A(19):2532–2537

168. Leventopoulos G, Kitsiou-Tzeli S, Kritikos K et al (2009) A clinical study of sotos syndrome patients with review of the literature. Pediatr Neurol 40(5):357–364

169. Tatton-Brown K, Rahman N (2007) Sotos syndrome. Eur J Hum Genet 15(3):264–271

170. Hanks S, Coleman K, Reid S et al (2004) Constitutional aneuploidy and cancer predisposition caused by biallelic mutations in BUB1B. Nat Genet 36(11):1159–1161

171. D'Angio GJ (2007) The National Wilms Tumor Study: a 40 year perspective. Lifetime Data Anal 13(4):463–470

172. Green DM, Breslow NE, Beckwith JB, Norkool P (1993) Screening of children with hemihypertrophy, aniridia, and Beckwith-Wiedemann syndrome in patients with Wilms tumor: a report from the National Wilms Tumor Study. Med Pediatr Oncol 21(3):188–192

173. McNeil DE, Langer JC, Choyke P, DeBaun MR (2002) Feasibility of partial nephrectomy for Wilms' tumor in children with Beckwith-Wiedemann syndrome who have been screened with abdominal ultrasonography. J Pediatr Surg 37(1):57–60

174. Beckwith JB (1998) Children at increased risk for Wilms tumor: monitoring issues. J Pediatr 132(3 Pt 1):377–379

175. Coppes MJ, Arnold M, Beckwith JB et al (1999) Factors affecting the risk of contralateral Wilms tumor development: a report from the National Wilms Tumor Study Group. Cancer 85(7): 1616–1625

176. Choyke PL, Siegel MJ, Craft AW, Green DM, DeBaun MR (1999) Screening for Wilms tumor in children with Beckwith-Wiedemann syndrome or idiopathic hemihypertrophy. Med Pediatr Oncol 32(3):196–200

177. Surveillance, Epidemiology, and End Results (SEER) Program (2001) Public Use Data (1973–1998), National Cancer Institute, DCCPS, Surveillance Research Program, Cancer Statistics Branch, Bethesda, MD

178. Gronskov K, Olsen JH, Sand A et al (2001) Population-based risk estimates of Wilms tumor in sporadic aniridia. A comprehensive mutation screening procedure of PAX6 identifies 80% of mutations in aniridia. Hum Genet 109(1):11–18

179. Craft AW, Parker L, Stiller C, Cole M (1995) Screening for Wilms' tumour in patients with aniridia, Beckwith syndrome, or hemihypertrophy. Med Pediatr Oncol 24(4):231–234

180. Scott RH, Walker L, Olsen OE et al (2006) Surveillance for Wilms tumour in at-risk children: pragmatic recommendations for best practice. Arch Dis Child 91(12):995–999

181. Niemitz EL, Feinberg AP, Brandenburg SA, Grundy PE, DeBaun MR (2005) Children with idiopathic hemihypertrophy and beckwith-wiedemann syndrome have different constitutional epigenotypes associated with wilms tumor. Am J Hum Genet 77(5): 887–891

182. Gylys-Morin V, Hoffer FA, Kozakewich H, Shamberger RC (1993) Wilms tumor and nephroblastomatosis: imaging characteristics at gadolinium-enhanced MR imaging. Radiology 188(2):517–521

183. Choyke PL, Siegel MJ, Oz O, Sotelo-Avila C, DeBaun MR (1998) Nonmalignant renal disease in pediatric patients with Beckwith-Wiedemann syndrome. AJR Am J Roentgenol 171(3):733–737

184. Han JW, Kwon SY, Won SC, Shin YJ, Ko JH, Lyu CJ (2009) Comprehensive clinical follow-up of late effects in childhood cancer survivors shows the need for early and well-timed intervention. Ann Oncol 20(7):1170–1177

185. Cotton CA, Peterson S, Norkool PA, Takashima J, Grigoriev Y, Breslow NE (2009) Early and late mortality after diagnosis of Wilms' tumor. J Clin Oncol 27(8):1304–1309

186. Shaw NJ, Eden OB, Jenney ME et al (1991) Pulmonary function in survivors of Wilms' tumor. Pediatr Hematol Oncol 8(2):131–137

187. Green DM, Peabody EM, Nan B, Peterson S, Kalapurakal JA, Breslow NE (2002) Pregnancy outcome after treatment for Wilms tumor: a report from the National Wilms Tumor Study Group. J Clin Oncol 20(10):2506–2513

188. Byrne J, Mulvihill JJ, Connelly RR et al (1988) Reproductive problems and birth defects in survivors of Wilms' tumor and their relatives. Med Pediatr Oncol 16(4):233–240

Chapter 13
Neurofibromatosis and Schwannomatosis

Miriam J. Smith and Scott R. Plotkin

Keywords Neurofibromatosis • Schwannomatosis • NF1 • NF2 • Neurofibroma • Café-au-lait spot • Mosaicism • Schwannoma

Introduction

Neurofibromatosis type 1 (NF1), NF2, and schwannomatosis constitute a group of related tumor suppressor syndromes unified by the predisposition to nerve sheath tumors. These patients harbor germline inactivating mutations in tumor suppressor genes ("first-hit") and develop tumors when tissues acquire a second somatic mutation in the remaining allele ("second-hit"). Despite the overlap between these disorders, there are many differences in the phenotype and management of these patients. This chapter reviews the clinical and genetic aspects of these related disorders.

Neurofibromatosis 1

Clinical Features and Diagnostic Criteria

Neurofibromatosis type 1 (NF1), previously known as von Recklinghausen's disease or peripheral neurofibromatosis, is the most common neurogenetic disorder with a birth prevalence of 1 in 3,000 [1]. NF1 is a tumor suppressor syndrome with multisystem involvement. The disorder is characterized by the age-dependent development of dermatologic, neurologic, and skeletal manifestations. NF1 is transmitted in an autosomal dominant fashion with full penetrance. Thus, the risk of NF1 in each offspring of an affected parent is 50%.

Importantly, NF1 shows extreme phenotypic variability, even within families. Siblings with the same mutation may develop different clinical manifestations, and parents with mild symptoms can have children with severe expression of the disease (and vice versa). The *NF1* gene has a high rate of mutation and roughly 50% of patients encountered in the clinic are founders, with new germline mutations and clinically unaffected parents.

The diagnostic criteria developed by the NIH Consensus Conference in 1987 and updated in 1997 (Table 13.1) determined that two or more of the following clinical features confirms a diagnosis of NF1: six or more café-au-lait macules greater than 1.5 cm in postpubertal individuals, or greater than 0.5 cm in prepubertal individuals; two or more neurofibromas or one plexiform neurofibroma; freckling in the axillary or inguinal regions; optic pathway glioma; two or more Lisch nodules of the iris; a distinctive bony lesion such as sphenoid dysplasia or thinning of the long bone cortex; or a first-degree relative with NF1 [2, 3]. By age 2, 50% of individuals with NF1 will fulfill diagnostic criteria; by age 8, this number increases to 97%, and by age 20, essentially all patients with classic NF1 meet diagnostic criteria [4].

Tumor Manifestations

The hallmark tumor of NF1 is the neurofibroma, a benign tumor derived from the nerve sheath. Neurofibromas contain multiple cell types, including Schwann cells, perineurial fibroblasts, and mast cells, embedded in extracellular matrix and collagen. Unlike schwannomas, which grow eccentrically to the nerves and are usually well encapsulated, neurofibromas grow within the nerve bundle and do not usually have a surrounding capsule. By puberty, more than 80% of NF1 patients develop neurofibromas [4, 5]. Neurofibromas may be cutaneous, subcutaneous, or deep in location. Cutaneous tumors increase in number with age and may cause psychological distress, although their potential for malignant transformation is nil.

Plexiform neurofibromas are a subset of neurofibromas affecting multiple nerve fascicles, often taking the gross

S.R. Plotkin (✉)
Department of Neurology and Cancer Center,
Massachusetts General Hospital, Boston, MA, USA
e-mail: splotkin@partners.org

Table 13.1 Diagnostic criteria for NF1, NF2 and schwannomatosis

NF1	NF2	Definite schwannomatosis
Two or more of the following: • ≥6 Café-au-lait macules >1.5 cm in postpubertal individuals, OR >0.5 cm in prepubertal individuals • ≥2 Neurofibromas OR one plexiform neurofibroma • Freckling in the axillary or inguinal regions • Optic glioma • ≥2 Lisch nodules • Distinctive bony lesion such as sphenoid dysplasia OR thinning of the long bone cortex • A first-degree relative with NF1	• The presence of bilateral vestibular schwannomas OR a family history of NF2 AND • Either a unilateral vestibular schwannoma or any two of the following tumors: schwannoma, meningioma, neurofibroma, glioma, juvenile posterior subcapsular lenticular opacity	• Age >30 years AND • ≥2 Nonintradermal schwannomas, at least 1 with histologic confirmation AND • No evidence of vestibular tumor on high-quality MRI scan AND • No known constitutional NF2 mutation OR one pathologically confirmed nonvestibular schwannoma plus a first-degree relative who meets above criteria

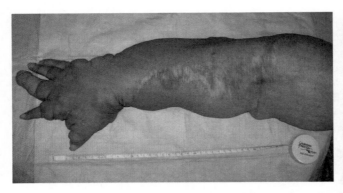
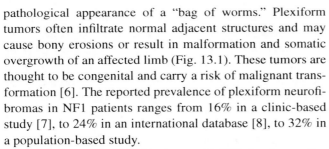

Fig. 13.1 Photograph of the arm of an NF1 patients affected by plexiform neurofibroma. Note the tissue overgrowth that may occur in the setting of this infiltrative tumor

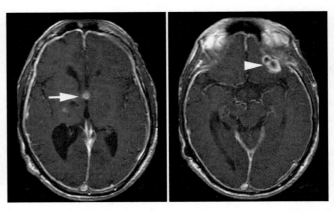

Fig. 13.2 Postcontrast axial T1-weighted image of an NF1 patient with multiple non-optic gliomas. The patient has a low grade glioma (*arrow*) and biopsy-proven glioblastoma (*arrowhead*)

pathological appearance of a "bag of worms." Plexiform tumors often infiltrate normal adjacent structures and may cause bony erosions or result in malformation and somatic overgrowth of an affected limb (Fig. 13.1). These tumors are thought to be congenital and carry a risk of malignant transformation [6]. The reported prevalence of plexiform neurofibromas in NF1 patients ranges from 16% in a clinic-based study [7], to 24% in an international database [8], to 32% in a population-based study.

Approximately 10% of patients with NF1 develop malignant peripheral nerve sheath tumors (MPNST) during their lifetime [9, 10]. Patients with internal plexiform neurofibromas are 20 times more likely to develop MPNSTs than those without, supporting the theory that they can arise from existing plexiform neurofibromas [11]. The overall survival for patients with MPNSTs is poor with 5-year survival rates ranging from 21 to 32% [9, 12].

Around 15% of patients demonstrate radiographic evidence of lesions in the optic nerve, chiasm, or tract consistent with optic pathway glioma [4]. These lesions usually appear during childhood and, in most cases, are not progressive [3]. Symptomatic optic glioma occurs in approximately 4% of patients. Nonoptic gliomas also occur at increased frequency in patients with NF1 [13]. Low-grade tumors involving the brainstem or cortex are the most common [14], but

high-grade tumors such as glioblastomas are also encountered (Fig. 13.2) [5, 15].

NF1 is associated with an increased risk of other tumors, including gastrointestinal stromal tumors, pheochromocytomas, and myeloproliferative diseases. Schwannomas are rarely, if ever, seen in NF1 patients: if a schwannoma is found by an experienced pathologist, this should prompt reevaluation of the diagnosis.

Non-tumor Manifestations

Café-au-lait spots are flat, uniformly hyperpigmented macules, which may also be found in unaffected individuals. They are usually present at birth, but may increase in number, size, and conspicuousness until puberty; in some persons, they may be better visualized using an ultraviolet or Wood's lamp. Lisch nodules are found in more than 70% of patients and usually appear around puberty. These melanocytic hamartomas occur on the iris and may be useful for diagnosing NF1, but do not cause any ophthalmologic symptoms [3]. Learning disability with or without attention-deficit disorder is present in one-third to two-thirds of patients, mental retardation in 4–8% of patients, and seizure disorder in about 5% of patients [16, 17]. In this population, there appears to be a higher incidence of psychiatric manifestations, such as depression, anxiety, personality disorder, or schizophrenia. Peripheral neuropathy is rare in NF1. Other nontumorous manifestations include headache, vasculopathy, osseous dysplasias, pseudoarthrosis, disorders of growth and development (most commonly short stature and precocious or delayed puberty), and hypertension.

Genetics and Molecular Biology

The *NF1* gene is found on chromosome 17q11.2. It covers approximately 335 kilobases of genomic DNA and contains 57 constitutive exons [18]. A germline mutation in the *NF1* gene can be identified in more than 95% of classically affected individuals [19]. The demonstration of a second somatic *NF1* mutation in NF1-related tumors has been technically difficult. A complicating factor in mutational analyses of these benign tumors is their heterogeneous pathological composition. The mixed cell population suggests that *NF1* acts as a tumor suppressor in a single cell, which then recruits other wild-type elements into the tumor. Supporting this hypothesis, loss of *NF1* in Schwann cells alone has been shown to be sufficient to generate tumors in mice [20]. When tissue culture is used to separate the Schwann cell and fibroblast components of benign tumors, loss of *NF1* can be demonstrated in the Schwann cells but not in the fibroblasts [21]. Similarly, loss of *NF1* can be demonstrated in melanocytes isolated from café-au-lait macules of NF1 patients [22].

Thus far, no particular mutation hot spot has been identified in the *NF1* gene and most unrelated patients carry distinct mutations, including nonsense (~37%), splice-site (~28%), frameshift (~18%), and missense mutations (~9%) [19]. Despite intense investigation, few discrete genotype–phenotype relationships have been described. Deletion of the entire gene is associated with a more severe phenotype. Specifically, patients with large deletions have fewer cutaneous neurofibromas, but higher degrees of dysmorphism and increased rates of mental retardation and MPNST compared with NF1 patients in general [23, 24]. It is not yet clear whether this phenotype is due to the deletion of flanking elements, or to the influence of other intragenic factors. In addition, absence of cutaneous neurofibromas has been associated with a 3-bp in-frame deletion in exon 17 of the *NF1* gene [25].

Mosaic NF1 is caused by postzygotic mutation of the *NF1* gene [26]. The clinical phenotype depends on the timing of the mutation and the cell types affected. Mutations occurring early in development will lead to a mild, generalized form of NF1, similar to patients with an inherited mutation. Mutations occurring at a later stage of development, in a more specialized

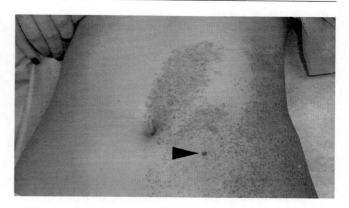

Fig. 13.3 Photograph of a patient with segmental NF1 showed anatomically limited freckling and a cutaneous neurofibroma (*arrowhead*). Segmental disease is a manifestation of genetic mosaicism and is caused by postzygotic mutation of the *NF1* gene

cell type lead to segmental disease, localized to one region, quadrant or half of the body (Fig. 13.3). Loss of *NF1* in Schwann cells causes the formation of neurofibromas, whereas loss of *NF1* in melanocytes leads to the development of café-au-lait macules [26].

Gonadal mosaicism occurs when only the gametes are affected. This is rare and can only be diagnosed when clinically unaffected parents have 2 or more affected offspring [27]. It is important to be able to identify mosaic forms of the disease as the risk of transmitting the affected gene is lower than the 50% chance of transmission in those with an inherited germline mutation.

The most common product of the *NF1* gene is a 2,818 amino acid protein, neurofibromin, which has a GTPase-activating protein (GAP) domain that negatively regulates the proto-oncogene Ras. There are many splice variants of *NF1*, not associated with disease [28]. In addition, intron 27 of the *NF1* gene contains 3 smaller genes including the oligodendrocyte myelin glycoprotein gene (*OMGP*), and *EV12A* and *EV12B* genes, whose functions are unknown. These three genes are all transcribed in the opposite orientation to the *NF1* [29]. Loss of function mutations of the *NF1* gene are associated with increased Ras activity and with the occurrence of benign and malignant tumors in neural crest-derived tissues [30]. The mammalian target of the rapamycin (mTOR) pathway is aberrantly activated in both *NF1*-deficient primary cells and in human tumors [31, 32], and its activation is mediated by the phosphorylation and inactivation of the TSC2-encoded protein, tuberin. *NF1* gene inactivation in mouse neural stem cells results in neural stem cell proliferation and survival of morphologically abnormal, immature astroglial cells in vitro, whereas, in vivo, it increases the numbers of astroglial progenitors and proliferating cells in both embryonic and adult brains. Both aberrant survival advantage and differentiation are rescued by expression of the Ras-GTPase activating protein domain of neurofibromin [33].

Genetic Testing

At the present time, genetic testing is not used to confirm a clinical diagnosis of NF1. The role of genetic testing in individuals with some features of NF1 but who do not meet criteria is controversial. Some clinicians recommend genetic testing for children with multiple café-au-lait macules and clinically unaffected parents while other clinicians monitor these patients clinically. In contrast, genetic testing is appropriate for affected individuals who wish to receive prenatal diagnosis or preimplantation genetic diagnosis (PGD). A germline mutation can be identified in more than 95% of classically affected individuals [19], and this can be useful for genetic counseling. If a causative mutation can be identified through genetic testing, molecular probes can be generated to assist in screening of potential offspring. Prenatal diagnosis is typically performed at 11–14 weeks gestation on samples acquired through amniocentesis or chorionic villus sampling. PGD is performed on single blastomeres, obtained from 3-day-old in vitro fertilization embryos and is used as an alternative to therapeutic termination of pregnancy after prenatal diagnosis. Multiplex polymerase chain reaction (PCR) of microsatellite markers in the *NF1* region have been developed to screen blastomeres from the IVF embryos, so that only embryos without the affected gene are transferred to the mother [34].

Management of Patients with NF1

Initial evaluation of a patient with known or suspected NF1 requires a detailed developmental history, review of growth charts in children, and family history of all first degree relatives. Physical examination should include measurements of growth and blood pressure, detailed skin inspection using a Wood's lamp, and age-appropriate neurological examination. Once a diagnosis is established, patients with NF1 should receive neurological and blood pressure evaluations annually. Children should also have a developmental assessment and review of growth and sexual development. An annual ophthalmologic exam should also be performed from 2 to 7 years of age to screen for symptomatic optic glioma. Routine laboratory investigations are not needed for NF1 patients, and imaging studies of the brain and spine should be reserved for those with unexplained or progressive neurological symptoms [3].

Current therapy for NF1 remains primarily surgical. Spinal tumors should only be resected when they produce progressive neurological symptoms with or without radiographic progression. Many patients request plastic surgery intervention for cutaneous tumors, especially large deforming plexiform tumors. Complex and repeated surgical interventions are often best accomplished in a multidisciplinary neurofibromatosis center. Patients with rapidly enlarging masses or new occurrence of severe pain may harbor occult MPNST. In these patients, positron emission tomography (PET) scanning may be helpful in defining areas of malignant degeneration within large plexiform lesions. Biopsy can be targeted to lesions with elevated uptake of 2-fluoro-2-deoxy-D-glucose (FDG) [35, 36].

MRI findings consistent with optic pathway gliomas are identified in about 15% of children with NF1; importantly, only a minority is symptomatic. Asymptomatic lesions should be followed with serial MRI scans and visual testing without intervention. Symptomatic lesions should be monitored closely with therapy generally reserved for progressive lesions. Surgery is indicated in patients with visual loss and pain or deformity related to mass effect. While radiotherapy is often used to treat sporadic optic pathway gliomas, NF1 patients who receive radiation are at increased the risk of developing new primary tumors, which may be malignant [37]. Thus, radiation should be reserved for NF1 patients with optic pathway gliomas that progress despite treatment with chemotherapy.

The recent finding that the mTOR pathway may be involved in the development of tumors in NF1 has raised interest in investigating a possible therapeutic role for mTOR inhibitors such as rapamycin (sirolimus), which is currently approved for use as an immunosuppressant.

Relationship Between Sporadic and NF1-Related Tumors

Tumors associated with NF1 also occur in patients without an underlying genetic disorder. In some sporadic tumors, the *NF1* gene is inactivated, suggesting a central role for the NF1 pathway in tumorigenesis. In other tumors, the *NF1* gene is unaffected and alternative genetic mechanisms give rise to tumor formation.

Neurofibroma

There is little published data on the mechanism of development for sporadic neurofibromas. Biallelic inactivation of the *NF1* gene is the initiating event in NF1-related neurofibromas [30, 38]. A single report on sporadic neurofibromas suggests that biallelic inactivation of the NF1 pathway is responsible for these tumors as well [39].

Leukemia

Hyperactivation of the Ras pathway is a causative feature in juvenile myelomonocytic leukemia (JMML), and children with NF1 carry an increased risk of developing JMML [40]. Mutations in the *N-Ras* and *K-Ras2* genes are found in non-NF1 linked cases of JMML, but not in NF1-related cases [41]. The *NF1* product, neurofibromin, is an Ras-GAP, suggesting that the same pathway is deregulated in both sporadic and NF1-related cases of JMML.

Pheochromocytoma

Pheochromocytoma occurs in association with NF1 and von Hipple Lindau disease (VHL), as well as in sporadic patients. NF1-associated pheochromocytomas harbor germline *NF1* mutations and demonstrate loss-of-heterozygosity at the *NF1* locus, suggesting that pheochromocytoma is a true complication of NF1 [42]. Sporadic pheochromocytomas have been shown to have mutations in a variety of genes, including the oncogene *RET*, the metabolic regulatory genes succinate dehydrogenase subunit B (*SDHB*) and succinate dehydrogenase subunit D (*SDHD*), and the tumor suppressor genes *VHL* and *NF1* [43, 44]. These findings suggesting that a variety of pathways are involved in pheochromocytoma formation.

Optic Pathway Glioma

Optic pathway gliomas constitute 1–5% of intracranial neoplasms in children and are the most common brain tumor in patients with NF1. NF1-related optic pathway gliomas tend to be located in the optic nerve and chiasm, whereas sporadic tumors tend to occur in the optic chiasm or postchiasm [45]. In NF1-related tumors, the chemokine, CXCL12, functions cooperatively with loss of neurofibromin in astrocytes to promote tumor growth [46]. In contrast, mutation of the *EF-1α2* gene appears to be involved in the formation of sporadic tumors [47], suggesting an alternative pathway in these tumors.

Gastrointestinal Stromal Tumor

Gastrointestinal stromal tumors (GIST) occur in both sporadic and NF1 patients. In sporadic patients, somatic mutations in the c-KIT and PDGF receptor genes have been identified [48, 49]. Treatment with drugs that inhibit these receptors (e.g., imatinib and sunitinib) have shown clinical benefit [50, 51].

In contrast, molecular analysis of NF1-related GISTs indicates that mutations in c-KIT and PDGF receptor are not present [52]. Instead, mitotic recombination of the germline alteration has been identified in a small number of NF1-related GISTS. Not surprisingly, treatment with imatinib or sunitinib has shown little benefit in these patients [53]. Together, these findings suggest that alternative molecular pathways are involved in sporadic and NF1-related tumors.

Malignant Peripheral Nerve Sheath Tumor

Approximately 50% of all MPNSTs occur in patients with NF1 [54]. The 5-year survival rate for MPNSTs is lower in NF1 patients, which may be related to earlier detection in sporadic cases [55]. Hyperactive Ras signaling has been implicated in the formation and progression of NF1-related MPNSTs as levels of Ras have been shown to be raised in NF1 linked MPNSTs [56], but not in non-NF1 related MPNSTs. However, the mTORC1 inhibitor, RAD001, reduces growth of both NF1-linked and sporadic MPNST cells in preclinical studies [56].

Neurofibromatosis 2

Clinical Features and Diagnostic Criteria

NF2, previously called central neurofibromatosis, is less common than NF1 with a birth prevalence of 1 in 25,000 [12]. As with NF1, NF2 is transmitted in an autosomal dominant fashion with full penetrance, and the risk of NF2 in each offspring of an affected parent is 50%. About 50% of NF2 patients are founders with new mutations and clinically unaffected parents. NF2 is characterized by the predisposition to develop multiple tumors, including schwannomas, meningiomas, and spinal cord gliomas. The average age of onset of symptoms is between 17 and 21 and typically precedes a formal diagnosis of NF2 by 5–8 years. Younger patients normally present with cranial nerve dysfunction, peripheral nerve dysfunction, myelopathy, seizures, skin tumors, café-au-lait macules, and juvenile cataracts. In adults, the most common presenting symptoms are due to eighth cranial nerve dysfunction (deafness, tinnitus, or imbalance).

The NIH clinical criteria for the diagnosis of NF2 (Table 13.1) is based on either (1) the presence of bilateral vestibular schwannomas or (2) a family history of NF2 and either a unilateral vestibular schwannoma or any two of the following tumors: schwannoma, meningioma, neurofibroma, glioma, juvenile posterior subcapsular lenticular opacity [2, 57]. Thus, only patients with bilateral vestibular schwannomas or a family history can qualify for a diagnosis under NIH criteria. Patients who do not fulfill these criteria but have multiple features associated with NF2 represent a diagnostic dilemma. For this reason, revised criteria were proposed by the Manchester group in 1992 and by the National Neurofibromatosis Foundation (NNFF) in 1997. The relative merits of these criteria continue to be debated by researchers.

Tumor Manifestations

Bilateral vestibular schwannomas (VS) are the hallmark of NF2 and invariably develop in patients with the disorder (Fig. 13.4). Schwannomas of nonvestibular cranial nerves and spinal nerves are also common. NF2-related schwannomas are histologically benign, but malignant peripheral nerve sheath tumors may occur in patients who have received prior radiation therapy. About 50% of all patients with NF2 develop intracranial meningiomas (Fig. 13.5). Optic sheath meningiomas occur in 4–8% of patients with NF2 and are a disproportionate cause of decreased visual acuity. Meningiomas associated with NF2 are almost universally benign histologically. Spinal ependymomas and astrocytomas in patients with NF2 present as intramedullary spinal cord lesions and occur in up to 50% of patients [58, 59]. Two-thirds of patients with ependymomas have multiple tumors. The cervicomedullary junction or cervical spine is most commonly involved (63–82%) followed by the thoracic spine (36–44%) [58, 59]. The brain and lumbar spine, common sites for sporadic

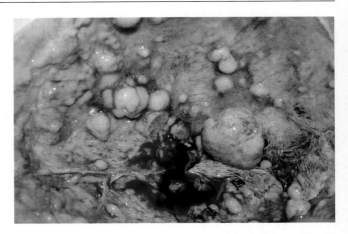

Fig. 13.5 Photograph of the skull base from an NF2 patient taken at autopsy showing multiple meningiomas

ependymomas, are rarely involved. Radiographic evidence of tumor progression occurs in less than 10% of patients and progressive neurologic dysfunction requiring surgical intervention occurs in 12–20% of patients [58, 59].

Nontumor Manifestations

Presenile cataracts are the most common nontumor manifestation in NF2, occurring in approximately 70% of cases [60, 61]. In some patients, this may be the first sign of NF2. Neuropathy occurs in NF2 at a frequency of between 6 and 48% [62, 63] and up to 67% when electrophysiological findings are studied [63]. It is more common in patients with a more severe phenotype and is thought to be due to reduced *NF2* gene dosage in affected peripheral nerves [64]. Focal amyotrophy is a rare complication of NF2, but has been reported to precede tumor manifestations in a small number of cases [65]. However, the underlying pathogenic pathway is unknown.

Genetics and Molecular Biology

The *NF2* gene was mapped to chromosome 22 in 1987 [66, 67] and then identified by two independent groups in 1993 [68, 69]. The *NF2* gene is composed of 17 exons spanning 110 kb. There are three alternative messenger RNA species (7, 4.4, and 2.6 kb) due to variable length of the 3′untranslated region. The predominant *NF2* gene product is a 595 amino acid protein and is a member of the 4.1 family of cytoskeletal proteins, named Merlin (moesin, ezrin, radixin-like protein) to emphasize its relationship to other cytoskeletal proteins. Merlin links membrane-associated proteins to

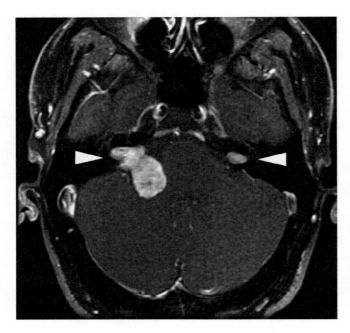

Fig. 13.4 Postcontrast axial T1-weighted image of an NF2 patient with bilateral vestibular schwannomas (*arrowheads*)

the actin cytoskeleton, thereby acting as an interface with the extracellular environment [70].

Constitutional mutations of the *NF2* gene include nonsense (29–39%), splice-site (~25%), frameshift (25–27%), and missense mutations (5–7%) [71, 72]. Hot spots have been identified at CpG dinucleotides that leading to TGA nonsense mutations, particularly in exons 2, 6, 8 and 11 [71]. To date, no strong genotype–phenotype correlations have been identified, although truncating mutations are more common in severely affected patients [73] and non-truncating mutations are associated with mildly affected patients [74].

The NF2 protein is a true tumor suppressor, as biallelic loss of the gene results in tumor growth. Inactivation of the *NF2* gene can be detected in the vast majority of sporadic schwannomas [75] and in about 50–60% of sporadic meningiomas [76]. Despite significant progress in understanding the role of the *NF2* gene product, the molecular mechanism by which loss of Merlin leads to tumorigenesis has not been fully elucidated. Multiple binding partners have been identified for Merlin with implications in a variety of signaling pathways involved in maintenance of contact-dependent inhibition of growth and proliferation, stabilization of adherens junctions and the regulation of receptor tyrosine kinases at the cell surface [70].

Mosaic NF2 is caused by postzygotic mutation of the *NF2* gene. As with NF1, the clinical phenotype includes a mild, generalized form of NF2 with bilateral vestibular schwannomas and segmental disease with unilateral vestibular schwannomas and other tumors associated with NF2 [77]. Patients with mosaic NF2 account for about 25–33% of patients with bilateral vestibular schwannomas. Importantly, the risk of transmission to offspring is reduced compared with patients with non-mosaic disease [78, 80].

Genetic Testing

Comprehensive mutational analysis of the *NF2* gene identifies a causative mutation in about 70–90% of affected individuals [79]. The presence of large deletions, mutations in promoter or intronic regions, and somatic mosaicism contributes to the difficulty in identifying a mutation in all patients. The introduction of improved detection methods has increased mutation detection rates. Currently, an *NF2* alteration is identified in 33% of mosaic patients presenting with bilateral vestibular schwannomas and in 60% of patients presenting with unilateral vestibular schwannomas [80].

Genetic counseling is an essential component of the care of the patient with NF2. As for NF1, genetic testing can be used for family planning (i.e., prenatal or preimplantation genetic diagnosis) or for presymptomatic diagnosis of individuals at risk but should not be used to confirm a clinical

diagnosis. If a causative mutation in the *NF2* gene can be identified, molecular testing with 100% specificity will be available for that family.

Mosaicism is a common cause of noninformative testing in sporadic NF2 patients who meet clinical criteria, but have no family history and no detectable germline mutation in blood lymphocytes. For these individuals, tumor specimens should be frozen for molecular analysis of the *NF2* gene. If two genetic alterations (e.g., one mutation and one allele loss of the *NF2* gene) can be identified in a tumor, one is inferred to be the constitutional mutation. Haplotype analysis can then be used to screen at risk individuals for the mutation in constitutional DNA [81]. In families with two or more affected individuals, linkage analysis using intragenic markers or markers flanking the *NF2* gene can be used for presymptomatic diagnosis with >99% certainty of affected status.

Management of Patients with NF2

Initial evaluation of patients who have, or are at risk for, NF2 should include testing to confirm a diagnosis and to identify potential problems. A medical history should include questions about auditory and vestibular function, focal neurologic symptoms, skin tumors, seizures, headache, and visual symptoms. A family history should explore unexplained neurological and audiological symptoms in all first-degree relatives. MR imaging of the brain should include gadolinium and include axial and coronal thin cuts (3 mm) through the brainstem to identify vestibular schwannomas. MR imaging of the cervical spine should also be performed given the predilection of ependymomas for this site. Some clinicians recommend imaging of the thoracic and lumbar spine, whereas others reserve these exams for patients with neurologic symptoms referable to these locations. Ophthalmologic examination serves to identify characteristic lesions such as lens opacities, retinal hamartomas, or epiretinal membranes. A complete neurological examination serves as a baseline for future comparison and may assist in the selection of sites within the nervous system that require further imaging studies. Audiological examination (including pure tone threshold and word recognition) and brainstem evoked responses document eighth cranial nerve dysfunction related to vestibular schwannomas and set a baseline for future comparisons.

After initial diagnosis, patients should be seen approximately every 3–6 months until the growth rate and biologic behavior of tumors is determined. Consultation with an experienced surgeon after initial diagnosis is often helpful for presymptomatic patients (i.e., those with normal hearing) to discuss the feasibility of hearing-sparing surgery. Most patients without acute problems can be followed on an annual basis. Evaluation at these visits should include complete neurological examination, MR imaging of the brain with thin cuts (3 mm) through the brainstem, and MR imaging of symptomatic lesions outside the brain if present. Ophthalmologic evaluation should be performed in selected patients with visual impairment or facial weakness. Yearly audiology serves to document changes in pure tone threshold and word recognition. This information can be helpful in planning early surgical intervention for vestibular schwannomas and in counseling patients about possible complete hearing loss. The frequency with which routine spinal imaging is obtained varies among clinics, but is clearly indicated in patients with new or progressive symptoms referable to the spinal cord.

The approach to management of NF2-associated tumors differs from that of sporadic tumors. Surgery is the mainstay for treatment of NF2-related tumors. However, the surgical removal of every lesion is not possible or advisable, and the primary goal is to preserve function and maximize quality of life. Surgery is clearly indicated for patients with significant brainstem or spinal cord compression or with obstructive hydrocephalus. In patients with little or no neurologic dysfunction related to their tumors, watchful waiting may allow patients to retain neurologic function for many years [82].

Indications for surgical resection of other tumors are less well defined. Surgical resection in these patients should be reserved for those with unacceptable neurologic symptoms or rapid tumor growth. Patients with meningiomas typically have more than one tumor, and resection of all lesions is often not advisable. The benefit of surgery must be carefully weighed against potential complications. As a general rule, indications for resection include rapid tumor growth and worsening neurologic symptoms. Intervention for spinal cord tumors is necessary in a minority of patients [58]. Surgery is more often required in patients with extramedullary tumors (59%) than for intramedullary tumors (12%) [59].

Radiation is often used as adjuvant therapy for treatment of sporadic brain tumors. Treatment outcomes for patients with NF2-related vestibular schwannomas are worse than for patients with sporadic tumors [83]. More recently, fractionated stereotactic radiotherapy has been advocated to minimize the risk of hearing loss. The actuarial 5-year local control rate using this technique is 93% and the hearing-preservation rate is 64% [84]. The role of adjuvant radiation in other tumors such as meningiomas and ependymomas is not established, but the majority of these tumors is histologically benign and can be controlled surgically. No case series have been published on treatment of NF2-related meningiomas.

Most clinicians prefer surgical extirpation of tumors when possible and reserve radiation treatment for tumors that are not surgically accessible. This practice is based on the experience that radiation therapy makes subsequent resection of VS and function of auditory brainstem implants more difficult [85]. In addition, there are reports of malignant transformation of NF2-associated schwannomas after radiation treatment and indirect evidence of increased numbers of malignancy in NF2 patients who have received radiation [86, 87]. The role of chemotherapy for NF2-related tumors is evolving, and reports of response to targeted agents have been published [88].

Relationship Between Sporadic and NF2-Related Tumors

Schwannomas and meningiomas are common in the general population and comprise approximately 40% of tumors in the Central Brain Tumor Registry of the United States [89]. Biallelic inactivation of the NF2 gene is the causative event in both sporadic and NF2-related vestibular schwannomas [75]. However, the mutation spectrum differs between NF2-related and sporadic schwannomas. The detection rate is higher in sporadic tumors than in NF2-related tumors. Point mutations are more common in NF2-related tumors, whereas small deletions are more common in sporadic tumors [90].

Meningiomas are found in approximately 50% of NF2 patients [62] and truncating mutations of the NF2 gene can be found in up to 60% of sporadic tumors [76], with different rates of detection depending on the type of meningioma. Fibroblastic and transitional meningiomas showed a much higher rate of detection (70 and 83%) than meningothelial meningiomas (25%), suggesting that this subtype may involve a different molecular pathway. The mechanism of tumor progression is not well understood, but may involve loss of the DAL-1/4.1B gene [91].

Loss of heterozygosity of chromosome 22 is a frequent occurrence in ependymomas in adults, but not in children [92]. Spinal ependymomas, which tend to be found in adults, are found in patients with NF2, and mutations in the NF2 gene have been found in sporadic cases of spinal ependymomas, but not cranial ependymomas. Other genes involved in ependymoma formation have yet to be determined. However, studies show that other genes on chromosome 22 may be involved [93, 94].

Mutation of the NF2 gene has been found in 40% of sporadic mesothelioma cases and disruption of the NF2 signaling pathway is necessary for mesothelioma development [95]. Interestingly, mesothelioma is not present at increased frequency in NF2 patients. Deficiency in the ink4a/ARF gene has also been shown to be essential for mesothelioma progression [96]. In mesothelial tumors without NF2 mutations, downstream effectors of the NF2 pathway are dysregulated by mutation of genes involved in regulation of the Merlin protein, via CPI-17 [95].

Schwannomatosis

Clinical Features and Diagnostic Criteria

Schwannomatosis is a third major form of neurofibromatosis. It is thought to be as prevalent as NF2, affecting approximately 1 in 40,000 people [97]. The true prevalence is likely higher given the difficulty in ascertaining individuals affected by schwannomatosis. Unlike patients with NF1 who have characteristic dermatologic findings and patients with NF2 who have 8th cranial nerve dysfunction at a young age, patients with schwannomatosis have nonspecific symptoms that may not lead to medical evaluation. Familial schwannomatosis accounts for 15% of cases and is transmitted in autosomal dominant fashion with incomplete penetrance. In these families, the risk of transmitting the affected allele to each offspring of an affected parent is 50%. Sporadic schwannomatosis accounts for the remaining 85% of patients who have clinically unaffected parents. The risk of transmitting the affected allele in sporadic patients is significantly less than 50%, although the exact figure is not known due to incomplete penetrance.

Schwannomatosis is characterized by the predisposition to develop multiple schwannomas. In contrast to patients with NF2, patients with schwannomatosis do not have vestibular or intradermal schwannomas. Patients with schwannomatosis most commonly develop symptoms in the second or third decade of life. Pain is the hallmark of schwannomatosis and is the most common initial complaint. Neurologic dysfunction related to schwannomas is uncommon and, when present, is often a complication of surgery. One-third of patients with schwannomatosis have evidence of anatomically limited, or segmental, disease. The radiographic appearance of schwannomatosis is characterized by multiple, discrete lesions along peripheral or spinal nerves (Fig. 13.6). Pathologically, schwannomas in patients with schwannomatosis resemble those from patients with NF2 and sporadic lesions. Although no single feature can reliably distinguish schwannomatosis-associated schwannomas, they tend to have more peritumoral edema in the adjacent nerve, intratumoral myxoid changes, and intraneural growth patterns than other schwannomas [98].

Consensus criteria for diagnosis of schwannomatosis (Table 13.1) have been published [98]. The diagnostic criteria for schwannomatosis are organized hierarchically and patients may be labeled as having definite or possible schwannomatosis. The criteria for definite schwannomatosis include: age greater than 30 years with two or more nonintradermal schwannomas (at least 1 with histologic confirmation) and no evidence of vestibular tumor on high-quality MRI scan, and no known constitutional NF2 mutation; or one pathologically confirmed nonvestibular schwannoma plus a first-degree relative who meets above criteria.

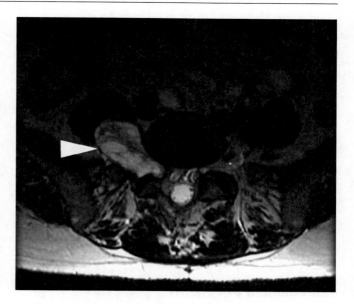

Fig. 13.6 Axial T2-weighted image of the lumbar spine of a schwannomatosis patient showing a schwannoma exiting the neural foramen and extending into the psoas muscle (*arrowhead*)

Genetics and Molecular Biology

The pathogenesis of schwannomatosis is an area of active research. A minority of patients who fulfill research criteria for sporadic schwannomatosis have been shown to have mosaic NF2 [99]. Truncating mutations in the *NF2* gene are present in the vast majority of schwannomatosis-associated schwannomas. However, multiple tumors from the same patient do not share a common mutation, indicating that mutation of the *NF2* gene is not the germline event in familial schwannomatosis [100]. Schwannomatosis is now classified as a separate condition with a distinct molecular and clinical pathology [98]. The underlying cause for somatic instability in the *NF2* gene in schwannomatosis is not known.

The first candidate for a causative gene in familial schwannomatosis was identified in 2007 [101]. The SWI/hSNF5 matrix-associated actin-dependent regulator of chromatin family B member 1 (*SMARCB1*) gene (also termed *INI1*, *hSNF5*, and *BAF47*) is located on chromosome 22, centromeric to the *NF2* gene. *SMARCB1/INI1* is a core subunit of the SWI/SNF transcriptional complex that normally contains between nine and twelve subunits [102]. Together, the components of this complex activate and repress transcription of target genes throughout the genome by remodeling chromatin. Germline mutations and second somatic mutation in tumors have been identified in 33–68% of familial cases tested, but only 8–10% of sporadic cases of schwannomatosis in which no family history is present [101, 103–105]. *SMARCB1* is a known tumor suppressor in other cancer syndromes, including its biallelic inactivation in the aggressive pediatric syndrome atypical teratoid/rhabdoid tumor (AT/RT). However, the reason for the difference in phenotypes of these disparate conditions remains unclear.

Genetic Testing

Although germline alterations in *SMARCB1/INI1* have been identified in patients with familial schwannomatosis and sporadic schwannomatosis (i.e., those without a family history), clinical testing is not routinely performed in these patients. Genetic testing remains largely for research purposed at the present time.

Management of Patients with Schwannomatosis

Initial evaluation of patients who have or are at risk for schwannomatosis should include testing to confirm a diagnosis (usually exclusion of NF1 and NF2) and to identify potential problems. A medical history should include questions about auditory and vestibular function, focal neurologic symptoms, skin tumors or hyperpigmented lesions, seizures, headache, and visual symptoms. A family history should explore unexplained neurological, dermatological, and audiological symptoms in all first-degree relatives. MRI scans of the brain with attention to the internal auditory canals should be performed to exclude vestibular schwannomas. MRI scans of other body parts should be obtained based on the history and clinical exam. A combination of MRI scan and pathologic analysis is used to establish a diagnosis of definite or possible schwannomatosis. Management of patients with schwannomatosis is primarily symptom oriented. As noted above, pain is the hallmark of this disorder. Surgery should be reserved for patients with symptomatic tumors or rapidly expanding lesions in the spinal cord. Most patients require pain medication; these patients may benefit from referral to a Pain Clinic with experience in managing neuropathic pain.

Relationship Between Sporadic, and Schwannomatosis-Related Tumors

A single immunohistochemical study on familial (i.e., NF2- or schwannomatosis-related) and sporadic schwannomas suggests that *SMARCB1* is inactivated in a mosaic pattern in familial tumors. In contrast, inactivation of *SMARCB1* has not been found in sporadic schwannomas, suggesting an alternative pathway in these tumors [106]. The occurrence of meningioma in schwannomatosis is rare, but mutation of *SMARCB1* has been reported in a minority of meningiomas [107, 108].

Atypical teratoid/rhabdoid tumors (AT/RTs) are aggressive malignancies with a poor prognosis. These tumors are associated with the homozygous deletion of *SMARCB1* [109]. In contrast, schwannomatosis-related schwannomas, show a mosaic pattern of staining for *SMARCB1* protein [106]. A report of the co-occurrence of AT/RT and schwannomatosis in the same family has been reported and is linked to a common *SMARCB1* mutation [110]. However, the mechanistic differences that lead to development of familial schwannomatosis rather than familial AT/RT are not known. It has been suggested that there is a window of opportunity for the development of AT/RT in children and that if it fails to develop there may be the opportunity to develop schwannomas in later life [105, 110, 111].

Summary

NF1, NF2, and schwannomatosis are distinct tumor suppressor syndromes characterized by the predisposition to nerve sheath tumors. Table 13.2 highlights important differences

Table 13.2 Comparison of selected genetic and clinical features of NF1, NF2 and schwannomatosis

	NF1	NF2	Schwannomatosis
Causative gene	*NF1*	*NF2*	*SMARCB1/INI1*
Inheritance pattern	Autosomal dominant	Autosomal dominant	Autosomal dominant
% Familial	50%	50%	15%
Penetrance	Complete	Complete	Incomplete
Genetic testing availability	Clinical	Clinical	Research
Hallmark tumor	Neurofibroma	Schwannoma	Schwannoma
Age at diagnosis	1st decade	2–3rd decade	3–4th decade
Presenting symptoms	Café-au-lait macule	Hearing loss	Pain
Hearing loss	No	Yes	No
Ophthalmic features	Lisch nodules	Cataracts	None
Risk of malignancy	10% lifetime risk	No	No

among these disorders. Prompt recognition of neurofibromatosis and schwannomatosis is critical to provide optimal clinical care and genetic counseling to affected patients and their families. Identification of the genetic defects responsible for these relatively uncommon disorders has broadened the understanding of critical molecular pathways in tumorgenesis.

References

1. Lammert M, Friedman JM, Kluwe L, Mautner VF (2005) Prevalence of neurofibromatosis 1 in German children at elementary school enrollment. Arch Dermatol 141(1):71–74
2. NIH Consensus Conference (1988) Neurofibromatosis. Conference statement. National Institutes of Health Consensus Development Conference. Arch Neurol 45(5):575–578
3. Gutmann DH, Aylsworth A, Carey JC et al (1997) The diagnostic evaluation and multidisciplinary management of neurofibromatosis 1 and neurofibromatosis 2. JAMA 278(1):51–57
4. DeBella K, Szudek J, Friedman JM (2000) Use of the national institutes of health criteria for diagnosis of neurofibromatosis 1 in children. Pediatrics 105(3 Pt 1):608–614
5. Leonard JR, Perry A, Rubin JB, King AA, Chicoine MR, Gutmann DH (2006) The role of surgical biopsy in the diagnosis of glioma in individuals with neurofibromatosis-1. Neurology 67(8):1509–1512
6. Huson SM, Harper PS, Compston DA (1988) Von Recklinghausen neurofibromatosis. A clinical and population study in south–east Wales. Brain 111(Pt 6):1355–1381
7. Waggoner DJ, Towbin J, Gottesman G, Gutmann DH (2000) Clinic-based study of plexiform neurofibromas in neurofibromatosis 1. Am J Med Genet 92(2):132–135
8. Friedman JM, Birch PH (1997) Type 1 neurofibromatosis: a descriptive analysis of the disorder in 1, 728 patients. Am J Med Genet 70(2):138–143
9. Evans DG, Baser ME, McGaughran J, Sharif S, Howard E, Moran A (2002) Malignant peripheral nerve sheath tumours in neurofibromatosis 1. J Med Genet 39(5):311–314
10. McCaughan JA, Holloway SM, Davidson R, Lam WW (2007) Further evidence of the increased risk for malignant peripheral nerve sheath tumour from a Scottish cohort of patients with neurofibromatosis type 1. J Med Genet 44(7):463–466
11. Tucker T, Wolkenstein P, Revuz J, Zeller J, Friedman JM (2005) Association between benign and malignant peripheral nerve sheath tumors in NF1. Neurology 65(2):205–211
12. Evans DG, Moran A, King A, Saeed S, Gurusinghe N, Ramsden R (2005) Incidence of vestibular schwannoma and neurofibromatosis 2 in the North West of England over a 10-year period: higher incidence than previously thought. Otol Neurotol 26(1):93–97
13. Gutmann DH, Rasmussen SA, Wolkenstein P et al (2002) Gliomas presenting after age 10 in individuals with neurofibromatosis type 1 (NF1). Neurology 59(5):759–761
14. Guillamo JS, Creange A, Kalifa C et al (2003) Prognostic factors of CNS tumours in Neurofibromatosis 1 (NF1): a retrospective study of 104 patients. Brain 126(Pt 1):152–160
15. Miyata S, Sugimoto T, Kodama T et al (2005) Adenoid glioblastoma arising in a patient with neurofibromatosis type-1. Pathol Int 55(6):348–352
16. North K, Hyman S, Barton B (2002) Cognitive deficits in neurofibromatosis 1. J Child Neurol 17(8):605–612
17. Creange A, Zeller J, Rostaing-Rigattieri S et al (1999) Neurological complications of neurofibromatosis type 1 in adulthood. Brain 122(Pt 3):473–481
18. Li Y, O'Connell P, Breidenbach HH et al (1995) Genomic organization of the neurofibromatosis 1 gene (NF1). Genomics 25(1):9–18
19. Messiaen LM, Callens T, Mortier G et al (2000) Exhaustive mutation analysis of the NF1 gene allows identification of 95% of mutations and reveals a high frequency of unusual splicing defects. Hum Mutat 15(6):541–555
20. Zhu Y, Ghosh P, Charnay P, Burns DK, Parada LF (2002) Neurofibromas in NF1: Schwann cell origin and role of tumor environment. Science 296(5569):920–922
21. Serra E, Rosenbaum T, Winner U et al (2000) Schwann cells harbor the somatic NF1 mutation in neurofibromas: evidence of two different Schwann cell subpopulations. Hum Mol Genet 9(20):3055–3064
22. De SS, Maertens O, Callens T, Naeyaert JM, Lambert J, Messiaen L (2008) Somatic mutation analysis in NF1 cafe au lait spots reveals two NF1 hits in the melanocytes. J Invest Dermatol 128(4):1050–1053
23. Cnossen MH, van der Est MN, Breuning MH et al (1997) Deletions spanning the neurofibromatosis type 1 gene: implications for genotype–phenotype correlations in neurofibromatosis type 1? Hum Mutat 9(5):458–464
24. Kehrer-Sawatzki H, Kluwe L, Funsterer C, Mautner VF (2005) Extensively high load of internal tumors determined by whole body MRI scanning in a patient with neurofibromatosis type 1 and a non-LCR-mediated 2-Mb deletion in 17q11.2. Hum Genet 116(6):466–475
25. Upadhyaya M, Huson SM, Davies M et al (2007) An absence of cutaneous neurofibromas associated with a 3-bp inframe deletion in exon 17 of the NF1 gene (c.2970-2972 delAAT): evidence of a clinically significant NF1 genotype–phenotype correlation. Am J Hum Genet 80(1):140–151
26. Maertens O, De SS, Vandesompele J et al (2007) Molecular dissection of isolated disease features in mosaic neurofibromatosis type 1. Am J Hum Genet 81(2):243–251
27. Ruggieri M, Huson SM (2001) The clinical and diagnostic implications of mosaicism in the neurofibromatoses. Neurology 56(11):1433–1443
28. Vandenbroucke I, Callens T, De PA, Messiaen L (2002) Complex splicing pattern generates great diversity in human NF1 transcripts. BMC Genomics 3(1):13
29. Viskochil D, Cawthon R, O'Connell P et al (1991) The gene encoding the oligodendrocyte-myelin glycoprotein is embedded within the neurofibromatosis type 1 gene. Mol Cell Biol 11(2):906–912
30. Serra E, Puig S, Otero D et al (1997) Confirmation of a double-hit model for the NF1 gene in benign neurofibromas. Am J Hum Genet 61(3):512–519
31. Dasgupta B, Yi Y, Chen DY, Weber JD, Gutmann DH (2005) Proteomic analysis reveals hyperactivation of the mammalian target of rapamycin pathway in neurofibromatosis 1-associated human and mouse brain tumors. Cancer Res 65(7):2755–2760
32. Johannessen CM, Reczek EE, James MF, Brems H, Legius E, Cichowski K (2005) The NF1 tumor suppressor critically regulates TSC2 and mTOR. Proc Natl Acad Sci USA 102(24):8573–8578
33. Dasgupta B, Li W, Perry A, Gutmann DH (2005) Glioma formation in neurofibromatosis 1 reflects preferential activation of K-Ras in astrocytes. Cancer Res 65(1):236–245
34. Spits C, De RM, Van RN et al (2005) Preimplantation genetic diagnosis for neurofibromatosis type 1. Mol Hum Reprod 11(5):381–387
35. Ferner RE, Lucas JD, O'Doherty MJ et al (2000) Evaluation of (18)fluorodeoxyglucose positron emission tomography ((18)FDG PET) in the detection of malignant peripheral nerve sheath tumours arising from within plexiform neurofibromas in neurofibromatosis 1. J Neurol Neurosurg Psychiatr 68(3):353–357
36. Bredella MA, Torriani M, Hornicek F et al (2007) Value of PET in the assessment of patients with neurofibromatosis type 1. AJR Am J Roentgenol 189(4):928–935

37. Sharif S, Ferner R, Birch JM et al (2006) Second primary tumors in neurofibromatosis 1 patients treated for optic glioma: substantial risks after radiotherapy. J Clin Oncol 24(16):2570–2575

38. Colman SD, Williams CA, Wallace MR (1995) Benign neurofibromas in type 1 neurofibromatosis (NF1) show somatic deletions of the NF1 gene. Nat Genet 11(1):90–92

39. Storlazzi CT, Von Steyern FV, Domanski HA, Mandahl N, Mertens F (2005) Biallelic somatic inactivation of the NF1 gene through chromosomal translocations in a sporadic neurofibroma. Int J Cancer 117(6):1055–1057

40. Bader JL, Miller RW (1978) Neurofibromatosis and childhood leukemia. J Pediatr 92(6):925–929

41. Kalra R, Paderanga DC, Olson K, Shannon KM (1994) Genetic analysis is consistent with the hypothesis that NF1 limits myeloid cell growth through p21Ras. Blood 84(10):3435–3439

42. Bausch B, Borozdin W, Mautner VF et al (2007) Germline NF1 mutational spectra and loss-of-heterozygosity analyses in patients with pheochromocytoma and neurofibromatosis type 1. J Clin Endocrinol Metab 92(7):2784–2792

43. Opocher G, Conton P, Schiavi F, Macino B, Mantero F (2005) Pheochromocytoma in von Hippel-Lindau disease and neurofibromatosis type 1. Fam Cancer 4(1):13–16

44. Neumann HP, Bausch B, McWhinney SR et al (2002) Germ-line mutations in nonsyndromic pheochromocytoma. N Engl J Med 346(19):1459–1466

45. Chateil JF, Soussotte C, Pedespan JM, Brun M, Le MC, Diard F (2001) MRI and clinical differences between optic pathway tumours in children with and without neurofibromatosis. Br J Radiol 74(877):24–31

46. Warrington NM, Woerner BM, Daginakatte GC et al (2007) Spatiotemporal differences in CXCL12 expression and cyclic AMP underlie the unique pattern of optic glioma growth in neurofibromatosis type 1. Cancer Res 67(18):8588–8595

47. Gutmann DH, Hedrick NM, Li J, Nagarajan R, Perry A, Watson MA (2002) Comparative gene expression profile analysis of neurofibromatosis 1-associated and sporadic pilocytic astrocytomas. Cancer Res 62(7):2085–2091

48. Hirota S, Isozaki K, Moriyama Y et al (1998) Gain-of-function mutations of c-kit in human gastrointestinal stromal tumors. Science 279(5350):577–580

49. Heinrich MC, Corless CL, Duensing A et al (2003) PDGFRA activating mutations in gastrointestinal stromal tumors. Science 299(5607):708–710

50. Verweij J, Casali PG, Zalcberg J et al (2004) Progression-free survival in gastrointestinal stromal tumours with high-dose imatinib: randomised trial. Lancet 364(9440):1127–1134

51. Demetri GD, van Oosterom AT, Garrett CR et al (2006) Efficacy and safety of sunitinib in patients with advanced gastrointestinal stromal tumour after failure of imatinib: a randomised controlled trial. Lancet 368(9544):1329–1338

52. Stewart DR, Corless CL, Rubin BP et al (2007) Mitotic recombination as evidence of alternative pathogenesis of gastrointestinal stromal tumours in neurofibromatosis type 1. J Med Genet 44(1):e61

53. Mussi C, Schildhaus HU, Gronchi A, Wardelmann E, Hohenberger P (2008) Therapeutic consequences from molecular biology for gastrointestinal stromal tumor patients affected by neurofibromatosis type 1. Clin Cancer Res 14(14):4550–4555

54. Doorn PF, Molenaar WM, Buter J, Hoekstra HJ (1995) Malignant peripheral nerve sheath tumors in patients with and without neurofibromatosis. Eur J Surg Oncol 21(1):78–82

55. Carli M, Ferrari A, Mattke A et al (2005) Pediatric malignant peripheral nerve sheath tumor: the Italian and German soft tissue sarcoma cooperative group. J Clin Oncol 23(33):8422–8430

56. Johansson G, Mahller YY, Collins MH et al (2008) Effective in vivo targeting of the mammalian target of rapamycin pathway in malignant peripheral nerve sheath tumors. Mol Cancer Ther 7(5):1237–1245

57. Mulvihill JJ, Parry DM, Sherman JL, Pikus A, Kaiser-Kupfer MI, Eldridge R (1990) NIH conference. Neurofibromatosis 1 (Recklinghausen disease) and neurofibromatosis 2 (bilateral acoustic neurofibromatosis). An update. Ann Intern Med 113(1):39–52

58. Mautner VF, Tatagiba M, Lindenau M et al (1995) Spinal tumors in patients with neurofibromatosis type 2: MR imaging study of frequency, multiplicity, and variety. AJR Am J Roentgenol 165(4):951–955

59. Patronas NJ, Courcoutsakis N, Bromley CM, Katzman GL, MacCollin M, Parry DM (2001) Intramedullary and spinal canal tumors in patients with neurofibromatosis 2: MR imaging findings and correlation with genotype. Radiology 218(2):434–442

60. Parry DM, Eldridge R, Kaiser-Kupfer MI, Bouzas EA, Pikus A, Patronas N (1994) Neurofibromatosis 2 (NF2): clinical characteristics of 63 affected individuals and clinical evidence for heterogeneity. Am J Med Genet 52(4):450–461

61. Ragge NK, Baser ME, Klein J et al (1995) Ocular abnormalities in neurofibromatosis 2. Am J Ophthalmol 120(5):634–641

62. Evans DG, Huson SM, Donnai D et al (1992) A genetic study of type 2 neurofibromatosis in the United Kingdom. I. Prevalence, mutation rate, fitness, and confirmation of maternal transmission effect on severity. J Med Genet 29(12):841–846

63. Sperfeld AD, Hein C, Schroder JM, Ludolph AC, Hanemann CO (2002) Occurrence and characterization of peripheral nerve involvement in neurofibromatosis type 2. Brain 125(5):996–1004

64. Hanemann CO, Diebold R, Kaufmann D (2007) Role of NF2 haploinsufficiency in NF2-associated polyneuropathy. Brain Pathol 17(4):371–376

65. Trivedi R, Byrne J, Huson SM, Donaghy M (2000) Focal amyotrophy in neurofibromatosis 2. J Neurol Neurosurg Psychiatr 69(2):257–261

66. Rouleau GA, Wertelecki W, Haines JL et al (1987) Genetic linkage of bilateral acoustic neurofibromatosis to a DNA marker on chromosome 22. Nature 329(6136):246–248

67. Wertelecki W, Rouleau GA, Superneau DW et al (1988) Neurofibromatosis 2: clinical and DNA linkage studies of a large kindred. N Engl J Med 319(5):278–283

68. Trofatter JA, MacCollin MM, Rutter JL et al (1993) A novel moesin-, ezrin-, radixin-like gene is a candidate for the neurofibromatosis 2 tumor suppressor. Cell 75(4):826

69. Rouleau GA, Merel P, Lutchman M et al (1993) Alteration in a new gene encoding a putative membrane-organizing protein causes neuro-fibromatosis type 2. Nature 363(6429):515–521

70. McClatchey AI, Giovannini M (2005) Membrane organization and tumorigenesis – the NF2 tumor suppressor, Merlin. Genes Dev 19(19):2265–2277

71. Ahronowitz I, Xin W, Kiely R, Sims K, MacCollin M, Nunes FP (2007) Mutational spectrum of the NF2 gene: a meta-analysis of 12 years of research and diagnostic laboratory findings. Hum Mutat 28(1):1–12

72. Baser ME (2006) The distribution of constitutional and somatic mutations in the neurofibromatosis 2 gene. Hum Mutat 27(4):297–306

73. MacCollin M, Braverman N, Viskochil D et al (1996) A point mutation associated with a severe phenotype of neurofibromatosis 2. Ann Neurol 40(3):440–445

74. Ruttledge MH, Andermann AA, Phelan CM et al (1996) Type of mutation in the neurofibromatosis type 2 gene (NF2) frequently determines severity of disease. Am J Hum Genet 59(2):331–342

75. Jacoby LB, MacCollin M, Barone R, Ramesh V, Gusella JF (1996) Frequency and distribution of NF2 mutations in schwannomas. Genes Chromosomes Cancer 17(1):45–55

76. Wellenreuther R, Kraus JA, Lenartz D et al (1995) Analysis of the neurofibromatosis 2 gene reveals molecular variants of meningioma. Am J Pathol 146(4):827–832

77. Aghi M, Kluwe L, Webster MT et al (2006) Unilateral vestibular schwannoma with other neurofibromatosis Type 2-related tumors: clinical and molecular study of a unique phenotype. J Neurosurg 104:201–207

78. Kluwe L, Mautner V, Heinrich B et al (2003) Molecular study of frequency of mosaicism in neurofibromatosis 2 patients with bilateral vestibular schwannomas. J Med Genet 40(2):109–114

79. Wallace AJ, Watson CJ, Oward E, Evans DG, Elles RG (2004) Mutation scanning of the NF2 gene: an improved service based on meta-PCR/sequencing, dosage analysis, and loss of heterozygosity analysis. Genet Test 8(4):368–380

80. Evans DG, Ramsden RT, Shenton A et al (2007) Mosaicism in neurofibromatosis type 2: an update of risk based on uni/bilaterality of vestibular schwannoma at presentation and sensitive mutation analysis including multiple ligation-dependent probe amplification. J Med Genet 44(7):424–428

81. Kluwe L, Friedrich RE, Tatagiba M, Mautner VF (2002) Presymptomatic diagnosis for children of sporadic neurofibromatosis 2 patients: a method based on tumor analysis. Genet Med 4(1):27–30

82. Liu R, Fagan P (2001) Facial nerve schwannoma: surgical excision versus conservative management. Ann Otol Rhinol Laryngol 110(11):1025–1029

83. Fuss M, Debus J, Lohr F et al (2000) Conventionally fractionated stereotactic radiotherapy (FSRT) for acoustic neuromas. Int J Radiat Oncol Biol Phys 48(5):1381–1387

84. Combs SE, Volk S, Schulz-Ertner D, Huber PE, Thilmann C, Debus J (2005) Management of acoustic neuromas with fractionated stereotactic radiotherapy (FSRT): long-term results in 106 patients treated in a single institution. Int J Radiat Oncol Biol Phys 63(1):75–81

85. Slattery WH III, Brackmann DE (1995) Results of surgery following stereotactic irradiation for acoustic neuromas. Am J Otol 16(3):315–319

86. Baser ME, Evans DG, Jackler RK, Sujansky E, Rubenstein A (2000) Neurofibromatosis 2, radiosurgery and malignant nervous system tumours. Br J Cancer 82(4):998

87. Thomsen J, Mirz F, Wetke R, Astrup J, Bojsen-Moller M, Nielsen E (2000) Intracranial sarcoma in a patient with neurofibromatosis type 2 treated with gamma knife radiosurgery for vestibular schwannoma. Am J Otol 21(3):364–370

88. Plotkin SR, Singh MA, O'Donnell CC, Harris GJ, McClatchey AI, Halpin C (2008) Audiologic and radiographic response of NF2-related vestibular schwannoma to erlotinib therapy. Nat Clin Pract Oncol 5(8):487–491

89. CBTRUS (2005) Statistical report: primary brain tumors in the United States, 1998–2002

90. Welling DB, Guida M, Goll F et al (1996) Mutational spectrum in the neurofibromatosis type 2 gene in sporadic and familial schwannomas. Hum Genet 98(2):189–193

91. Nunes F, Shen Y, Niida Y et al (2005) Inactivation patterns of NF2 and DAL-1/4.1B (EPB41L3) in sporadic meningioma. Cancer Genet Cytogenet 162(2):135–139

92. von Haken MS, White EC, Neshvar-Shyesther L et al (1996) Molecular genetic analysis of chromosome arm 17p and chromosome arm 22q DNA sequences in sporadic pediatric ependymomas. Genes Chromosomes Cancer 17(1):37–44

93. Ammerlaan AC, De BC, Ararou A et al (2005) Localization of a putative low-penetrance ependymoma susceptibility locus to 22q11 using a chromosome 22 tiling-path genomic microarray. Genes Chromosomes Cancer 43(4):329–338

94. Hulsebos TJ, Oskam NT, Bijleveld EH et al (1999) Evidence for an ependymoma tumour suppressor gene in chromosome region 22pter-22q11.2. Br J Cancer 81(7):1150–1154

95. Thurneysen C, Opitz I, Kurtz S, Weder W, Stahel RA, Felley-Bosco E (2009) Functional inactivation of NF2/merlin in human mesothelioma. Lung Cancer 64(2):140–147

96. Jongsma J, van ME, Vooijs M et al (2008) A conditional mouse model for malignant mesothelioma. Cancer Cell 13(3):261–271

97. Antinheimo J, Sankila R, Carpen O, Pukkala E, Sainio M, Jaaskelainen J (2000) Population-based analysis of sporadic and type 2 neurofibromatosis-associated meningiomas and schwannomas. Neurology 54(1):71

98. MacCollin M, Chiocca EA, Evans DG et al (2005) Diagnostic criteria for schwannomatosis. Neurology 64(11):1838–1845

99. Jacoby LB, Jones D, Davis K et al (1997) Molecular analysis of the NF2 tumor-suppressor gene in schwannomatosis. Am J Hum Genet 61(6):1293–1302

100. MacCollin M, Willett C, Heinrich B et al (2003) Familial schwannomatosis: exclusion of the NF2 locus as the germline event. Neurology 60(12):1968–1974

101. Hulsebos TJ, Plomp AS, Wolterman RA, Robanus-Maandag EC, Baas F, Wesseling P (2007) Germline mutation of INI1/SMARCB1 in familial schwannomatosis. Am J Hum Genet 80(4):805–810

102. Roberts CW, Orkin SH (2004) The SWI/SNF complex–chromatin and cancer. Nat Rev Cancer 4(2):133–142

103. Sestini R, Bacci C, Provenzano A, Genuardi M, Papi L (2008) Evidence of a four-hit mechanism involving SMARCB1 and NF2 in schwannomatosis-associated schwannomas. Hum Mutat 29(2):227–231

104. Hadfield KD, Newman WG, Bowers NL et al (2008) Molecular characterisation of SMARCB1 and NF2 in familial and sporadic schwannomatosis. J Med Genet 45(6):332–339

105. Boyd C, Smith MJ, Kluwe L, Balogh A, MacCollin M, Plotkin SR (2008) Alterations in the SMARCB1 (INI1) tumor suppressor gene in familial schwannomatosis. Clin Genet 74(4):358–366

106. Patil S, Perry A, MacCollin M et al (2008) Immunohistochemical analysis supports a role for INI1/SMARCB1 in hereditary forms of schwannomas, but not in solitary, sporadic schwannomas. Brain Pathol 18(4):517–519

107. Rieske P, Zakrzewska M, Piaskowski S et al (2003) Molecular heterogeneity of meningioma with INI1 mutation. Mol Pathol 56(5):299–301

108. Schmitz U, Mueller W, Weber M, Sevenet N, Delattre O, von DA (2001) INI1 mutations in meningiomas at a potential hotspot in exon 9. Br J Cancer 84(2):199–201

109. Versteege I, Sevenet N, Lange J et al (1998) Truncating mutations of hSNF5/INI1 in aggressive paediatric cancer. Nature 394(6689):203–206

110. Swensen JJ, Keyser J, Coffin CM, Biegel JA, Viskochil DH, Williams MS (2009) Familial occurrence of schwannomas and malignant rhabdoid tumour associated with a duplication in SMARCB1. J Med Genet 46(1):68–72

111. Janson K, Nedzi LA, David O et al (2006) Predisposition to atypical teratoid/rhabdoid tumor due to an inherited INI1 mutation. Pediatr Blood Cancer 47(3):279–284

Chapter 14
The HapMap Project and Low-Penetrance Cancer Susceptibility Alleles

Edwin Choy and David Altshuler

Keywords Haplotype • HapMap • Single-nucleotide polymorphism • Genome-wide association study • Allele • Linkage

Introduction

Previous chapters in this book (Chaps. 3 and 5–13) describe hereditary cancer syndromes that confer a substantial increase in risk for developing a particular malignancy. Such syndromes are considered to be Mendelian diseases, as the pattern of affected patients within an extended family closely follows the pattern of transmission of genes in a diploid organism as understood by Mendel's laws of inheritance. DNA variants – or mutations – that underlie Mendelian diseases or traits are highly penetrant. That is, by inheriting the disease mutation or allele, an individual has a very high chance of developing the disease in question.

As transmission of the DNA variant, known as alleles, closely track with the inheritance of Mendelian disease – that is, having a particular genotype confers a near 100% chance of developing a particular disease – genes underlying familial cancer syndromes can be identified using a genetic analysis tool referred to as linkage analysis. The human genome is approximately 3.3 billion base pairs long and has scattered within a large number of polymorphic loci consisting of repeating units of 1–6 base pairs in length. These loci are known as microsatellites, and they serve as genomic markers to identify a location on the chromosome. During reproductive meiosis, the chances of recombination between any two sites along a chromosome are proportional to the distance between the sites. Linkage analysis takes advantage of the fact that markers located near the disease causing mutation

will be transmitted to the offspring more frequently than markers distant to the mutation, a phenomenon termed linkage disequilibrium (LD) [1].

For example, Fig. 14.1 is an illustration of several versions of a region on chromosome 6 that existed in a specific population several generations ago [2]. These versions are identified by polymorphic variations within various HLA genes, HLA-DR and HLA-A. A disease causing mutation (green star) in the hemochromatosis gene (HFE) originates in the ancestral chromosome that carries the genetic variants HLA-DR4 and A3. However, over time, recombination between HFE and HLA-A occurs so rarely that the HFE mutation is still associated with A3 in 70% of cases. Because DR4 is further away from HFE than is A3, recombination between HFE and HLA-DR occurs more frequently than between HFE and HLA-A. Therefore, HFE is linked with DR4 in only 45% of the cases.

During reproduction, meiotic recombination would lead to greater cotransmission of the disease-causing mutation with HLA-A alleles rather than with HLA-DR alleles. Therefore, HLA-A3 would be cotransmitted with disease to offspring at a significantly higher frequency than with HLA-DR4 and markers on other chromosomes, linking the disease-causing mutation closely with the chromosomal region around HLA-A. By studying the patterns of cancer and marker transmission in large families with a significantly high frequency of a highly penetrant mutation for a particular cancer, the chromosomal region for that disease-causing mutation can be identified. Such techniques are not as well powered to identify poorly penetrant alleles, as the lower association of the disease-causing mutation with disease leads to significant reductions in associating nearby markers with disease.

Although identification of several cancer-causing mutations have led to great advances in our understanding of the biologic basis of certain cancers and ability to predict risk for patients who carry those mutations, the genetic basis for the overwhelming majority of cancers has not been identified [3–7]. Furthermore, even for patients with cancer caused by a known mutations, those alleles only partially explain the increased risk of disease that is observed. For example,

E. Choy (✉)
Department of Medicine, Massachusetts General Hospital, Boston, MA, USA
e-mail: echoy@partners.org

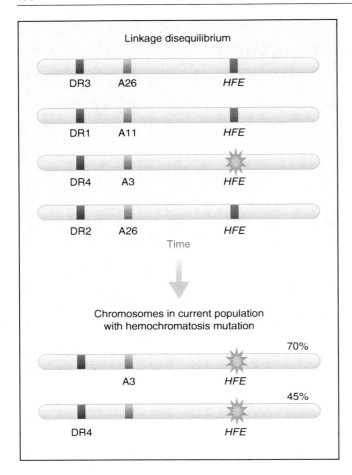

Linkage disequilibrium

DR3   A26   HFE

DR1   A11   HFE

DR4   A3   HFE

DR2   A26   HFE

Time

Chromosomes in current population
with hemochromatosis mutation

70%

A3   HFE

45%

DR4   HFE

Fig. 14.1 Example of linkage disequilibrium (from Guttmacher and Collins [2]. Copyright © 2002 Massachusetts Medical Society. All rights reserved)

mutations in BRCA1 and BRCA2 explain only 20% of the twofold excess risk in relatives of the BRCA+ breast cancer patient [8].

As illustrated in Fig. 14.2, most of the familial excess in breast and colorectal cancer remains unaccounted for, and this excess can be attributed to other low-penetrance alleles that can each contribute a small genotypic risk that can combine to confer a broad range of susceptibility in the population [4]. However, for reasons stated above, such low-penetrance alleles only partially correlate with disease traits, and even the largest of family-based linkage studies would not have the statistical power to detect the risk-conferring allele.

In this chapter, we describe the historical advent of theory and technology that allows for a genome-wide search for low-penetrance cancer susceptibility alleles. We will then describe where the field is in 2009, describing examples from GWAS of several of the most common cancers, and where the next generation of discoveries is to be made. Finally, we will discuss the value of such discoveries to biology, medicine, and society.

SNPs

Although linkage analysis using microsatellite markers led to the identification of many important cancer susceptibility alleles, such alleles were extremely rare in population, as these strongly deleterious mutations conferred a selective disadvantage to the individuals' chances of surviving long enough to pass on these alleles to their offspring – a process called purifying selection. However, the less penetrant cancer susceptibility alleles would not necessarily impact an individual's ability to survive to parenthood and may exist more commonly in population. Such alleles can quickly increase in frequency in populations that undergo rapid expansion [9]. In order to identify alleles that confer cancer risk more generally, population based studies involving many thousands of subjects, rather than studies of family-based transmission of traits and alleles, would be required, as such family studies by nature will be very limited in size.

Microsatellite markers are unsatisfactory for population based studies as only 5,000 such markers exist genome-wide [10], leaving, on the average, 660 Kb between markers. Any two unrelated individuals are likely separated by hundreds, if not thousands, of meiotic events, and the linkage between a putative disease causing allele and the nearest microsatellite would typically break down completely at that genomic distance.

Single nucleotide polymorphisms, or SNPs, are instances in the genome where, across populations, there is variation at a given DNA position (see Fig. 14.3). SNPs can exist within genes as missense, nonsense, or conservative mutations, or they can exist in nongenic regions as regulatory or nonfunctional mutations. SNPs are just one of several types of DNA variations, which also include insertions and deletions of single nucleotide bases, duplications or deletions of larger numbers of DNA bases (copy number variations), and polymorphic repeats of DNA sequences (such as microsatellites).

Figure 14.3 is an illustration of SNPs at position 3, 4, and 5 (in orange) interspersed with invariant nucleotide bases (in gray) along genomic DNA. Here, SNPs at positions 3 and 4 appear to be linked; that is, where there is a guanine nucleotide (G) at position SNP3, there is a cytosine nucleotide (C) at position SNP4; and where there is a thymine nucleotide (T) at position SNP3, there is a T at position SNP4. Such regions of sequentially linked SNPs are referred to as haplotype blocks. SNP5, on the other hand, appears unlinked to SNPs 3 and 4, as a T at position SNP5 can be associated with both versions of haplotypes defined by SNP positions at 3 and 4.

What made SNPs particularly useful was that they were several orders more frequent within the genome than microsatellites. As the heterogeneity rate for SNPs is approximately one every 1,000 bases [11], if a dense enough catalog of SNPs can be tested, there likely exists an SNP that is nearby any given disease causing allele. Furthermore, technology was developed that enabled SNPs to be genotyped at increasingly higher

Fig. 14.2 Most of the familial excess in breast and colorectal cancers is due to unknown genes (reprinted by permission from Macmillan Publishers Ltd: Oncogene 23:6471–6476, copyright 2004)

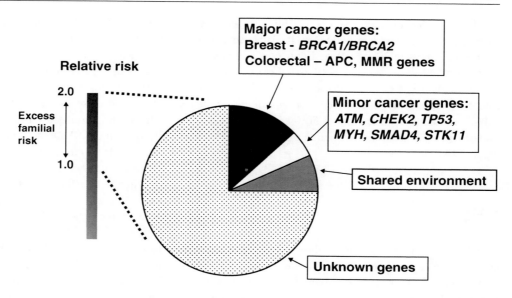

Fig. 14.3 The nature of genomic variation: SNPs (from Christensen K, Murray JC (2007) What genome-wide association studies can do for medicine. N Engl J Med 356:1094–1097. Copyright © 2007 Massachusetts Medical Society. All rights reserved)

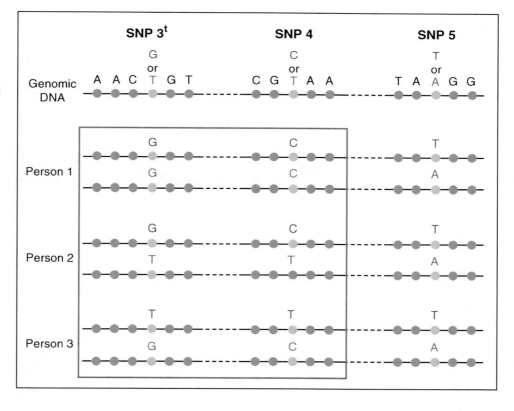

accuracy and throughput at vanishingly lower cost. Currently, a number of platforms are available, capable of genotyping one to one million SNPs for one to 384 patients per assay plate: Taqman, Sequenom, and SNPlex platforms can genotype one to 48 SNPs in 384 samples per run. Affymetrix and Illumina-Infinium platforms can genotype 950,000 to one million SNPs in one sample per run. Understandably, throughput decreases with increasing number of SNPs analyzed.

The SNP Consortium (TSC) is a public–private partnership that cataloged all identified SNPs. Its database contained 1.4 million SNPs in 2001 [12], and now contains more than 10 million SNPs [13]. At each SNP loci, there exists an allele that is more frequent in population (major allele) than the minor allele. For any given SNP, the minor allele frequency (MAF) can be as high just under 50% and as rare as a fraction of 1%. By convention, we define a common SNP as having an MAF of greater than 1%.

HapMap

Which of the millions of SNPs should investigators use to correlate DNA variation to cancers? The answer to this question depended upon three variables: (1) the frequency of a given SNP; (2) the degree of LD around a given SNP, indicating how strongly population variation of an SNP would correlate to population variation of a putative disease causing mutation, and (3) the genomic region being studied. In 2002, the International HapMap Project (IHP) was launched to understand the first two of the variables above [14].

The project initially genotyped approximately one million SNPs in 90 individuals each from populations of Asia,

West Africa, and Caucasians of European descent [15]. Simultaneously, a private company, Perlegen Sciences, used a proprietary platform to genotype 1,586,383 SNPs in 71 Americans of European, African, and Asian ancestry [16]. By 2007, the project had genotyped more than three million SNPs in each of these 270 individuals [17]. By improving knowledge of the frequencies and LD structure of SNPs across the genome, the IHP allowed for rational selection of SNPs for association studies. Furthermore, software was developed and made publicly available to analyze and display HapMap data in a fashion that would be readily usable by investigators. One example of such open source software, Haploview [18], is available on http://www.broad.mit.edu/mpg/haploview/. Haploview provides a common interface to perform a variety of tasks related to analyzing HapMap and Perlegen data. In addition to performing and visualizing LD and haplotype block analysis, Haploview contains functionalities to estimate haplotype population frequency, perform single SNP and haplotype association tests, perform permutation testing to determine significance of associations observed, use SNP selection algorithms to select for high yield SNPs, and visualize results of whole genome association results.

Figure 14.4 illustrates an example of Haploview results for a magnified region of a chromosome. Each black dot represents a SNP with two allelic possibilities. At the intersection

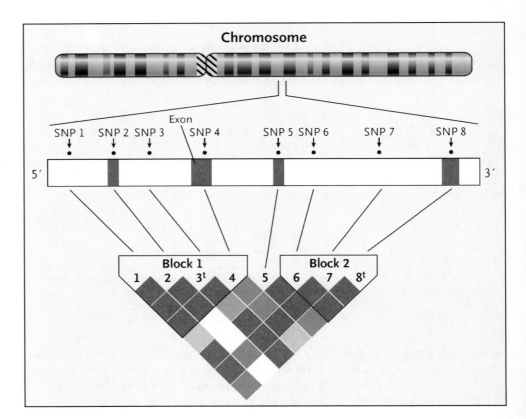

Fig. 14.4 Mapping the relationships among SNPs (from Christensen K, Murray JC (2007) What genome-wide association studies can do for medicine. N Engl J Med 356:1094–1097. Copyright © 2007 Massachusetts Medical Society. All rights reserved)

between any two SNPs (shown in red, pink, or white squares), the degree of correlation between SNPs can be strong (red), weak (pink), or nonexistent (white). Such a schema can reveal blocks of strong association (haplotype block) separated by areas of little association. Certain SNPs – such as SNPs 3 and 8 in this illustration – can serve as "tagging" or surrogate SNPs for the haplotype block, as testing for such SNPs can highly predict for the genotypes of all of the other SNPs within the block.

Figure 14.5 is a Haploview diagram of actual data from the International HapMap Project showing 420 genetic variants in a 500 kb region on chromosome 5q31. (Typically, microsatellite data would capture only one polymorphism in such a region.) Looking at the Haploview plot of pairwise correlations, blocks of strong correlations can be discerned (outlined in black).

Figure 14.6 is a more detailed illustration of DNA variations than Fig. 14.4, demonstrating a range of variations seen in the human genome. Here, ten individuals are represented with 20 distinct copies of the human genome. For each individual, a 5 kb region of genome centered on a chromosomal region of frequent recombination (a recombination hotspot) is represented by 12 common variations – including ten SNPs, one insertion/deletion polymorphism, and a repeat polymorphism of a four nucleotide sequence. At the left of the recombination hotspot, six DNA variants are strongly correlated. Additionally, other rarer variants are illustrated in Fig. 14.5, including five rare SNPs (in red) and a large area of deletion (second from the bottom chromosome).

Although six polymorphisms, with two alleles at each site, can theoretically yield $2^6 = 64$ possibilities, only three possibilities are actually observed (in blocks of pink, green, and orange). Each of these patterns are haplotypes seen in real population. Likewise, to the right of the recombination hotspot, only two haplotypes are seen (illustrated in blocks of blue and purple). In the triangular Haploview illustration below, the pairwise correlations between linked SNPs are shown in red, while unlinked SNPs are shown is white.

Initially, SNPs and HapMap data were initially useful for performing candidate gene association studies [19–23]. Observations in basic science laboratory experiments would implicate a single gene or group of genes to be potentially important in predisposing an individual to a given disease. Known DNA variants would be genotyped both within and around the candidate gene in cohorts of individuals with disease, and the frequency of SNPS were compared to a cohort of individuals without disease – an approach known as the association study.

Using this approach, numerous claims of genotype–phenotype associations were made [24]. However, very few such associates bore out in replication studies [25].

This failure to replicate associations was due to several factors. Many studies were susceptible to confounding by unaccounted differences in the genetic background of the case/control cohorts being compared [26, 27]. Importantly, early association studies did not appreciate how small the effects of disease causing alleles would be, and as a result, most such studies were underpowered with respect to study size to identify disease causing variants. Another reason for failing to identify disease causing alleles was that current biological knowledge was simply inadequate to identify an accurate chromosomal region to perform the association study [28]. We will show below that the low-penetrance cancer susceptibility alleles that were identified in genome wide

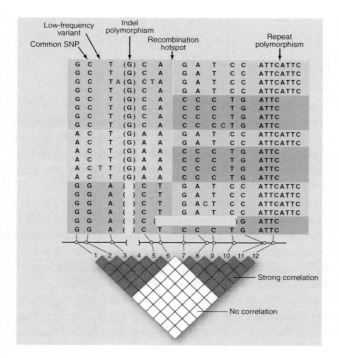

Fig. 14.5 Haploview diagram of observed data from the International HapMap Project (from Altshuler et al. [28])

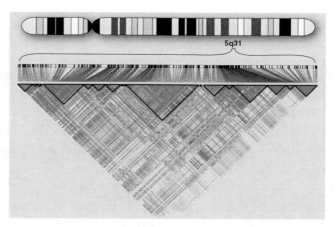

Fig. 14.6 Common and rare genetic variation in ten individuals, carrying 20 distinct copies of the human genome (from Altshuler et al. [28])

association studies mostly lie in regions previously unappreciated by modern biology.

Genome-Wide Association Studies

As SNP genotyping – initially costing approximately $1 per measurement – became more affordable, accurate, and high throughput, massively parallel genotyping was made possible. Several technologies exist that enable one million SNPs representing regions across the entire genome to be genotyped simultaneously at >99% accuracy and completeness, costing less than $0.001 per SNP.

This technology, combined with the advances in statistical design, analysis, and interpretation resulting from the HapMap Project, has enabled the performance of numerous genome-wide association studies (GWAS) unbiased by prior biological suppositions.

Breast Cancer

Figure 14.7 demonstrates the relationship between the effect size of the breast cancer causing mutation linked to an SNP, the frequency of SNPs linked to cancer, and the ability to detect such SNPs given a variety of genetic tools [3]. The highly penetrant mutations leading to several fold increase in risk, although rare in population, can be identified by studying families with breast cancer syndromes. The more moderate-risk alleles are more frequent in population and can be identified by sequencing candidate genes in patients with breast cancer. The bulk of low-risk alleles are very common

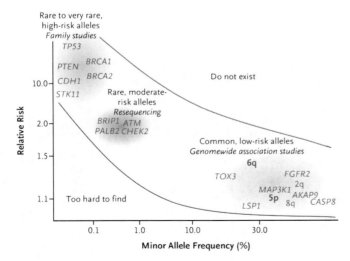

Fig. 14.7 Breast cancer susceptibility loci and genes (from Foulkes [3]. Copyright © 2008 Massachusetts Medical Society. All rights reserved)

in population, each contributing a very small increase in overall risk for cancer and requiring a very large association study to be discovered.

One of the early successful GWAS in cancer was performed in breast cancer by a consortium of international investigators led by groups from the UK and Australia [29]. The group conducted a two-stage GWAS in which 227,876 SNPs were genotyped in 4,398 individuals with breast cancer and 4,316 controls. Thirty of the most significant SNPs derived from this GWAS were further tested for replication in 21,860 individuals with breast cancer and 22,578 controls. Of the 30 genes tested, six SNPs proved to have genome-wide statistical significance ($P < 10^{-7}$). One of these SNPs did not lie near any known gene. Five of these SNPs were either within genes or within LD range of a known gene (FGFR2, TNRC9, MAP3K1, and LSP1, see Fig. 14.8). Of these genes, only one (FGFR2) has prior relevance to breast cancer. Most previously identified cancer susceptibility genes lie within the DNA repair and sex hormone synthesis or metabolism pathway, but none of the genes identified in this GWAS are implicated in these pathways.

This study highlighted the importance of study size in GWAS and reminded us that prior biological knowledge is quite incomplete. The authors estimate that when the relative risks for all five loci are combined in a multiplicative genetic model, this study explains only an additional 3.6% of the excess familial risk of breast cancer. This is in addition to the 25% of familial risk that is explained by the high-penetrance alleles such as BRCA1, BRCA2, CHEK2, ATM, and others. 71.4% of the excess familial risk of breast cancer remains unexplained.

Prostate Cancer

In another multiple-staged GWAS design, another international consortia of investigators led by groups in the US genotyped 527,869 SNPs in 1,172 individuals with prostate cancer and 1,157 controls. 26,958 SNPs were selected from the first stage and genotyped in 3,941 cases and 3,964 controls [30].

This group confirmed two previously reported loci on chromosome 8q24 and one locus in chromosome 17 in the HNF1B gene (also called TCF2). The study also identified three novel loci with genome-wide significance at or near genes on chromosomes 7 (JAZF1) and 10 (CTBP2 and MSMB), and one loci on chromosome 11 that is not close to any known gene. Interestingly, most of the SNPs that achieved genome-wide significance were not among the top 1,000 most significant SNPs after the first stage of the study. As with the breast cancer GWAS, most of the loci are not in LD with any gene previously implicated in risk for prostate cancer.

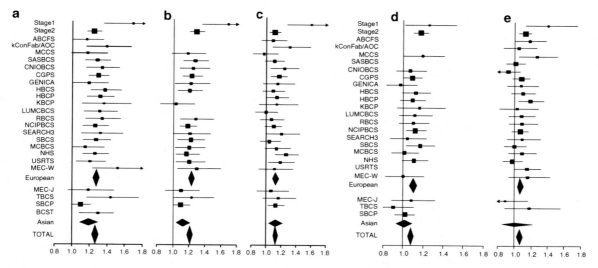

Fig. 14.8 Forest plots of the per-allele odds ratios for each of the five SNPs reaching genome-wide significance (Reprinted by permission from Macmillan Publishers Ltd: Nature 447:1087–1093, copyright 2007)

Colorectal Cancer

An international group of investigators led by groups from Oxford conducted a meta-analysis of GWAS for colorectal cancer [31]. The meta-analysis analyzed 38,710 SNPs genotyped in 13,315 individuals. Results were replicated on 27,418 individuals, and four previously unreported risk loci were identified. One locus was not near any known gene. The other loci were at or near BMP4, CDH1, and RHPN2.

A repeating lesson learned from each GWAS is that the effect sizes for each cancer-causing DNA variant is quite small and, as a result, the power to detect these alleles was low in previous studies. For the loci that are identified, most do not involve previous candidate genes or pathways and therefore immediately suggest new biologic hypothesis for further investigation. Additionally, a substantial portion of new loci discovered are not near any known genes, suggesting a need for a radically new understanding of genome biology or gene regulation.

Summary of Results

Taken together, the GWAS described above, as well as others, demonstrate that GWAS is an effective approach to identifying novel loci and confirming previously described loci linked to disease causing inherited mutations. A comprehensive list of GWAS for cancers and other diseases can be found in the National Human Genome Research Institute catalog of published GWA studies (http://www.genome. gov/26525384). As of March 24, 2009, there have been 278 GWAS publications on breast cancer.

As depicted in Table 14.1, cancer-risk alleles appear to fall into three categories of high, moderate, and low relative risk. As the high-risk alleles likely confer a reproductive disadvantage to the carrier, these alleles are extremely rare in population. Alternatively, although low-risk alleles do not individually confer any practical degree of risk to the carriers, their high prevalence in population makes them biologically important mutations.

Future Studies

Although GWAS studies have identified numerous novel loci, in all cases, the disease causing inherited mutation has not been identified. As done for linkage analysis, identification of the deleterious mutation requires "fine-mapping," by genotyping at many more SNPs or even sequencing within the loci for a large number of cases and controls. If the causal variant is genotyped, its association to cancer should be higher than other SNPs, unless one or more SNPs are completely linked to the causal SNP.

Even after the causal variant is identified, much work will be needed to understand its functional significance. Highly penetrant alleles were likely to induce significant changes in protein structure or function by alterations in amino acid sequence or truncating the protein. Low-penetrance alleles, however, are likely to act by altering regulation of gene expression. Loci that are not near any known genes (gene desert) are even more difficult to study in functional assays.

Table 14.1 Genes and loci implicated in the inheritance of common cancers, according to the risk among heterozygotes[a]

Cancer site	Relative risk ≥5.0	Relative risk ≥1.5 and <5.0	Relative risk ≥1.01 and <1.5
	Gene (% of cancers caused by mutation in this gene)	Genes or loci	
Lung	*RB1* (<0.1), *TP53* (<0.1)	No convincing examples	rs1051730, rs8034191; *CHRNA3*, *CHRNB4*, *CHRNA5* are candidate genes
Breast	*BRCA1* (1–5)[b], *BRCA2* (1–5)[b], *TP53* (<0.5), *PTEN* (<0.5), *STK11* (<0.1), *CDH1* (<0.1)	*CHEK2*, *ATM*, *PALB2*, *BRIP1*	*CASP8*[c], *FGFR2*[d], *MAP3K1*, loci on 8q24, 5p[d], *TOX3*[d], 2q[d], 6q22[e], *LSP1*
Colon and rectum	*APC* (0.5–1.0), *MLH1* (1–2), *MSH2* (1–2), *MSH6* (<1), *PMS2* (<1)	*APC* (I1307K), *BLM* (*BLM*[Ash])	*MUTYH*[f], *CASP8*[c], 8q24loci, 8q23 (*EIF3H*), 10p14, 11q23, *CRAC1*, *SMAD7*[g]
Prostate	*BRCA2* (<0.1)	8q24 loci[h]	*rs6501455* (and other adjacent loci), *rs721048*, *NBS1*, *EHBP1*, *TCF2*, *CTBP2*, *JAZF1*, *MSMB*, *LMTK2*, *KLK3*, *SLC22A3*[i]
Pancreas	*BRCA2* (<0.5), *CDKN2A* (<0.1), *STK11* (<0.1), *TP53* (<0.1), *PRSS1* (<0.1), *SPINK1*[j] (<0.1)	*BRCA1*, *MSH2*, *MLH1*	No convincing examples

[a]In the high-risk category, risk alleles are rare (<0.1–0.01%) or very rare (<0.01%). In the moderate-risk category, most risk alleles are very rare and a few risk alleles are common. In the low-risk category, most risk alleles are common (>10%). The population attributable risk percentage is not indicated because it is a misleading number (i.e., it can sum to more than 100%)

[b]This percentage is closer to 1% in most populations and closer to 5% in the Ashkenazi Jewish population

[c]Variants in *CASP8* are associated with a decreased risk of breast, colorectal, and other cancers

[d]These loci only contribute to the risk of estrogen-receptor-positive breast cancer

[e]The effects of this locus appear to be restricted to the Ashkenazi Jewish population

[f]Biallelic mutations in *MUTYH* result in a distinct syndrome, *MUTYH*-associated polyposis, which is akin to attenuated or classic familial adenomatous polyposis

[g]The pooled odds ratio for the association between the *SMAD7* intron 3 SNP rs4939827 and the risk of colorectal cancer is 0.87 (95% confidence interval (CI), 0.80–0.95). The rs12953717 is also in intron 3 of *SMAD7* and is associated with an increased risk of colorectal cancer (odds ratio, 1.11; 95% CI, 1.03–1.20)

[h]The alleles associated with increased risk are remarkably frequent in blacks (approximately 40% of blacks carry one or more of these variants). The allele at rs1447295 is also frequent in this population, but it does not appear to be associated with an increased risk of prostate cancer

[i]Apart from *NBS1*, for all other cases in this group, the named gene is only the most likely candidate to be implicated in prostate cancer. The strength of each candidate varies. *MSMB* encodes a secreted protein. *KLK3* encodes prostate-specific antigen, and therefore it may have nothing to do with prostate-cancer susceptibility itself. *LMTK2* encodes a cyclin-dependent kinase

[j]Mutations in *STK11* cause Peutz–Jeghers syndrome, whereas *PRSS1* and *SPINK1* mutations are responsible for a sizable fraction of cases of hereditary pancreatitis

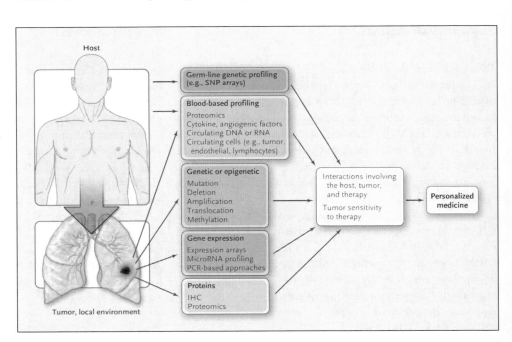

Fig. 14.9 Molecular-profiling approaches to the development of personalized therapy (from Herbst et al. [32]. Copyright © 2008 Massachusetts Medical Society. All rights reserved)

Summary

The ultimate goal of medical genetic studies in oncology would be personalized medical care. Rather than treating all patients with a particular subtype of cancer with the same drugs, patients would be characterized individually to include detailed profiles of many protein, RNA, and DNA variations in malignancies as well as further genetic and environmental characteristics of the patient (see Fig. 14.9). In searching for low-penetrance cancer alleles, another hope is to enable better prognostication for an individual's likelihood to develop a particular type of cancer. By understanding one's own genetic risk, an individual can adapt their behavior and environment in specific ways to minimize the chances of developing cancer.

Preliminary findings from the cancer GWAS described above indicate that such fine tuned prognostication and personalized medicine is not likely to significantly benefit most patients. For example, the additional five low-penetrance alleles discovered by Easton et al. for breast cancer only explain an additional 3.6% of the excess familial risk of breast cancer. Clinically, being able to tell a patient that his or her risk is increased 3.6% over the average risk typically does little in terms of practical benefit. Furthermore, there is little evidence that such prognostication actually alters patient behavior in any significant manner. Currently, the biggest factor that increases the risk for many cancers is tobacco use, which currently contributes to several-fold higher risks for cancer than any known low-penetrance genetic risk allele.

The real benefit to discovering low-penetrance alleles is in the contribution of such data to understanding the biological basis of cancer. To use an example outside of cancer research, GWASs have recently identified common genetic variations in enzymes involved in cholesterol metabolism that each has small effects on cholesterol levels. However, drugs that target a particular cholesterol metabolism enzyme, HMGCR, have a much larger effect on cholesterol levels and thereby significantly reduce incidence of heart disease. By developing such drugs that pharmacologically amplify the phenotype of low-penetrance alleles, human physiology and propensity to develop a disease can be dramatically modified. The hope in cancer genetics is that by discovering new genes that contribute – albeit at low risk – to the development of cancer, we can better understand, both scientifically and clinically, what is needed to improve prevention and treatment.

References

1. Reich DE, Cargill M, Bolk S et al (2001) Linkage disequilibrium in the human genome. Nature 411:199–204
2. Guttmacher AE, Collins FS (2002) Genomic medicine – a primer. N Engl J Med 347:1512–1520
3. Foulkes WD (2008) Inherited susceptibility to common cancers. N Engl J Med 359:2143–2153
4. Houlston RS, Peto J (2004) The search for low-penetrance cancer susceptibility alleles. Oncogene 23:6471–6476
5. Hunter DJ, Altshuler D, Rader DJ (2008) From Darwin's finches to canaries in the coal mine – mining the genome for new biology. N Engl J Med 358:2760–2763
6. Ponder BA (2001) Cancer genetics. Nature 411:336–341
7. Stratton MR, Rahman N (2008) The emerging landscape of breast cancer susceptibility. Nat Genet 40:17–22
8. (2000) Prevalence and penetrance of BRCA1 and BRCA2 mutations in a population-based series of breast cancer cases. Anglian Breast Cancer Study Group. Br J Cancer 83:1301–1308
9. Reich DE, Lander ES (2001) On the allelic spectrum of human disease. Trends Genet 17:502–510
10. Dib C, Faure S, Fizames C et al (1996) A comprehensive genetic map of the human genome based on 5,264 microsatellites. Nature 380:152–154
11. Li WH, Sadler LA (1991) Low nucleotide diversity in man. Genetics 129:513–523
12. Sachidanandam R, Weissman D, Schmidt SC et al (2001) A map of human genome sequence variation containing 1.42 million single nucleotide polymorphisms. Nature 409:928–933
13. Entrez SNP, http://www.ncbi.nlm.nih.gov/sites/entrez?db=snp.
14. The International HapMap Consortium (2003) The International HapMap Project. Nature 426:789–796
15. International HapMap Consortium (2005) A haplotype map of the human genome. Nature 437:1299–1320
16. Hinds DA, Stuve LL, Nilsen GB et al (2005) Whole-genome patterns of common DNA variation in three human populations. Science 307:1072–1079
17. Frazer KA, Ballinger DG, Cox DR et al (2007) A second generation human haplotype map of over 3.1 million SNPs. Nature 449:851–861
18. Barrett JC, Fry B, Maller J, Daly MJ (2005) Haploview: analysis and visualization of LD and haplotype maps. Bioinformatics 21:263–265
19. Hunter DJ, Riboli E, Haiman CA et al (2005) A candidate gene approach to searching for low-penetrance breast and prostate cancer genes. Nat Rev Cancer 5:977–985
20. Chen YC, Kraft P, Bretsky P et al (2007) Sequence variants of estrogen receptor beta and risk of prostate cancer in the National Cancer Institute Breast and Prostate Cancer Cohort Consortium. Cancer Epidemiol Biomarkers Prev 16:1973–1981
21. Feigelson HS, Cox DG, Cann HM et al (2006) Haplotype analysis of the HSD17B1 gene and risk of breast cancer: a comprehensive approach to multicenter analyses of prospective cohort studies. Cancer Res 66:2468–2475
22. Kraft P, Pharoah P, Chanock SJ et al (2005) Genetic variation in the HSD17B1 gene and risk of prostate cancer. PLoS Genet 1:e68
23. Freedman ML, Penney KL, Stram DO et al (2005) A haplotype-based case-control study of BRCA1 and sporadic breast cancer risk. Cancer Res 65:7516–7522
24. Lohmueller KE, Pearce CL, Pike M, Lander ES, Hirschhorn JN (2003) Meta-analysis of genetic association studies supports a contribution of common variants to susceptibility to common disease. Nat Genet 33:177–182
25. Hirschhorn JN, Lohmueller K, Byrne E, Hirschhorn K (2002) A comprehensive review of genetic association studies. Genet Med 4:45–61
26. Freedman ML, Reich D, Penney KL et al (2004) Assessing the impact of population stratification on genetic association studies. Nat Genet 36:388–393
27. Campbell CD, Ogburn EL, Lunetta KL et al (2005) Demonstrating stratification in a European American population. Nat Genet 37:868–872
28. Altshuler D, Daly MJ, Lander ES (2008) Genetic mapping in human disease. Science 322:881–888

29. Easton DF, Pooley KA, Dunning AM et al (2007) Genome-wide association study identifies novel breast cancer susceptibility loci. Nature 447:1087–1093

30. Thomas G, Jacobs KB, Yeager M et al (2008) Multiple loci identified in a genome-wide association study of prostate cancer. Nat Genet 40:310–315

31. Houlston RS, Webb E, Broderick P et al (2008) Meta-analysis of genome-wide association data identifies four new susceptibility loci for colorectal cancer. Nat Genet 40: 1426–1435

32. Herbst RS, Heymach JV, Lippman SM (2008) Lung cancer. N Engl J Med 359:1367–1380

Chapter 15

Somatic Genetic Alterations and Implications for Targeted Therapies in Cancer (GIST, CML, Lung Cancer)

Alice T. Shaw, Eyal C. Attar, Edwin Choy, and Jeffrey Engelman

Keywords Tyrosine kinase • Tyrosine kinase inhibitor • Gastrointestinal stromal tumor • Chronic myelogenous leukemia • Lung cancer • Imatinib • EGFR inhibitor • Philadelphia chromosome • c-KIT • Stem cell factor • Fluorescence in situ hybridization

Introduction

The last decade has witnessed tremendous advances in the treatment of patients with cancer. Chief among these is the discovery and successful development of new, targeted cancer therapies. These therapies are highly effective in genetically defined subsets of patients, i.e., patients whose tumors harbor specific genetic abnormalities. In contrast to previous chapters focusing on germline genetic alterations that increase the risk of cancer, this chapter will examine cancers with somatic genetic alterations that confer sensitivity to molecularly targeted therapies. Examples of targeted therapies include imatinib for chronic myelogenous leukemia and gastrointestinal stromal tumors, traztuzumab and lapatinib for *HER2*-amplified breast cancer, and erlotinib, a tyrosine kinase inhibitor (TKI) targeting epidermal growth factor receptor (EGFR), for *EGFR*-mutant nonsmall cell lung cancer (see Table 15.1).

In this chapter, we will focus on three of the four major cancer types listed above: chronic myelogenous leukemia, gastrointestinal stromal tumor, and non-small cell lung cancer. For each type of cancer, we will discuss the underlying genetic mutations that drive the carcinogenic process and how knowledge of these mutations has led to the successful development of molecularly targeted agents. In lung cancer, both EGFR and ALK (anaplastic lymphoma kinase) have been validated as therapeutic targets (Table 15.1) and will be discussed separately. While the impact of targeted therapies has been enormous for select subsets of cancer patients, much more work remains to be done. In particular, as described below, resistance to targeted agents is inevitable for the vast majority of patients with advanced disease. Identifying and targeting pathways mediating resistance will be essential to developing more effective and more durable treatments for these patients.

Chronic Myeloid Leukemia

Chronic myeloid leukemia (CML) is a clonal myeloproliferative disorder rooted in primitive hematopoietic stem cells [1]. It accounts for approximately 20% of adult leukemias. Chronic myeloid leukemia is divided into three stages: (1) the chronic phase, which is characterized by an increase in the pool of myeloid progenitors with resulting peripheral blood leukocytosis and thrombocytosis, (2) an intermediate phase termed accelerated phase, and (3) a more rapidly advancing phase akin to acute leukemia known as blast crisis. Left untreated, CML in chronic phase ultimately develops into blast crisis over a period of 3–5 years.

Targeting BCR-ABL in CML

CML represents a paradigm for the development of molecularly targeted therapies in malignancy. More than 95% of patients have a translocation between chromosomes 9 and 22 involving rearrangement of the breakpoint cluster region (*BCR*) on chromosome 22 with the *c-ABL* proto-oncogene on chromosome 9 (Fig. 15.1) [2]. The truncated chromosome 22, known as the Philadelphia chromosome, results in generation of a chimeric oncoprotein known as *BCR-ABL*, which is principally responsible for driving cell autonomous proliferation. CML was once treated with allogeneic stem cell transplantation, though this procedure was not available

A.T. Shaw (✉)
Massachusetts General Hospital Cancer Center,
Harvard Medical School, Boston, MA, USA
e-mail: ashaw1@partners.org

Table 15.1 Summary of cancers with molecular targeted therapies

Disease	Target	Targeted Rx	Incidence in US[a]
CML	BCR-ABL	Imatinib	5,000
Breast cancer	HER2	Traztuzumab, lapatinib	38,000
GIST	CKIT	Imatinib	4,000
Lung cancer	EGFR	Erlotinib, gefitinib	20,000
	EML4-ALK	PF-02341066	6,000

[a]Incidence is defined as the number of new cases per year in the United States

for all patients due to the lack of an available donor, comorbidities, or advanced age [3]. Thus, agents such as interferon, cytarabine, and hydroxyurea were utilized. Today, CML is currently treated using oral tyrosine kinase inhibitors, which have excellent response rates and are preferred to allografting as initial therapy [4]. However, tyrosine kinase inhibitors are most useful in patients with CML in chronic phase. While they are active in patients with accelerated and blastic forms of the disease, conventional chemotherapies and allogeneic stem cell transplantation are required for such advanced patients.

Imatinib was the first treatment for CML targeting the BCR-ABL oncoprotein [5]. Imatinib inhibits the constitutively active BCR-ABL tyrosine kinase and impairs the growth and proliferation of CML cells. Over time, this permits the resumption of normal hematopoiesis. While treatment modalities such as stem cell transplantation or chemotherapy agents were required in the past, imatinib has revolutionized the care of patients with CML. In patients with newly diagnosed CML in chronic phase, the complete cytogenetic rate (defined as the achievement of a bone marrow without detectable BCR-ABL-positive cells) at 18 months is 74%, compared with 9% in patients treated with interferon [6]. After 60 months of therapy, the complete cytogenetic rate in patients receiving imatinib is 87%, and 67% of patients originally randomized to receive imatinib maintained a complete cytogenetic remission [7]. The estimated rate of

60-month event-free survival is 83%, and 93% of patients have not progressed to accelerated phase or blast crisis.

Molecular Monitoring of Disease

The availability of a distinct molecular alteration present in most patients with the disease provides the opportunity for molecular monitoring. Various practice guidelines have been developed to provide guidance for treating patients with CML in the chronic phase receiving tyrosine kinase inhibitors (TKI). One such set of guidelines, provided by the National Comprehensive Cancer Network (http://www.nccn. org), describes milestones for monitoring of disease at 3, 6, 12, and 18 months and subsequently. For example, after 3 months of therapy with a TKI, patients with CML in chronic phase are expected to have achieved hematologic remission. After 6 months of therapy, at least a partial cytogenetic response is expected (i.e., less than 35% of bone marrow cells harbor the Philadelphia chromosome). After 12 months of therapy, patients are to have achieved a complete cytogenetic remission. A three-order log reduction in the BCR-ABL molecular transcript is expected after 18 months of therapy with a TKI.

Monitoring of therapy is facilitated using advanced molecular techniques. For example, bone marrow cytogenetic analysis takes place after 6, 12, and 18 months of therapy. Peripheral blood BCR-ABL transcript levels are measured at diagnosis and then every 3 months. Following a complete cytogenetic remission, the peripheral blood BCR-ABL transcript level may be measured every 3–6 months, and bone marrow cytogenetics are recommended as clinically indicated. When a patient develops an increasing BCR-ABL transcript level, further bone marrow testing is conducted to characterize the disease. This information is then used to determine if the TKI dose should be increased, if another TKI should be used for treatment, or if intensive chemotherapy and allogeneic stem cell transplantation is required.

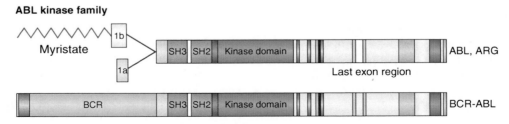

Fig. 15.1 Structural organization of the BCR-ABL fusion in CML. Reprinted by permission from Macmillan Publishers Ltd: Nature Reviews Drug Discovery. Quintas-Cardama A, Kantarjian H, Cortes J (2007) Flying under the radar: the new wave of BCR-ABL inhibitors. Nat Rev Drug Discov 6:834–848, copyright 2007

Mechanisms of Imatinib Resistance

As expected, resistance to tyrosine kinase inhibitors is an important clinical problem. In the IRIS trial, approximately 17% of patients relapsed and 7% of patients developed acquired resistance to imatinib [7]. Furthermore, rates of resistance are higher among patients with advanced and blast phase CML, even those who initially respond to treatment [8, 9]. Also, patients with aggressive phases of disease eventually relapse without allogeneic stem cell transplantation. For example, complete hematologic responses for patients with advanced and myeloid blast crisis CML enrolled in Phase II studies are 38 and 7%, respectively [10]. The complete cytogenetic response rates are 16 and 2%, respectively. These patients have limited overall survival rates. Thus, there is a major incentive to develop tyrosine kinase inhibitors capable of treating patients no longer responsive to imatinib or patients with advanced disease who have a limited duration of response.

There are a variety of imatinib resistance mechanisms which have been identified. Point mutations within the kinase domain of *BCR-ABL* are capable of preventing imatinib binding and are a frequent cause of imatinib resistance [11]. In patients with acquired resistance, the development of point mutations has been reported in 34–91% of patients [12]. Also, the risk of developing mutations increases as patients develop more clinically advanced disease [12, 13]. There are more than 40 different resistance-conferring mutations [14]. They generally fall within four regions of the ABL kinase domain. These include the ATP binding loop (P-loop), the contact site (example T315 and F317), the SH2 binding site (example M351), and the A-loop (Fig. 15.1) [15]. While mutations occur at different frequencies, those that confer higher degrees of resistance are preferentially selected. The most frequently occurring mutations (approximately 35%) are those within the P-loop, and these confer a very high level of resistance to imatinib. A highly feared mutation, T315I, is clinically significant because it renders complete resistance not only to imatinib [16] but also to the second-generation TKIs, nilotinib and dasatinib (see below [17]). Agents capable of inhibiting T315I are currently in development and are under active investigation.

At least three additional mechanisms of resistance to imatinib have been reported. First, BCR-ABL can be over-produced, either through genomic amplification [16, 18] or overexpression [19]. Second, activation of alternative signaling pathways can occur, bypassing the need for activation of BCR-ABL. These pathways include activation of SRC family kinases [20], in addition to activation of the PI3 kinase/AKT/MTOR pathway [21]. Third, intracellular levels of imatinib may be decreased due to altered expression or function of drug influx (OCT-1) [22] and efflux proteins (PGP) [23]. Finally, clonal evolution, with acquisition of new cytogenetic abnormalities, also represents a possible cause of imatinib resistance [24].

Role of Dasatinib and Nilotinib in Imatinib-Resistant CML

There are two BCR-ABL inhibitors available for clinical use in patients with resistance or patients who are intolerant to imatinib. Dasatinib is currently approved for patients with imatinib-resistant and intolerant CML in any phase in addition to Philadelphia chromosome-positive acute lymphoblastic leukemia (ALL). Nilotinib, an analog of imatinib, is approved for use in treatment of patients in chronic phase or accelerated phase CML for whom prior imatinib therapy has failed. Like imatinib, both agents have multiple molecular targets. For example, imatinib is capable of inhibiting platelet-derived growth factor receptor α and β (PDGFR-α and β) in addition to c-KIT. Dasatinib is a dual kinase inhibitor of both BCR-ABL and SRC-family kinases. Dasatinib is also active against c-KIT, PDGFR-α and β, and ephrin-A2 [25–27]. Nilotinib similarly targets multiple kinases with a spectrum similar to that of imatinib [17, 28]. Nilotinib is capable of inhibiting multidrug resistance proteins in addition to several metabolic enzymes including those in the family of glucuronosyltransferase that conjugate bilirubin and phenolic compounds and various CYP450 enzymes.

Preclinical studies indicate that both dasatinib and nilotinib have efficacy against most imatinib-resistant mutations. However, these agents have differential molecular properties. Compared to imatinib, both dasatinib and nilotinib inhibit BCR-ABL more potently. Dasatinib is highly potent against all mutations except T315I within a narrow concentration range. For nilotinib, the effective concentrations of BCR-ABL inhibition are at least tenfold lower than imatinib. The development of specific mutations provides an opportunity to select the ideal second-generation TKI. However, there is little clinical information regarding which is the best agent in patients with resistant disease. Both dasatinib and nilotinib have significant clinical activity in patients with imatinib-resistant or intolerant CML. For example, responses among patients with CML in chronic phase in Phase I and II clinical studies treated with nilotinib indicate that the complete cytogenetic rate was 40% in patients with imatinib resistance and sensitive mutations compared to 42% among patients without BCR-ABL mutations [29]. Conversely, however, no complete cytogenetic responses were observed in patients with mutations considered to have intermediate in vitro sensitivity (Y253H, E255K/V, and F359C/V).

Summary

Advances in CML demonstrate how nonspecific therapies such as interferon, cytarabine, hydroxyurea, and allogeneic stem cell transplantation have been largely replaced by the molecularly targeted therapy imatinib. In CML, the ability to both diagnose and treat patients is made possible by the specific pathogenesis of the disease, namely a single genetic lesion present in more than 95% of patients. Thus, approaches to treating as well as monitoring the disease are based on the underlying genetic rearrangement. Appropriate treatment of CML involves the use of a tyrosine kinase inhibitor. The most highly studied agent is imatinib though two second-generation tyrosine kinase inhibitors, dasatinib and nilotinib, are capable of inducing clinical responses in patients who have developed resistance to imatinib or who are intolerant to this agent. As all three agents have limited activity in patients with clinically advanced phases of CML, novel targeted approaches are needed for these patients.

Gastrointestinal Stromal Tumors

Gastrointestinal stromal tumors (GISTs) are malignancies of the Interstitial Cells of Cajal (ICCs), the autonomic cells, which initiate pacemaker activity in the gastrointestinal (GI) tract [30]. Although accounting for less than 1% of all GI malignancies, GISTs are the most common mesenchymal malignancies of the GI tract, occurring at an incidence of 10–20 per million in the population [31]. GISTs may occur anywhere along the GI tract, but are most commonly found in the stomach (60–70%). They can also occur in the esophagus (<5%), the small bowel (20–25%), and the colon or rectum (5%) [32]. Additionally, GISTs may also occur outside the GI tract in the omentum and mesenteric structures adjacent to but separate from the stomach and intestines [33].

The clinical spectrum of GISTs is broad, ranging from small, benign, incidentally found tumors to high-grade malignant tumors with metastasis at presentation [34]. Although only 20–30% of GISTS are overtly malignant, half of all patients with malignant GIST already have metastatic disease at initial presentation [34]. The rate of eventual metastatic spread increases proportionally with the size of the primary tumor and the frequency of mitosis observed histologically. The incidentally found small GISTs (<1 cm) rarely progress to develop malignant disease. The location of primary GISTs is also predictive for malignancy. Although benign GISTs outnumber malignant GISTs 3–5:1 when occurring in the stomach, most esophageal and colorectal GISTs are malignant. GISTs most frequently metastasize to the liver and intraabdominal lymph nodes, less frequently to the lung and bone [35].

Molecular Targets in GIST

C-KIT

GISTs almost universally (95%) maintain the cell surface expression of KIT (also known as CD117 [36] or stem cell factor receptor [37]) that is found on ICCs [32, 38]. The KIT protein is a 145-kD transmembrane glycoprotein that is a member of the receptor tyrosine kinase family of proteins structurally related to macrophage colony stimulating factor receptor (Fig. 15.2). Upon binding its ligand – stem cell factor – KIT homodimerizes and autophosphorylates tyrosine residues, leading to further binding and activation of signal transduction molecules leading to cellular proliferation. Approximately 80% of GISTs are hyperactivated at KIT [39, 40].

In a seminal paper by Hirota et al., the c-KIT gene that codes for the KIT protein was observed to be mutated in GISTs from five patients (Fig. 15.2) [41]. All of the corresponding KIT proteins were constitutively activated in a ligand-independent fashion. When mutant c-KIT cDNAs were stably transfected into murine lymphoid cell lines, malignant transformation was observed. The initial set of mutations was observed in exon 11, a region between the transmembrane and tyrosine kinase coding domains of c-KIT. Such mutations in exon 11 allow for receptor dimerization in the absence of ligand binding.

Subsequent studies have shown that approximately half of GISTs have mutations in exon 11 of c-KIT. Other mutations have been identified at lower frequency in exons 9, 13, and 17. Exon 9 mutations also result in constitutively active KIT. Interestingly, these mutations are found predominantly in small intestinal GISTs and are overrepresented in malignant tumors. Exon 13 mutations are found at very low frequency and are believed to cause ligand-independent activation of c-KIT by spontaneous receptor homodimerization. Finally, in exon 17, mutation in the activation loop of c-KIT has been observed in rare cases.

PDGFR-α

In approximately one-half of the subset of GISTs that are not KIT activated, cellular proliferation and tumorigenicity is driven by a related tyrosine kinase receptor – platelet-derived growth factor receptor α (PDGFR-α). In another seminal paper by Heinrich et al., the gene encoding PDGFR-α was observed to harbor activating mutations in approximately 35% of GISTs lacking c-KIT mutations [42]. In this study, to identify alternative receptor tyrosine kinases that might drive GIST tumorigenesis, the investigators used polyclonal antisera against peptides from regions of strong sequence conservation across the entire family of receptor

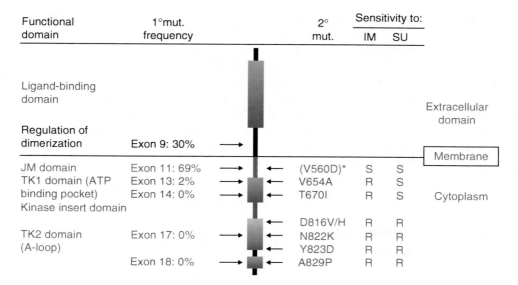

Functional domain	1°mut. frequency		2° mut.	Sensitivity to:	
				IM	SU
Ligand-binding domain					
					Extracellular domain
Regulation of dimerization	Exon 9: 30%	→			
					Membrane
JM domain	Exon 11: 69%	→	← (V560D)*	S	S
TK1 domain (ATP binding pocket)	Exon 13: 2%	→	← V654A	R	S
	Exon 14: 0%	→	← T670I	R	S	Cytoplasm
Kinase insert domain					
			← D816V/H	R	R
TK2 domain (A-loop)	Exon 17: 0%	→	← N822K	R	R
			← Y823D	R	R
	Exon 18: 0%	→	← A829P	R	R

Fig. 15.2 Schematic representation of CKIT showing functional domains, as well as location of both primary and secondary mutations. *S* sensitivity; *R* resistance; *IM* imatinib; *SU* sunitinib. From Gajiwala KS, Wu JC, Christensen J et al (2009) KIT kinase mutants show unique mechanisms of drug resistance to imatinib and sunitinib in gastrointestinal stromal tumor patients. Proc Natl Acad Sci USA 106:1542–1547. Copyright (2009) National Academy of Sciences, USA

tyrosine kinases (panRTK Ab) and performed immunoprecipitations on a collection of 40 GIST tumors *lacking c-KIT* mutations. Phosphotyrosine immunostaining of panRTK immunoprecipitates revealed phosphoproteins of 150 and 170 kD, representing immature and mature glycosylated PDGFR-α. PhosphoPDGFR-α expression was restricted to c-KIT wild-type GISTs (11 of 37 in WT C-KIT tumors, 0 of 36 in C-KIT mutant GISTs). Sequencing subsequently revealed two types of mutations in exon 18 of PDGFR-α, a missense mutation and in-frame deletions, both affecting ligand-dependent kinase activation. Finally, investigators showed that CHO cell lines transiently transfected with mutated PDGFR-α showed uniform activation of AKT, MAPK, and Stat1 and Stat3 – all signal transduction molecules that are also activated downstream of c-KIT.

While similar at the molecular level, PDGFR-α and C-KIT mutant GISTs have a number of clinicopathologic differences [43]. PDGFR-α mutant GISTs frequently have epithelioid morphology, stain weakly for KIT by immunohistochemistry, arise almost exclusively in the stomach (whereas c-KIT mutant GISTs can arise throughout the GI tract), and cluster separately from c-KIT mutant GISTs by gene expression profiling.

Targeting C-KIT and PDGFR-α in GIST

In 2000 and 2001, two groups independently showed that the small molecule compound imatinib – originally developed to inhibit BCR-ABL in CML as discussed above [5, 44–46] –

can inhibit c-KIT activation and subsequent signal transduction [47, 48]. Heinrich et al. used imatinib to treat a human myeloid leukemia cell line (M-07e) that expressed c-KIT [47]. They showed that imatinib inhibited ligand-induced KIT autophosphorylation, MAP kinase activation, and Akt phosphorylation at an EC50 of 100 nM. Imatinib also inhibited KIT induced phosphorylation in a human mast cell leukemia cell line (HMC-1) with a constitutively active mutant form of KIT. In a separate study using imatinib to inhibit c-KIT, Tuveson et al established a human GIST cell line (GIST882) with an activating c-KIT mutation [48]. Constitutive tyrosine phosphorylation by mutant KIT was completely abolished after incubation with imatinib. In addition, treated cells demonstrated decreased proliferation and, after prolonged incubation with imatinib, evidence of apoptosis. Taken together, these two studies suggested that imatinib might act as a potent inhibitor of activated KIT and thereby have a therapeutic role in patients with surgically inoperable GIST.

As predicted by the preclinical studies, c-KIT has been validated as a therapeutic target in the clinic. In 2001, Joensuu et al. described a dramatic and sustained response in a patient with metastatic GIST treated with imatinib [49]. In the phase I EORTC trial of 36 patients with GIST, 25 patients had partial responses of more than 20% tumor regression [50]. In a subsequent open label, randomized phase II trial, 147 patients were treated with 400 or 600 mg imatinib daily [51]. 120 patients (82%) had either partial response or stable disease and 20 patients demonstrated early resistance to treatment.

Because of the role of activated PDGFR-α in a subset of GISTs, inhibition of PDGFR-α was examined in patients who had progressed on imatinib. In a phase I/II study using sunitinib (SU11248, Sutent), a small molecule inhibitor of PDGFR-α as well as c-KIT, FLT3, RET, and other tyrosine kinase receptors, Demetri et al treated 98 patients with imatinib-refractory GIST. Sunitinib demonstrated a partial response or >6 month stable disease in 54% of evaluable patients, with 13% confirmed partial responses [52]. In a larger, international randomized phase III study using sunitinib in imatinib refractory GIST, the treatment group demonstrated a 7% partial response rate, but progression free survival was fourfold higher than the control group (27 vs. 6 weeks) [53].

Genotype–Phenotype Correlations and Mechanisms of Resistance

Several studies have analyzed the relationship between c-KIT mutation and patient outcome. In one study, most c-KIT mutations involved either exon 11 (76%) or exon 9 (21%), but mutations were also seen in exons 13 and 17. Patients with exon 11 mutations demonstrated a partial response rate of 83.5% whereas those with exon 9 mutations had a 47.8% response rate. In addition, patients with GISTs harboring exon 11 mutations were associated with longer event-free and overall survival compared to patients whose tumors did not harbor exon 11 mutations [54]. In a different study, Heinrich et al again found that exon 11 of c-KIT was the most frequent site of mutations and correlated with the best treatment outcome (72% response rate, time to progression of 25 months). Tumors with either no c-KIT mutation or c-KIT mutations in exon 9 had a response rate of 44% and time to progression of 12–17 months [55].

For GISTs that initially respond to imatinib but then acquire resistance, secondary mutations in *c-KIT* have been observed (Fig. 15.2) [55, 56]. Antonescu et al genotyped 15 GIST tumors with acquired resistance to imatinib and 13 tumors sensitive to imatinib. Although none of the imatinib-sensitive tumors demonstrated secondary mutations in either c-KIT or PDGFR-α, imatinib-resistant tumors demonstrated secondary mutations in 46% of tested samples. Each tumor had primary mutations in exon 11 of c-KIT, while most of the secondary mutations were seen in exon 17. Secondary mutations in exons 13 and 14 were also seen. Similarly, Heinrich et al. genotyped 33 tumors with acquired resistance to imatinib and found secondary mutations in 67% of samples. They also observed mutations in exons 17, 13, and 14. Of note, exon 13 and 14 mutations involve the KIT-adenosine triphosphate binding pocket, whereas exon 17 mutations involve the KIT activation loop.

As with imatinib, sunitinib response appears to correlate with particular tyrosine kinase genotypes. However, in contrast to imatinib, sunitinib induces a higher response rate in tumors with mutations in exon 9 (58% response rate) and with wild type KIT (56% response rate), compared with those harboring mutations in exon 11 (34% response rate). Progression free survival and overall survival were also higher for patients with either wild-type c-KIT or exon 9 mutations [57]. When resistant tumors were analyzed, patients with secondary mutations in exons 13 or 14 demonstrated longer progression free and overall survival than patients with secondary mutations in exons 17 or 18.

Summary

In the last decade, our scientific knowledge of GISTs has advanced from a vague pathological classification to an in-depth understanding of the genetic basis of tumorigenesis [58], including mechanisms of acquired drug resistance [59, 60]. This understanding has led to the development of specific kinase inhibitors that serve as effective therapy for patients who traditionally have had few treatment options. Activating *c-KIT* mutations have been identified in a handful of other tumor types, including other sarcomas such as dermatofibrosarcoma protuberans [61, 62] and melanomas [63–65], and confer sensitivity to treatment with imatinib [66–68]. Targeted therapy, as opposed to nonspecific cytotoxic therapy with DNA alkylating or intercalating agents, clearly holds the promise of safer, more effective therapies for GISTs and other c-KIT mutant tumors.

Non-small Cell Lung Cancers Harboring Activating EGFR Mutations

Advanced nonsmall cell lung cancer (NSCLC) is currently incurable. Traditional cytotoxic chemotherapy is modestly effective at best and produces a median survival of approximately 1 year [69]. Over the past several years, there have been substantial efforts to improve upon traditional cytotoxic chemotherapies by developing molecularly targeted therapies to treat these cancers. The EGFR TKIs, gefitinib and erlotinib, were developed for the treatment of NSCLC. Recent advances in the understanding of the genetic abnormalities and intracellular signaling cascades that promote lung carcinogenesis have lead to the development of strategies that aim to disrupt critical oncogenic mechanisms. The EGFR is one such target, as it is known to promote growth of cells, to function as an oncogene, and is expressed in 80–90% of NSCLCs [70–76].

The EGFR is one of the four members in the ErbB family of receptor tyrosine kinases (RTK). The other members are ErbB-2/HER2, ErbB-3, and ErbB-4. These receptors homo- or heterodimerize upon ligand binding. Upon dimerization, there is trans-autophosphorylation of the dimer partner (for reviews see refs. [77–79]). The tyrosine-phosphorylated proteins then serve as docking molecules to initiate intracellular signaling pathways including the Phosphoinositide 3-Kinase (PI3K)/Akt, Ras/Raf/Erk, and Jak/STAT pathways. These pathways are important in promoting and maintaining the transformed phenotype. In fact, activating mutations of several of these downstream signaling proteins have also been observed in NSCLC. The development of EGFR inhibitors was based on the idea that blocking EGFR activity in NSCLCs would downregulate these critical downstream signaling cascades, resulting in growth inhibition and/or apoptosis.

The proposal that inhibiting EGFR may serve as an effective cancer treatment has been around for decades and was further inspired by the work of Dr. Mendelsohn and colleagues who demonstrated that antibodies directed against the EGFR inhibit the growth of the A431 carcinoma cell line [80]. In the 1990s, a class of small molecule inhibitors of EGFR, anilinoquinazolones, was developed. These function as competitive TKIs by reversibly binding to the ATP binding site on EGFR. Two such quinazolones under clinical development are gefitinib (ZD1839, Iressa; Astrazeneca, London, UK) and erlotinib (OSI-774, Tarceva; Genentech, South San Francisco, CA and OSI Pharmaceuticals, Melville, NY).

EGFR Inhibitors in Unselected Patients with Advanced NSCLC

Gefitinib was shown to possess antitumor activity in preclinical tumor models as a single agent and in combination with cytotoxic chemotherapy or radiotherapy (reviewed in ref. [81]). These observations led to its clinical development for use in cancer patients. Phase I studies of gefitinib demonstrated that gefitinib was well tolerated by patients with most dose-limiting toxicities occurring at doses of ≥800 mg. At doses ≤600 mg, the most common adverse effects were diarrhea and acne-like rash, which were mild and usually manageable. In the three phase I trials of gefitinib conducted in Europe, Australia, and the USA, 77 patients with NSCLC were treated with gefitinib [82–84]. There were partial responses in five patients (6.5%) and prolonged stable disease ≥6 months in ten patients (13%). Rare patients with other tumor types also demonstrated prolonged stable disease ≥6 months with gefitinib treatment. In a Japanese phase I trial, 5/23 patients (22%) with NSCLC demonstrated partial responses [85].

The promising activity seen in the Phase I studies led to two large multicenter Phase II trials with gefitinib termed the Iressa Dose Evaluation in Advanced Lung Cancer (IDEAL)-1 and -2. IDEAL 1 was performed in Japan, Europe, Australia, and South Africa and included 210 patients with advanced

NSCLC who had previously been treated with one or two chemotherapy regimens, including one platinum-containing regimen [86]. The IDEAL 2 trial was performed in the U.S. and included 216 patients with advanced NSCLC who had previously received a minimum of two prior chemotherapy regimens, including a platinum combination and docetaxel [87]. The radiographic response rates were 18.4 and 10% respectively in the two trials.

However, the remarkable responses and symptomatic improvement observed in a minority of the patients treated on the Phase II gefitinib trials led to its approval by the Food and Drug Administration (FDA) for patients with NSCLC progressing after platinum and docetaxel containing chemotherapy regimens. Two phase III trials of single-agent EGFR TKIs versus placebo have been conducted. In one study, patients with NSCLC who had received 1 or 2 prior chemotherapy regimens were treated with either erlotinib or placebo [88]. Those treated with erlotinib had a response rate of 9% and a statistically significant increase in median (6.7 months vs. 4.7 months), and 1 year survivals (31% vs. 21%) compared to patients receiving placebo. This survival benefit served as the basis for the FDA approval of erlotinib in NSCLC patients who progress after 1 or more chemotherapy regimens. The results from a second phase III study comparing gefitinib to placebo, in patients failing 1 or 2 prior chemotherapy regimens, have recently been reported [89]. In this study of 1,692 patients, there was no statistically significant difference in median survival for gefitinib compared to placebo (5.6 vs. 5.1 months; $p=0.11$) in all patients or in patients with adenocarcinoma (6.3 vs. 5.4 months; $p=0.07$). However, there were statistically significant improvements in overall survival among nonsmokers and patients of Asian descent (8.9 vs. 6.1 months, $p=0.01$ and 9.5 vs. 5.5 months, $p=0.01$ respectively).

Clinical experience in the Phase II trials and the Astra-Zeneca gefitinib expanded access program had demonstrated that some patients have remarkable and durable responses to EGFR TKIs. However, these patients represented a small minority of patients. A major challenge was to determine the reason why only certain patients responded. Shared clinical characteristics of patients who responded to EGFR TKIs were sought in an effort to understand and predict who would benefit from this class of drugs. Further examination of patients with NSCLC benefitting from EGFR TKIs in these clinical trials and those treated under the Astra-Zeneca gefitinib expanded access program revealed clinical characteristics associated with the greatest degree of benefit as measured by either response rate or survival [86, 87, 90–95]. Patients most likely to obtain tumor shrinkage from EGFR TKIs were women, patients with adenocarcinomas, Japanese patients, and patients who were nonsmokers. These observations suggested that these tumors might represent a subset of biologically distinct tumors addicted to the EGFR signaling pathway.

This ultimately led to the sequencing of the EGFR and identification of EGFR mutations associated with sensitivity to EGFR TKIs [96, 97].

Somatic EGFR Mutations in Lung Cancer

In 2004, it was discovered that lung cancers with somatic mutations in *EGFR* were associated with dramatic tumor response upon treatment with gefitinib [96–98]. Somatic mutations in *EGFR* are found in ~10% of Caucasian and in 30–40% of Asian NSCLC patients. *EGFR* mutations are present more frequently in never-smokers, females, those with adenocarcinoma, and in patients of East Asian descent. These are the same groups of patients previously clinically identified as most likely to benefit from gefitinib or erlotinib [86–88]. Several prospective clinical trials treating chemotherapy naïve patients with *EGFR* mutations with gefitinib or erlotinib have been reported to date [99–103]. A recent phase III clinical trial demonstrated that *EGFR* mutant patients had superior outcomes with gefitinib treatment (as measured by response rate and progression free survival) compared to standard cytotoxic chemotherapy [104]. Given the dramatic outcomes for patients with *EGFR* mutations treated with either gefitinib or erlotinib, there is a significant focus on clinical development of these agents in chemotherapy-naïve patients. Thus, there are now increasing efforts to determine the EGFR mutational status of newly diagnosed patients so that they can be treated with an EGFR TKI in the first-line setting.

EGFR mutations associated with increased response to gefitinib and erlotinib are found in the first four exons (18-21) of the tyrosine kinase domain of EGFR (Fig. 15.3). There are two types of mutations that are most common and most closely linked to sensitivity to gefitinib and erlotinib: ~45% are deletions involving at least 12 nucleotides in exon 19, eliminating a conserved LREA motif, and ~40% are a single point mutation in exon 21 (L858R). The subset of lung cancers with exon 19 deletions or L858R mutation demonstrates high response rates to EGFR TKIs, approaching 80% [99–103]. Additionally, amplification of the *EGFR* gene has been associated with benefit from EGFR TKIs [105].

The Biology of EGFR Oncogene Addiction

The past 20 years have provided numerous studies demonstrating that most epithelial cancers require certain intracellular signaling pathways for their proliferation and survival. The PI3K and extracellular signal-regulated kinase (ERK) (also termed p42/44 mitogen-activated protein kinase (MAPK))

pathways appear to be highly activated in many epithelial cancers, and there are many ways for a cell to activate these pathways. In fact, there appears to be an intimate relationship between oncogene addiction to a receptor tyrosine kinase and regulation of these pathways. When a cancer is susceptible to a specific targeted therapy, PI3K and ERK are under strict regulation by the target. Indeed, cancers that are sensitive to EGFR inhibitors utilize EGFR to regulate PI3K and ERK [106–108]. The same holds true for cancers that are sensitive to other receptor tyrosine kinases such as MET inhibitors [109] and HER2 inhibitors. In other terms, for a cancer to be sensitive to a particular targeted therapy, the cancer must be "addicted" to the target, and thus the target regulates critical growth and survival signals, especially the PI3K and ERK pathways (reviewed in ref. [110]). Thus, when the cancer is treated with the appropriate tyrosine kinase inhibitor, both PI3K and ERK signaling are turned off and the cells undergo apoptosis and cell growth arrest [110–113].

Acquired Resistance to Gefitinib/Erlotinib In EGFR Mutant Lung Cancer

Despite the initial clinical benefits of gefitinib/erlotinib in NSCLC patients harboring *EGFR* mutations, most, if not all, patients ultimately develop progressive cancer while receiving therapy with these agents. Recent studies have shown that when a cancer becomes resistant to EGFR TKIs, it essentially finds a way to circumvent the ability of the TKI to downregulate downstream signaling. In other words, the resistant cancers re-activate the downstream signaling pathways, especially the PI3K pathway in the presence of the EGFR TKI (reviewed in refs. [114, 115]). Initial studies of relapsed specimens identified a secondary *EGFR* mutation, T790M, that renders gefitinib and erlotinib ineffective inhibitors of EGFR kinase activity (Fig. 15.3), and thus EGFR is able to maintain activation of downstream signaling in cancers that acquire this mutation [116, 117]. Subsequent studies have demonstrated that the *EGFR* T790M mutation is found in approximately 50% of tumors (24/48) from patients that have developed acquired resistance to gefitinib or erlotinib [106, 118, 119].

This amino acid is often referred to as the "gatekeeper" residue in tyrosine kinases, and is analogous to resistance mutations observed in *BCR-ABL* and *c-KIT* in imatinib-resistant CML and GISTs, respectively [16, 56]. Accordingly, in vitro studies have clearly shown that EGFR T790M mutation is not inhibited by gefitinib or erlotinib at concentrations >10 mM [116, 120, 121]. Additionally, ectopic expression of the T790M resistance mutation is sufficient to render EGFR mutant cancer cell lines resistant to gefitinib [107], and transgenic mice with EGFR L858R-T790M induced lung

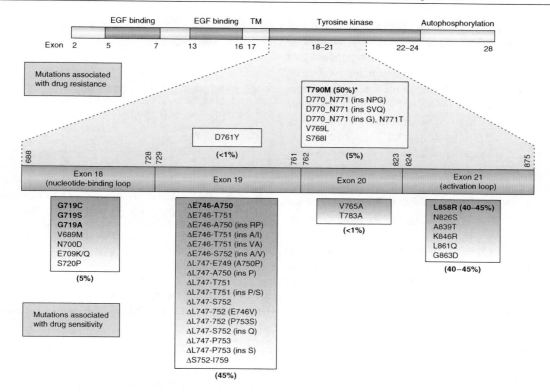

Fig. 15.3 Overview of *EGFR* mutations in NSCLC. The *EGFR* TKI-sensitizing mutations are found in exons 18–21 and are depicted in the magenta boxes. Mutations associated with resistance to EGFR TKIs are shown in the yellow boxes, and include the secondary mutation T790M in exon 20. Reprinted by permission from Macmillan Publishers Ltd: Nature Reviews Cancer. Sharma SV, Bell DW, Settleman J et al (2007) Epidermal growth factor receptor mutations in lung cancer. Nat Rev Cancer 7:169–181, copyright 2007

adenocarcinomas are resistant to erlotinib [122, 123]. In fact, when the highly sensitive *EGFR* mutant and amplified NSCLC-derived cell lines, PC-9 and H3255, were grown in the presence of gefitinib to model acquired resistance, they acquired a T790M mutation [107, 124].

In contrast to activating EGFR mutations, the T790M resistance mutation is often difficult to detect on standard sequence tracings from resistant biopsy specimens and can only be detected using more sensitive techniques [107, 118, 120]. It is possible that only a small percentage of resistant cancer cells in a biopsy have T790M-mediated resistance. Alternatively, since many *EGFR* mutant cancers also have high copy numbers of the *EGFR* gene [125], only a small percentage of the *EGFR* alleles per cell may harbor the T790M mutation (termed "allelic dilution"), as was observed in a cell line model of acquired resistance. A limited number of T790M alleles per cell may be sufficient since the T790M mutation significantly further enhances the activity and transforming capacity of EGFR proteins with activating mutations [121, 126, 127]. In fact, a recent report identified a family with inherited susceptibility to lung cancer that was correlated with a germline T790M mutation [128]. Moreover, in a few cases, the T790M mutation has been identified in lung cancers that had never been exposed to a TKI [129].

These findings underscore the importance of considering the T790M detection method when evaluating mechanisms of acquired resistance.

The *EGFR* T790M resistance mutation can be overcome by a new generation of irreversible EGFR inhibitors. These are ATP-mimetics that differ from gefitinib and erlotinib (both reversible inhibitors) because they covalently bind EGFR at cys-773. This property likely increases their local concentration near the EGFR active site by several orders of magnitude accounting for their ability to inhibit EGFR T790M. Studies have shown that irreversible EGFR inhibitors, such as EKB-569, PF00299804, and HKI-272, can inhibit phosphorylation of EGFR T790M and the growth of *EGFR* mutant NSCLC cell lines harboring the T790M mutation [116, 120, 130]. Additionally, preliminary clinical experience with this class of agents demonstrates that single-agent irreversible EGFR inhibitors have activity in a small proportion of patients with acquired resistance to erlotinib, but their activity is of modest duration [131].

We have recently identified other mechanisms of resistance to EGFR TKIs that do not involve acquisition of a T790M. These were identified by exposing EGFR TKI sensitive lung cancer cell lines to increasing concentrations of gefitinib until resistance developed. The first one identified was the amplification of the *MET* oncogene [106]. Amplification of *MET* leads to resistance because when MET is overexpressed, it activates downstream signaling independently of EGFR (or HER2), and thus is able to maintain downstream signaling (both PI3K and ERK) in the presence of gefitinib. Initially, amplification of MET in 4/18 (22%) of patients with acquired resistance to gefitinib or erlotinib. In addition, a study led by Dr. Pao also identified MET amplification in ~20% of cases of acquired resistance [132]. Importantly, treatment of the *MET* amplified resistant cells with a combination of MET and EGFR inhibitors induced massive apoptosis in the resistant cancers, and these findings serve as the basis for the development of combinatorial strategies currently in clinical trials.

One of the patients that we examined for acquired resistance mechanisms was from an autopsy series. In this special case, we were able to analyze two different resistant lesions from the same patient [106]. One lesion had a T790M and the other had *MET* amplification. Thus, this raises the humbling possibility that different resistant metastatic sites (or even different cells in the same lesion) may have different mechanisms of resistance (i.e., heterogeneity of resistance). This may partially explain the low response rates of single-agent irreversible EGFR inhibitors in this patient population despite the detection of T790M in ~50% of resistant lesions. Thus, the combination of irreversible EGFR inhibitors and MET inhibitors may be necessary to overcome resistance in a large subset of patients.

Nonsmall Cell Lung Cancers Harboring Translocations of Anaplastic Lymphoma Kinase

The *EML4-ALK* fusion oncogene represents one of the newest molecular targets in NSCLC. First described in 2007 [133, 134], the fusion results from a small inversion within chromosome 2p, leading to expression of a chimeric tyrosine kinase in which the N-terminal half of EML4 (echinoderm microtubule-associated protein-like 4) is fused to the intracellular kinase domain of ALK (anaplastic lymphoma kinase) (Fig. 15.4). Translocations involving *ALK* have been identified in other cancers, including anaplastic large cell lymphomas (ALCLs), neuroblastomas, and inflammatory myofibroblastic tumors (IMTs) [135]. In all cases, including EML4-ALK, the fusion partner mediates dimerization or oligomerization of ALK, resulting in constitutive kinase activity [134]. In cell culture systems, EML4-ALK has been shown to possess potent oncogenic activity [133]. In transgenic mouse models, expression of EML4-ALK leads to the development of lung adenocarcinomas [136]. The oncogenic activity of EML4-ALK can be effectively blocked both in vitro and in vivo by

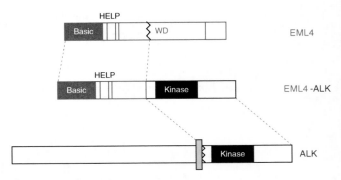

Fig. 15.4 Schematic representation of the *EML4-ALK* translocation in NSCLC. Note that the translocation site within ALK is highly conserved among all ALK fusions. *TM* transmembrane domain. Adapted by permission from Macmillan Publishers Ltd: Nature. Soda et al. [133], copyright 2007

a variety of small molecule inhibitors targeting ALK [136–138], supporting a role for EML4-ALK as a key driver of lung tumorigenesis.

Clinicopathologic Features of EML4-ALK-Positive NSCLC

Several studies have examined the frequency of *EML4-ALK* in NSCLC patients and cell lines. In the original report of *EML4-ALK*, 5 of 75 lung tumors, all derived from Japanese patients, demonstrated expression of the fusion transcript, corresponding to a frequency of 6.7% [133]. In subsequent studies involving primarily Asian patients with early-stage, resectable disease, *EML4-ALK* has been detected in a lower percentage of cases, ranging from 1 to 4.9% [134, 137, 139–144]. These findings suggest that in unselected NSCLC populations, the *EML4-ALK* rearrangement is a relatively rare event.

Recently, the key pathologic, epidemiologic, and demographic features associated with *EML4-ALK* have been identified. One of the most striking features of EML4-ALK-positive lung cancer is young age of onset. In the largest study of EML4-ALK positive NSCLC to date, patients harboring this translocation were significantly younger than nonALK positive patients, with a median age of 53 years compared with 66 [145]. Among the 19 patients with *EML4-ALK*, four were under 40 years old. A recent study of *EML4-ALK* in NSCLC patients from Hong Kong also noted a trend toward younger median age, though the difference in median age between *EML4-ALK* positive and negative patients was only 5 years and did not reach statistical significance [144]. Interestingly, other cancers known to harbor *ALK* rearrangements, such as ALCLs and IMTs, are also associated with younger age, and are in fact most common in children and young adults. Future studies should explore whether, independent of tumor type, there are common predisposing factors to *ALK* rearrangements in the young.

The presence of *EML4-ALK* in NSCLC is also strongly associated with never or light smoking history. In the first report of *EML4-ALK* in NSCLC, the chromosomal inversion was detected in five patients, two of whom were noted to have a smoking history [133]. In several follow-up studies, *EML4-ALK* was variably detected in both smokers and non-smokers [134, 137, 142, 143], suggesting a lack of association between smoking history and presence of *EML4-ALK*. However, two recent studies suggest that *EML4-ALK* is in fact strongly associated with never or light smoking history. In one study, 19 of 85 patients classified as either never or light (≤10 pack-years) cigarette smokers were positive for *EML4-ALK*, whereas all 56 patients with a smoking history (>10 pack-years) were negative for the *ALK* rearrangement [145].

At the histologic level, the vast majority of lung tumors harboring *EML4-ALK* are adenocarcinomas. However, *EML4-ALK*-positive cases from Caucasian patients are significantly more likely than *EGFR* mutant or WT/WT tumors to have abundant signet ring cells [145]. Signet ring cells are frequently found in gastric cancers, and rarely in cancers of other organs such as the lung. Several small case series suggest that signet ring cells may be associated with an aggressive clinical course and a poor prognosis [146–148]. Whether the presence of signet ring cells in *EML4-ALK* mutant lung cancer has biological or clinical significance remains to be determined. Of note, other studies of *EML4-ALK* in NSCLC have not reported an association with signet ring cells, though these studies have involved only patients of Asian descent. This discrepancy may reflect differences in pathologic interpretation or ethnic differences in patients with *EML4-ALK* positive lung cancer.

While the overall frequency of *EML4-ALK* in the general NSCLC population is low, knowledge of the clinicopathologic features enables enrichment for this genetically defined subset. In one study, patients were selected for genetic screening based on clinical features commonly associated with *EGFR* mutation, including never/light smoking status and adenocarcinoma histology [145]. In this select subpopulation of Caucasian patients, the frequency of *EML4-ALK* was significantly higher than that reported for unselected patients. Among the 141 patients screened, there were 19 with *EML4-ALK* and 31 with *EGFR* mutation, corresponding to frequencies of 13 and 22%, respectively. Within the group of never or light smokers in this study, the frequencies of *EML4-ALK* and *EGFR* were 22 and 32%, respectively; among never or light smokers without *EGFR* mutation, the frequency of *EML4-ALK* was 33%. These findings suggest that in NSCLC patients with clinical characteristics associated with *EGFR* mutation but with negative *EGFR* testing, as many as one in three may harbor *EML4-ALK* [145].

Diagnostic Testing

Several different diagnostic modalities have been developed to identify tumors harboring an *ALK* rearrangement. The gold standard assay is fluorescence in situ hybridization (FISH), performed on formalin-fixed, paraffin-embedded tumor tissues. FISH can be performed using a break-apart probe to the *ALK* gene, in which two differently-colored probes flank the conserved translocation breakpoint within *ALK* [145]. A second diagnostic assay commonly used is RT-PCR for the *EML4-ALK* fusion transcript. This technique is complicated by the fact that there are at least seven different *EML4-ALK* variant cDNAs and at least two other fusion partners in addition to EML4. A third diagnostic assay that is under development is immunohistochemistry for ALK protein expression. As ALK is normally not expressed within the lung except when present as a fusion protein, detection of ALK by IHC may serve as a sensitive assay for the presence of ALK rearrangement. Of note, both FISH and IHC can establish that an ALK rearrangement has occurred, but neither test identifies the fusion partner or the precise fusion itself.

Clinical Outcome with Standard Therapies

To date, only one study has examined the treatment response and clinical outcome of *EML4-ALK* patients with NSCLC [145]. In this retrospective study, patients with tumors harboring either *EML4-ALK* or *EGFR*, or neither genetic alteration (WT/WT) were compared in terms of response rate, time to progression (TTP) and overall survival. Among metastatic patients who received any platinum-based combination, *EML4-ALK* positive patients showed similar response rates and TTP as WT/WT patients. *EGFR* mutation-positive patients demonstrated a slightly higher response rate than either *EML4-ALK* or WT/WT patients, consistent with previous studies including the recently presented IPASS study in which the objective response rate to carboplatin/taxol was 47.3 and 23.5% in EGFR mutation-positive and mutation-negative patients, respectively [104].

In contrast to *EGFR* patients, *EML4-ALK* patients do not appear to respond to EGFR TKIs such as erlotinib [145]. Approved by the FDA for the second and third line treatment of metastatic NSCLC, erlotinib is frequently used in patients who have relapsed after platinum-based chemotherapy. Within the *EML4-ALK* cohort in the retrospective study described above, there were no clinical responses to EGFR TKIs, and the median time to progression was only 5 months. These findings are consistent with preclinical studies showing that the *EML4-ALK*-containing NSCLC cell line H3122 is resistant to erlotinib [137]. By contrast, the response rate among patients with EGFR mutations was 70% with a median time to progression of 17 months. Of note, patients without either *ALK* rearrangement or *EGFR* mutation showed a poor response to EGFR TKIs, similar to *EML4-ALK* patients. The distinction between EML4-ALK and EGFR mutant cases therefore has important therapeutic implications. In the absence of genetic testing, *EML4-ALK* patients are likely to be treated like *EGFR* mutant patients based on never/light smoking history, but clearly will not derive significant benefit from EGFR-directed therapies. These results illustrate the importance of pretreatment, genetic testing in order to guide clinical treatment recommendations, especially with regards to EGFR TKIs [145].

Clinical Outcome with Targeted Therapies

The first ALK inhibitor tested in patients is PF-02341066, a selective, ATP-competitive, small molecule targeting both the ALK and MET/HGF (hepatocyte growth factor) receptor tyrosine kinases [149]. A phase 1 dose-escalation trial has recently been conducted to investigate the safety and PK/PD in patients with advanced cancer [150]. PF-02341066 was administered orally twice a day at doses ranging from 50 mg daily to 300 mg twice a day. The most common side effects were fatigue, nausea/vomiting, and diarrhea. NSCLC patients whose tumors harbor EML4-ALK were recruited into an expanded cohort at the recommended phase 2 dose of 250 mg twice daily. Many of these patients were included in the retrospective case series described above. These patients were never or light smokers, had metastatic disease, and had failed on average two prior treatments. Remarkably, the response rate among these patients was approximately 50%, with an impressive disease control rate of over 75%. In a number of cases, patients reported symptomatic improvement within 1–2 weeks, reminiscent of the effect of erlotinib in patients with EGFR mutant lung cancer. The marked activity of PF-02341066 in EML4-ALK patients is consistent with the notion of oncogene addiction, and validates ALK as a therapeutic target in a small, but important, subset of NSCLC patients.

Summary and Future Directions

In conclusion, *EML4-ALK* defines a new molecular subset of NSCLC with distinct clinical and pathologic features. The patients most likely to harbor *EML4-ALK* are the young, never or light smokers with adenocarcinoma. As some of these features are also associated with *EGFR* mutation, it is essential to screen patients by genetic testing and not rely solely on the presence of clinical predictors. The results of genetic screening will then enable treatment with the appropriate targeted therapy. Preclinical studies have shown that *EML4-ALK* confers sensitivity to ALK inhibitors both in vitro and in vivo, and suggest that patients with this chromosomal translocation may derive clinical benefit from specific ALK inhibition. Indeed, preliminary results from a phase 1 study demonstrate that the ALK inhibitor PF-02341066 is active in patients whose tumors harbor *EML4-ALK* [150]. A phase 3 study is currently underway to prove definitively that PF-02341066 is superior to standard chemotherapy. Studies are also underway to begin to define mechanisms of resistance, both intrinsic and acquired. As with *EGFR* mutant lung cancer, the key to treating *EML4-ALK*-positive lung cancer may lie in combinatorial strategies aimed at targeting the oncogene as well as blocking the emergence of resistance.

References

1. Sawyers CL (1999) Chronic myeloid leukemia. N Engl J Med 340:1330–1340
2. Faderl S, Talpaz M, Estrov Z et al (1999) The biology of chronic myeloid leukemia. N Engl J Med 341:164–172
3. Gratwohl A, Brand R, Apperley J et al (2006) Allogeneic hematopoietic stem cell transplantation for chronic myeloid leukemia in Europe 2006: transplant activity, long-term data and current results. An analysis by the Chronic Leukemia Working Party of the European Group for Blood and Marrow Transplantation (EBMT). Haematologica 91:513–521
4. Hehlmann R, Berger U, Pfirrmann M et al (2007) Drug treatment is superior to allografting as first-line therapy in chronic myeloid leukemia. Blood 109:4686–4692
5. Druker BJ, Tamura S, Buchdunger E et al (1996) Effects of a selective inhibitor of the Abl tyrosine kinase on the growth of Bcr-Abl positive cells. Nat Med 2:561–566
6. O'Brien SG, Guilhot F, Larson RA et al (2003) Imatinib compared with interferon and low-dose cytarabine for newly diagnosed chronic-phase chronic myeloid leukemia. N Engl J Med 348:994–1004
7. Druker BJ, Guilhot F, O'Brien SG et al (2006) Five-year follow-up of patients receiving imatinib for chronic myeloid leukemia. N Engl J Med 355:2408–2417
8. Sawyers CL, Hochhaus A, Feldman E et al (2002) Imatinib induces hematologic and cytogenetic responses in patients with chronic myelogenous leukemia in myeloid blast crisis: results of a phase II study. Blood 99:3530–3539
9. Talpaz M, Silver RT, Druker BJ et al (2002) Imatinib induces durable hematologic and cytogenetic responses in patients with accelerated phase chronic myeloid leukemia: results of a phase 2 study. Blood 99:1928–1937
10. Novartis (2007) Imatinib prescribing information. Novartis, East Hanover, NJ
11. O'Hare T, Eide CA, Deininger MW (2007) Bcr-Abl kinase domain mutations, drug resistance, and the road to a cure for chronic myeloid leukemia. Blood 110:2242–2249
12. Soverini S, Colarossi S, Gnani A et al (2006) Contribution of ABL kinase domain mutations to imatinib resistance in different subsets of Philadelphia-positive patients: by the GIMEMA Working Party on Chronic Myeloid Leukemia. Clin Cancer Res 12:7374–7379

13. Branford S, Rudzki Z, Walsh S et al (2003) Detection of BCR-ABL mutations in patients with CML treated with imatinib is virtually always accompanied by clinical resistance, and mutations in the ATP phosphate-binding loop (P-loop) are associated with a poor prognosis. Blood 102:276–283

14. Hughes T, Deininger M, Hochhaus A et al (2006) Monitoring CML patients responding to treatment with tyrosine kinase inhibitors: review and recommendations for harmonizing current methodology for detecting BCR-ABL transcripts and kinase domain mutations and for expressing results. Blood 108:28–37

15. Deininger M, Buchdunger E, Druker BJ (2005) The development of imatinib as a therapeutic agent for chronic myeloid leukemia. Blood 105:2640–2653

16. Gorre ME, Mohammed M, Ellwood K et al (2001) Clinical resistance to STI-571 cancer therapy caused by BCR-ABL gene mutation or amplification. Science 293:876–880

17. O'Hare T, Walters DK, Stoffregen EP et al (2005) In vitro activity of Bcr-Abl inhibitors AMN107 and BMS-354825 against clinically relevant imatinib-resistant Abl kinase domain mutants. Cancer Res 65:4500–4505

18. Kantarjian HM, Talpaz M, Giles F et al (2006) New insights into the pathophysiology of chronic myeloid leukemia and imatinib resistance. Ann Intern Med 145:913–923

19. Hochhaus A, Kreil S, Corbin AS et al (2002) Molecular and chromosomal mechanisms of resistance to imatinib (STI571) therapy. Leukemia 16:2190–2196

20. Wu J, Meng F, Lu H et al (2008) Lyn regulates BCR-ABL and Gab2 tyrosine phosphorylation and c-Cbl protein stability in imatinib-resistant chronic myelogenous leukemia cells. Blood 111:3821–3829

21. Burchert A, Wang Y, Cai D et al (2005) Compensatory PI3-kinase/Akt/mTor activation regulates imatinib resistance development. Leukemia 19:1774–1782

22. Thomas J, Wang L, Clark RE et al (2004) Active transport of imatinib into and out of cells: implications for drug resistance. Blood 104:3739–3745

23. Zong Y, Zhou S, Sorrentino BP (2005) Loss of P-glycoprotein expression in hematopoietic stem cells does not improve responses to imatinib in a murine model of chronic myelogenous leukemia. Leukemia 19:1590–1596

24. Perel JM, McCarthy C, Walker O et al (2005) Clinical significance of development of Philadelphia-chromosome negative clones in patients with chronic myeloid leukemia treated with imatinib mesylate. Haematologica 90 Suppl:ECR25

25. Tokarski JS, Newitt JA, Chang CY et al (2006) The structure of Dasatinib (BMS-354825) bound to activated ABL kinase domain elucidates its inhibitory activity against imatinib-resistant ABL mutants. Cancer Res 66:5790–5797

26. Lombardo LJ, Lee FY, Chen P et al (2004) Discovery of N-(2-chloro-6-methyl- phenyl)-2-(6-(4-(2-hydroxyethyl)- piperazin-1-yl)-2-methylpyrimidin-4-ylamino)thiazole-5-carboxamide (BMS-354825), a dual Src/Abl kinase inhibitor with potent antitumor activity in preclinical assays. J Med Chem 47:6658–6661

27. Nam S, Kim D, Cheng JQ et al (2005) Action of the Src family kinase inhibitor, dasatinib (BMS-354825), on human prostate cancer cells. Cancer Res 65:9185–9189

28. Weisberg E, Manley PW, Breitenstein W et al (2005) Characterization of AMN107, a selective inhibitor of native and mutant Bcr-Abl. Cancer Cell 7:129–141

29. le Coutre P, Ottmann OG, Giles F et al (2008) Nilotinib (formerly AMN107), a highly selective BCR-ABL tyrosine kinase inhibitor, is active in patients with imatinib-resistant or -intolerant accelerated-phase chronic myelogenous leukemia. Blood 111:1834–1839

30. Miettinen M, Lasota J (2006) Gastrointestinal stromal tumors: review on morphology, molecular pathology, prognosis, and differential diagnosis. Arch Pathol Lab Med 130:1466–1478

31. Blanke CD, Eisenberg BL, Heinrich MC (2001) Gastrointestinal stromal tumors. Curr Treat Options Oncol 2:485–491

32. Corless CL, Fletcher JA, Heinrich MC (2004) Biology of gastrointestinal stromal tumors. J Clin Oncol 22:3813–3825

33. Miettinen M, Lasota J (2006) Gastrointestinal stromal tumors: pathology and prognosis at different sites. Semin Diagn Pathol 23:70–83

34. Rubin BP, Heinrich MC, Corless CL (2007) Gastrointestinal stromal tumour. Lancet 369:1731–1741

35. Somerhausen Nde S, Fletcher CD (1998) Gastrointestinal stromal tumours: an update. Sarcoma 2:133–141

36. Sarlomo-Rikala M, Kovatich AJ, Barusevicius A et al (1998) CD117: a sensitive marker for gastrointestinal stromal tumors that is more specific than CD34. Mod Pathol 11:728–734

37. Heinrich MC, Dooley DC, Freed AC et al (1993) Constitutive expression of steel factor gene by human stromal cells. Blood 82:771–783

38. Rubin BP, Singer S, Tsao C et al (2001) KIT activation is a ubiquitous feature of gastrointestinal stromal tumors. Cancer Res 61:8118–8121

39. Corless CL, Heinrich MC (2008) Molecular pathobiology of gastrointestinal stromal sarcomas. Annu Rev Pathol 3:557–586

40. Fletcher JA, Fletcher CD, Rubin BP et al (2002) KIT gene mutations in gastrointestinal stromal tumors: more complex than previously recognized? Am J Pathol 161:737–738, author reply 738–739

41. Hirota S, Isozaki K, Moriyama Y et al (1998) Gain-of-function mutations of c-kit in human gastrointestinal stromal tumors. Science 279:577–580

42. Heinrich MC, Corless CL, Duensing A et al (2003) PDGFRA activating mutations in gastrointestinal stromal tumors. Science 299:708–710

43. Lasota J, Stachura J, Miettinen M (2006) GISTs with PDGFRA exon 14 mutations represent subset of clinically favorable gastric tumors with epithelioid morphology. Lab Invest 86:94–100

44. Carroll M, Ohno-Jones S, Tamura S et al (1997) CGP 57148, a tyrosine kinase inhibitor, inhibits the growth of cells expressing BCR-ABL, TEL-ABL, and TEL-PDGFR fusion proteins. Blood 90:4947–4952

45. Druker BJ, Talpaz M, Resta DJ et al (2001) Efficacy and safety of a specific inhibitor of the BCR-ABL tyrosine kinase in chronic myeloid leukemia. N Engl J Med 344:1031–1037

46. Topaly J, Zeller WJ, Fruehauf S (2001) Synergistic activity of the new ABL-specific tyrosine kinase inhibitor STI571 and chemotherapeutic drugs on BCR-ABL-positive chronic myelogenous leukemia cells. Leukemia 15:342–347

47. Heinrich MC, Griffith DJ, Druker BJ et al (2000) Inhibition of c-kit receptor tyrosine kinase activity by STI 571, a selective tyrosine kinase inhibitor. Blood 96:925–932

48. Tuveson DA, Willis NA, Jacks T et al (2001) STI571 inactivation of the gastrointestinal stromal tumor c-KIT oncoprotein: biological and clinical implications. Oncogene 20:5054–5058

49. Joensuu H, Roberts PJ, Sarlomo-Rikala M et al (2001) Effect of the tyrosine kinase inhibitor STI571 in a patient with a metastatic gastrointestinal stromal tumor. N Engl J Med 344:1052–1056

50. van Oosterom AT, Judson I, Verweij J et al (2001) Safety and efficacy of imatinib (STI571) in metastatic gastrointestinal stromal tumours: a phase I study. Lancet 358:1421–1423

51. Blanke CD, Demetri GD, von Mehren M et al (2008) Long-term results from a randomized phase II trial of standard- versus higher-dose imatinib mesylate for patients with unresectable or metastatic gastrointestinal stromal tumors expressing KIT. J Clin Oncol 26:620–625

52. Demetri GD, Desai J, Fletcher JA et al (2004) SU11248, a multitargeted tyrosine kinase inhibitor, can overcome imatinib resistance caused by diverse genomic mechanisms in patients with

metastatic gastrointestinal stromal tumor. Proc Am Soc Clin Oncol 22:195s

53. Demetri GD, van Oosterom AT, Garrett CR et al (2006) Efficacy and safety of sunitinib in patients with advanced gastrointestinal stromal tumour after failure of imatinib: a randomised controlled trial. Lancet 368:1329–1338

54. Heinrich MC, Corless CL, Demetri GD et al (2003) Kinase mutations and imatinib response in patients with metastatic gastrointestinal stromal tumor. J Clin Oncol 21:4342–4349

55. Heinrich MC, Corless CL, Blanke CD et al (2006) Molecular correlates of imatinib resistance in gastrointestinal stromal tumors. J Clin Oncol 24:4764–4774

56. Antonescu CR, Besmer P, Guo T et al (2005) Acquired resistance to imatinib in gastrointestinal stromal tumor occurs through secondary gene mutation. Clin Cancer Res 11:4182–4190

57. Heinrich MC, Maki RG, Corless CL et al (2008) Primary and secondary kinase genotypes correlate with the biological and clinical activity of sunitinib in imatinib-resistant gastrointestinal stromal tumor. J Clin Oncol 26:5352–5359

58. Duensing A, Medeiros F, McConarty B et al (2004) Mechanisms of oncogenic KIT signal transduction in primary gastrointestinal stromal tumors (GISTs). Oncogene 23:3999–4006

59. Duensing A, Heinrich MC, Fletcher CD et al (2004) Biology of gastrointestinal stromal tumors: KIT mutations and beyond. Cancer Invest 22:106–116

60. Liegl B, Kepten I, Le C et al (2008) Heterogeneity of kinase inhibitor resistance mechanisms in GIST. J Pathol 216:64–74

61. McArthur GA, Demetri GD, van Oosterom A et al (2005) Molecular and clinical analysis of locally advanced dermatofibrosarcoma protuberans treated with imatinib: Imatinib Target Exploration Consortium Study B2225. J Clin Oncol 23:866–873

62. Mehrany K, Swanson NA, Heinrich MC et al (2006) Dermatofibrosarcoma protuberans: a partial response to imatinib therapy. Dermatol Surg 32:456–459

63. Beadling C, Jacobson-Dunlop E, Hodi FS et al (2008) KIT gene mutations and copy number in melanoma subtypes. Clin Cancer Res 14:6821–6828

64. Hodi FS, Friedlander P, Corless CL et al (2008) Major response to imatinib mesylate in KIT-mutated melanoma. J Clin Oncol 26:2046–2051

65. Jiang X, Zhou J, Yuen NK et al (2008) Imatinib targeting of KIT-mutant oncoprotein in melanoma. Clin Cancer Res 14:7726–7732

66. Heinrich MC, Corless CL (2004) Targeting mutant kinases in gastrointestinal stromal tumors: a paradigm for molecular therapy of other sarcomas. Cancer Treat Res 120:129–150

67. Demetri GD (2001) Targeting c-kit mutations in solid tumors: scientific rationale and novel therapeutic options. Semin Oncol 28:19–26

68. Heinrich MC, Blanke CD, Druker BJ et al (2002) Inhibition of KIT tyrosine kinase activity: a novel molecular approach to the treatment of KIT-positive malignancies. J Clin Oncol 20:1692–1703

69. Schiller JH, Harrington D, Belani CP et al (2002) Comparison of four chemotherapy regimens for advanced non-small-cell lung cancer. N Engl J Med 346:92–98

70. Laskin JJ, Sandler AB (2004) Epidermal growth factor receptor: a promising target in solid tumours. Cancer Treat Rev 30:1–17

71. Brabender J, Danenberg KD, Metzger R et al (2001) Epidermal growth factor receptor and HER2-neu mRNA expression in non-small cell lung cancer Is correlated with survival. Clin Cancer Res 7:1850–1855

72. Fontanini G, De Laurentiis M, Vignati S et al (1998) Evaluation of epidermal growth factor-related growth factors and receptors and of neoangiogenesis in completely resected stage I-IIIA non-small-cell lung cancer: amphiregulin and microvessel count are independent prognostic indicators of survival. Clin Cancer Res 4:241–249

73. Ohsaki Y, Tanno S, Fujita Y et al (2000) Epidermal growth factor receptor expression correlates with poor prognosis in non-small cell lung cancer patients with p53 overexpression. Oncol Rep 7:603–607

74. Rusch V, Baselga J, Cordon-Cardo C et al (1993) Differential expression of the epidermal growth factor receptor and its ligands in primary non-small cell lung cancers and adjacent benign lung. Cancer Res 53:2379–2385

75. Rusch V, Klimstra D, Venkatraman E et al (1997) Overexpression of the epidermal growth factor receptor and its ligand transforming growth factor alpha is frequent in resectable non-small cell lung cancer but does not predict tumor progression. Clin Cancer Res 3:515–522

76. Volm M, Rittgen W, Drings P (1998) Prognostic value of ERBB-1, VEGF, cyclin A, FOS, JUN and Myc in patients with squamous cell lung carcinomas. Br J Cancer 77:663–669

77. Carraway KL 3rd, Cantley LC (1994) A neu acquaintance for erbB3 and erbB4: a role for receptor heterodimerization in growth signaling. Cell 78:5–8

78. Riese DJ 2nd, Stern DF (1998) Specificity within the EGF family/ErbB receptor family signaling network. Bioessays 20:41–48

79. Roskoski R Jr (2004) The ErbB/HER receptor protein-tyrosine kinases and cancer. Biochem Biophys Res Commun 319:1–11

80. Kawamoto T, Sato JD, Le A et al (1983) Growth stimulation of A431 cells by epidermal growth factor: identification of high-affinity receptors for epidermal growth factor by an anti-receptor monoclonal antibody. Proc Natl Acad Sci USA 80:1337–1341

81. Sirotnak FM (2003) Studies with ZD1839 in preclinical models. Semin Oncol 30:12–20

82. Baselga J, Rischin D, Ranson M et al (2002) Phase I safety, pharmacokinetic, and pharmacodynamic trial of ZD1839, a selective oral epidermal growth factor receptor tyrosine kinase inhibitor, in patients with five selected solid tumor types. J Clin Oncol 20:4292–4302

83. Herbst RS, Maddox AM, Rothenberg ML et al (2002) Selective oral epidermal growth factor receptor tyrosine kinase inhibitor ZD1839 is generally well-tolerated and has activity in non-small-cell lung cancer and other solid tumors: results of a phase I trial. J Clin Oncol 20:3815–3825

84. Ranson M, Hammond LA, Ferry D et al (2002) ZD1839, a selective oral epidermal growth factor receptor-tyrosine kinase inhibitor, is well tolerated and active in patients with solid, malignant tumors: results of a phase I trial. J Clin Oncol 20:2240–2250

85. Nakagawa K, Tamura T, Negoro S et al (2003) Phase I pharmacokinetic trial of the selective oral epidermal growth factor receptor tyrosine kinase inhibitor gefitinib ('Iressa', ZD1839) in Japanese patients with solid malignant tumors. Ann Oncol 14:922–930

86. Fukuoka M, Yano S, Giaccone G et al (2003) Multi-institutional randomized phase II trial of gefitinib for previously treated patients with advanced non-small-cell lung cancer. J Clin Oncol 21:2237–2246

87. Kris MG, Natale RB, Herbst RS et al (2003) Efficacy of gefitinib, an inhibitor of the epidermal growth factor receptor tyrosine kinase, in symptomatic patients with non-small cell lung cancer: a randomized trial. JAMA 290:2149–2158

88. Shepherd FA, Pereira J, Ciuleanu TE et al (2004) A randomized placebo-controlled trial of erlotinib in patients with advanced non-small cell lung cancer (NSCLC) following failure of 1st line or 2nd line chemotherapy. A National Cancer Institute of Canada Clinical Trials Group (NCIC CTG) trial. Proc Am Soc Clin Oncol 622s

89. Thatcher N, Chang A, Parikh P et al (2005) Gefitinib plus best supportive care in previously treated patients with refractory advanced non-small-cell lung cancer: results from a randomised, placebo-controlled, multicentre study (Iressa Survival Evaluation in Lung Cancer). Lancet 366:1527–1537

90. Miller VA, Kris MG, Shah N et al (2004) Bronchioloalveolar pathologic subtype and smoking history predict sensitivity to gefitinib in advanced non-small-cell lung cancer. J Clin Oncol 22:1103–1109

91. Janne PA, Gurubhagavatula S, Yeap BY et al (2004) Outcomes of patients with advanced non-small cell lung cancer treated with gefitinib (ZD1839, 'Iressa') on an expanded access study. Lung Cancer 44:221–230

92. Haringhuizen A, van Tinteren H, Vaessen HF et al (2004) Gefitinib as a last treatment option for non-small-cell lung cancer: durable disease control in a subset of patients. Ann Oncol 15:786–792

93. Simon GR, Ruckdeschel JC, Williams C et al (2003) Gefitinib (ZD1839) in previously treated advanced non-small-cell lung cancer: experience from a single institution. Cancer Control 10:388–395

94. Argiris A, Mittal N (2004) Gefitinib as first-line, compassionate use therapy in patients with advanced non-small-cell lung cancer. Lung Cancer 43:317–322

95. Park J, Park BB, Kim JY et al (2004) Gefitinib (ZD1839) monotherapy as a salvage regimen for previously treated advanced non-small cell lung cancer. Clin Cancer Res 10:4383–4388

96. Lynch TJ, Bell DW, Sordella R et al (2004) Activating mutations in the epidermal growth factor receptor underlying responsiveness of non-small-cell lung cancer to gefitinib. N Engl J Med 350:2129–2139

97. Paez JG, Janne PA, Lee JC et al (2004) EGFR mutations in lung cancer: correlation with clinical response to gefitinib therapy. Science 304:1497–1500

98. Pao W, Miller V, Zakowski M et al (2004) EGF receptor gene mutations are common in lung cancers from "never smokers" and are associated with sensitivity of tumors to gefitinib and erlotinib. Proc Natl Acad Sci USA 101:13306–13311

99. Inoue A, Suzuki T, Fukuhara T et al (2006) Prospective phase II study of gefitinib for chemotherapy-naive patients with advanced non-small-cell lung cancer with epidermal growth factor receptor gene mutations. J Clin Oncol 24:3340–3346

100. Okamoto I, Kashii T, Urata Y et al (2006) EGFR mutation-based phase II multicenter trial of gefitinib in advanced non-small cell lung cancer (NSCLC) patients (pts): Results of West Japan Thoracic Oncology Group trial (WJTOG0403). J Clin Oncol 24:Absract 7073

101. Sutani A, Nagai Y, Udagawa K et al (2006) Phase II study of gefitinib for non-small cell lung cancer (NSCLC) patients with epidermal growth factor receptor (EGFR) gene mutations detected by PNA-LNA PCR clamp. J Clin Oncol 24:Abstract 7076

102. Morikawa N, Inoue A, Suzuki T et al (2006) Prospective analysis of the epidermal growth factor receptor gene mutations in non-small cell lung cancer in Japan. J Clin Oncol 24:Abstract 7077

103. Sequist LV, Martins RG, Spigel D et al (2008) First-line gefitinib in patients with advanced non-small-cell lung cancer harboring somatic EGFR mutations. J Clin Oncol 26:2442–2449

104. Mok T, Wu Y-L, Thongprasert S et al (2008) Phase III, randomised, open-label, first-line study of gefitinib vs carboplatin/paclitaxel in clinically selected patients with advanced non-small cell lung cancer (IPASS). 33rd ESMO congress, Stockholm

105. Tsao MS, Sakurada A, Cutz JC et al (2005) Erlotinib in lung cancer – molecular and clinical predictors of outcome. N Engl J Med 353:133–144

106. Engelman JA, Zejnullahu K, Mitsudomi T et al (2007) MET amplification leads to gefitinib resistance in lung cancer by activating ERBB3 signaling. Science 316:1039–1043

107. Engelman JA, Mukohara T, Zejnullahu K et al (2006) Allelic dilution obscures detection of a biologically significant resistance mutation in EGFR -amplified lung cancer. J Clin Invest 116:2695–2706

108. Tracy S, Mukohara T, Hansen M et al (2004) Gefitinib induces apoptosis in the EGFRL858R non-small cell lung cancer cell line H3255. Cancer Res 64:7241–7244

109. Smolen GA, Sordella R, Muir B et al (2006) Amplification of MET may identify a subset of cancers with extreme sensitivity to the selective tyrosine kinase inhibitor PHA-665752. Proc Natl Acad Sci USA 103:2316–2321

110. Engelman JA (2007) The role of phosphoinositide 3-kinase pathway inhibitors in the treatment of lung cancer. Clin Cancer Res 13:s4637–s4640

111. She Q, Solit D, Ye Q et al (2005) The BAD protein integrates survival signaling by EGFR/MAPK and PI3K/Akt kinase pathways in PTEN-deficient tumor cells. Cancer Cell 8:287–297

112. Mellinghoff IK, Wang MY, Vivanco I et al (2005) Molecular determinants of the response of glioblastomas to EGFR kinase inhibitors. N Engl J Med 353:2012–2024

113. Sharma SV, Fischbach MA, Haber DA et al (2006) "Oncogenic shock": explaining oncogene addiction through differential signal attenuation. Clin Cancer Res 12:4392s–4395s

114. Engelman JA, Settleman J (2008) Acquired resistance to tyrosine kinase inhibitors during cancer therapy. Curr Opin Genet Dev 18:73–79

115. Engelman JA, Janne PA (2008) Mechanisms of acquired resistance to epidermal growth factor receptor tyrosine kinase inhibitors in non-small cell lung cancer. Clin Cancer Res 14: 2895–2899

116. Kobayashi S, Boggon TJ, Dayaram T et al (2005) EGFR mutation and resistance of non-small-cell lung cancer to gefitinib. N Engl J Med 352:786–792

117. Pao W, Miller VA, Politi KA et al (2005) Acquired resistance of lung adenocarcinomas to gefitinib or erlotinib is associated with a second mutation in the EGFR kinase domain. PLoS Med 2:1–11

118. Kosaka T, Yatabe Y, Endoh H et al (2006) Analysis of epidermal growth factor receptor gene mutation in patients with non-small cell lung cancer and acquired resistance to gefitinib. Clin Cancer Res 12:5764–5769

119. Balak MN, Gong Y, Riely GJ et al (2006) Novel D761Y and common secondary T790M mutations in epidermal growth factor receptor-mutant lung adenocarcinomas with acquired resistance to kinase inhibitors. Clin Cancer Res 12:6494–6501

120. Kwak EL, Sordella R, Bell DW et al (2005) Irreversible inhibitors of the EGF receptor may circumvent acquired resistance to gefitinib. Proc Natl Acad Sci USA 102:7665–7670

121. Kobayashi S, Ji H, Yuza Y et al (2005) An alternative inhibitor overcomes resistance caused by a mutation of the epidermal growth factor receptor. Cancer Res 65:7096–7101

122. Li D, Shimamura T, Ji H et al (2007) Bronchial and peripheral murine lung carcinomas induced by T790M-L858R mutant EGFR respond to HKI-272 and rapamycin combination therapy. Cancer Cell 12:81–93

123. Regales L, Balak MN, Gong Y et al (2007) Development of new mouse lung tumor models expressing EGFR T790M mutants associated with clinical resistance to kinase inhibitors. PLoS One 2:e810

124. Ogino A, Kitao H, Hirano S et al (2007) Emergence of epidermal growth factor receptor T790M mutation during chronic exposure to gefitinib in a non small cell lung cancer cell line. Cancer Res 67:7807–7814

125. Cappuzzo F, Hirsch FR, Rossi E et al (2005) Epidermal growth factor receptor gene and protein and gefitinib sensitivity in non-small-cell lung cancer. J Natl Cancer Inst 97:643–655

126. Godin-Heymann N, Bryant I, Rivera MN et al (2007) Oncogenic activity of epidermal growth factor receptor kinase mutant alleles is enhanced by the T790M drug resistance mutation. Cancer Res 67:7319–7326

127. Greulich H, Chen TH, Feng W et al (2005) Oncogenic transformation by inhibitor-sensitive and -resistant EGFR mutants. PLoS Med 2:e313

128. Bell DW, Gore I, Okimoto RA et al (2005) Inherited susceptibility to lung cancer may be associated with the T790M drug resistance mutation in EGFR. Nat Genet 37:1315–1316

129. Kosaka T, Yatabe Y, Endoh H et al (2004) Mutations of the epidermal growth factor receptor gene in lung cancer: biological and clinical implications. Cancer Res 64:8919–8923

130. Engelman JA, Zejnullahu K, Gale CM et al (2007) PF00299804, an irreversible pan-ERBB inhibitor, is effective in lung cancer models with EGFR and ERBB2 mutations that are resistant to gefitinib. Cancer Res 67:11924–11932

131. Janne PA, Schellens JH, Engelman JA et al (2008) Preliminary activity and safety results from a phase I clinical trial of PF-00299804, an irreversible pan-HER inhibitor, in patients (pts) with NSCLC (Abstract #8027). J Clin Oncol 26:Abstract 8027

132. Bean J, Brennan C, Shih JY et al (2007) MET amplification occurs with or without T790M mutations in EGFR mutant lung tumors with acquired resistance to gefitinib or erlotinib. Proc Natl Acad Sci USA 104:20932–20937

133. Soda M, Choi YL, Enomoto M et al (2007) Identification of the transforming EML4-ALK fusion gene in non-small-cell lung cancer. Nature 448:561–566

134. Rikova K, Guo A, Zeng Q et al (2007) Global survey of phosphotyrosine signaling identifies oncogenic kinases in lung cancer. Cell 131:1190–1203

135. Chiarle R, Voena C, Ambrogio C et al (2008) The anaplastic lymphoma kinase in the pathogenesis of cancer. Nat Rev Cancer 8:11–23

136. Soda M, Takada S, Takeuchi K et al (2008) A mouse model for EML4-ALK-positive lung cancer. Proc Natl Acad Sci USA 105:19893–19897

137. Koivunen JP, Mermel C, Zejnullahu K et al (2008) EML4-ALK fusion gene and efficacy of an ALK kinase inhibitor in lung cancer. Clin Cancer Res 14:4275–4283

138. McDermott U, Iafrate AJ, Gray NS et al (2008) Genomic alterations of anaplastic lymphoma kinase may sensitize tumors to anaplastic lymphoma kinase inhibitors. Cancer Res 68:3389–3395

139. Fukuyoshi Y, Inoue H, Kita Y et al (2008) EML4-ALK fusion transcript is not found in gastrointestinal and breast cancers. Br J Cancer 98:1536–1539

140. Takeuchi K, Choi YL, Soda M et al (2008) Multiplex reverse transcription-PCR screening for EML4-ALK fusion transcripts. Clin Cancer Res 14:6618–6624

141. Perner S, Wagner PL, Demichelis F et al (2008) EML4-ALK fusion lung cancer: a rare acquired event. Neoplasia 10: 298–302

142. Inamura K, Takeuchi K, Togashi Y et al (2008) EML4-ALK fusion is linked to histological characteristics in a subset of lung cancers. J Thorac Oncol 3:13–17

143. Shinmura K, Kageyama S, Tao H et al (2008) EML4-ALK fusion transcripts, but no NPM-, TPM3-, CLTC-, ATIC-, or TFG-ALK fusion transcripts, in non-small cell lung carcinomas. Lung Cancer 61:163–169

144. Wong DW, Leung EL, So KK et al (2009) The EML4-ALK fusion gene is involved in various histologic types of lung cancers from nonsmokers with wild-type EGFR and KRAS. Cancer 115(8): 1723–1733

145. Shaw AT, Yeap BY, Mino-Kenudson M et al (2009) Clinical features and outcome of patients with non-small cell lung cancer harboring EML4-ALK. J Clin Oncol 27(26):4247–4253

146. Castro CY, Moran CA, Flieder DG et al (2001) Primary signet ring cell adenocarcinomas of the lung: a clinicopathological study of 15 cases. Histopathology 39:397–401

147. Tsuta K, Ishii G, Yoh K et al (2004) Primary lung carcinoma with signet-ring cell carcinoma components: clinicopathological analysis of 39 cases. Am J Surg Pathol 28:868–874

148. Iwasaki T, Ohta M, Lefor AT et al (2008) Signet-ring cell carcinoma component in primary lung adenocarcinoma: potential prognostic factor. Histopathology 52:639–640

149. Christensen JG, Zou HY, Arango ME et al (2007) Cytoreductive antitumor activity of PF-2341066, a novel inhibitor of anaplastic lymphoma kinase and c-Met, in experimental models of anaplastic large-cell lymphoma. Mol Cancer Ther 6:3314–3322

150. Kwak EL, Camidge DR, Clark J et al (2009) Clinical activity observed in a phase I dose-escalation trial of an oral c-Met and ALK inhibitor, PF-02341066. J Clin Oncol 27:15s

Index

A

Acute promyelocytic leukemia (APML), 5
Adenomatous polyposis syndromes
  familial adenomatous polyposis
    clinical features, 63–65
    extraintestinal malignancies, 65
    genetic testing, 66–67
    genetics, 65–66
    genotype/phenotype correlations, 66
    prevention strategies, 67
  MUTYH-associated polyposis
    colorectal cancers, 67, 68
    genetic testing, 68–69
    genotype/phenotype correlation, 69
    management implications, 69
    multiple adenomatous polyps, 67
    prevention strategies, 69
Adrenal cortical carcinoma (ACC), 46
All-trans retinoic acid (ATRA), 5
Alleles
  breast cancer, 200
  cancer-risk alleles, 201, 202
  SNPs, 196–198
Amsterdam criteria, 78. See also Lynch
      syndrome
Angiomyolipomas, 114
Atypical teratoid/rhabdoid tumors (AT/RTs), 190

B

Bannayan–Riley–Ruvalcaba (BRRS), 71
Beckwith Wiedemann syndrome (BWS),
      171–172
Beta-catenin mutations, 99
BHD. See Birt-Hogg-Dube syndrome
Bilateral prophylactic mastectomy (BPM)
  bilateral salpingo-oophorectomy, 54
  BRCA gene mutation carriers, 53
  clinical characteristics, 54
Bilateral salpingo-oophorectomy (BSO)
  BRCA gene mutation, 54
  risk-reducing efficacy, 59
Birt-Hogg-Dube syndrome (BHD)
  clinical presentation, 118–119
  molecular genetics, 119
BPM. See Bilateral prophylactic mastectomy
BSO. See Bilateral salpingo-oophorectomy
Breast cancer, 200, 201

C

Café-au-lait spots, 182
Carney complex, 159
Central nervous system (CNS), 65
Chromosome 13q14 deletion syndrome, 165–166, 168
Chronic myeloid leukemia (CML)
  BCR-ABL, 205–206
  dasatinib, 207
  imatinib resistance mechanisms, 207
  molecular monitoring, 206
  nilotinib, 207
Clinically atypical nevus (CAN), 130–131
CML. See Chronic myeloid leukemia
Colonic polyposis syndromes. See also Adenomatous polyposis
      syndromes; Hamartomatous polyposis syndromes;
      Hyperplastic polyposis syndrome
  adenomatous polyposis syndromes, 63–69
  hamartomatous polyposis syndromes, 69–72
  hyperplastic polyposis syndrome, 72–73
Colorectal cancer, 201
Congenital hypertrophy of the retinal epithelium (CHRPE), 65
Cowden syndrome (CS)
  clinical features and genetics
    consensus diagnostic criteria, 47
    PTEN gene, 48
  clinical management, 48
CpG island methylator phenotype (CIMP), 73
Cutaneous lichen amyloidosis (CLA), 151
Cyclin-dependent kinase 4 (CDK4), 134
Cyclin-dependent kinase inhibitor 2A (CDKN2A), 132
Cyclin-dependent kinases (CDKs), 9
Cystic fibrosis transmembrane receptor (CFTR), 92

D

Dasatinib, 207
Dihydrofolate reductase (DHFR), 17
Doorknob syndrome, 24
Dysplastic nevus (DN), 130–131

E

E-cadherin gene (CDH1), 48, 97
Education, genetics and cancer
  benefits, 30–31
  genes, tumorigenesis and inheritance patterns, 29
  limitations, 31
  possible test results, 30
  risk reduction options, 29

Endolymphatic sac tumors (ELST), 111
Entero-pancreatic neuroendocrine tumors, 155
Epidermal growth factor receptor (EGFR)), 2
Extracellular signal-regulated kinase (ERK), 212

F
Familial adenomatous polyposis (FAP)
    clinical features, 63–65
    extraintestinal malignancies, 65
    genetic testing, 66–67
    genetics, 65–66
    genotype/phenotype correlations, 66
    prevention strategies, 67
Familial atypical mole melanoma (FAMM) syndrome
    CDKN2A germline mutation, 134–135
    clinical features
        clinically atypical nevus (CAN), 130–131
        dysplastic nevus (DN), 130
        histopathological criteria, 129–130
    genetic counseling and testing
        limitations, 136
        pancreatic cancer screening, 137–138
        positive and negative result, 137
        psychological impact, 137
        regression models, 136–137
    genetics and genotypephenotype correlations
        cyclin-dependent kinase 4 (CDK4), 134
        melanocortin-1-receptor gene (MC1R), 134
        p16INK4A and p14ARF, 132–133
    management and prevention, 138–139
    Met53Ile mutation, 135
    ocular melanoma (OM), 135
    origin, 129
    pancreatic carcinoma (PC), 134–135
    sporadic vs. hereditary forms, 131–132
Familial medullary thyroid cancer (FMTC), 149–150
Familial pancreatic cancer, 92
Familial renal cell carcinoma
    BHD syndrome, 118–119
    constitutive translocations, chromosome 3,
        116–117
    hereditary leiomyomatosis with RCC (HLRCC), 118
    hereditary papillary RCC type 1, 117
    negative genetic test, 120–121
    referral and evaluation, 119–120
    succinate dehydrogenase B (SDHB), 117
    supernumerary nipple syndrome, 117
    tuberous sclerosis complex (TSC)
        clinical presentation, 114–115
        genetic testing, 115
        molecular genetics and therapeutic implications, 116
    VHL syndrome
        antiangiogenic agents, 112
        central nervous system hemangioblastomas, 110
        clinical presentation, 109–110
        genetic testing, 111
        molecular genetics, 113–114
        multiple and bilateral renal cysts, 110
        pancreatic lesions, 110–111
        papillary cystadenomas, 111
        pheochromocytomas, 110
        surveillance guidelines, 112–113
        treatment, 111
Familial Wilms' tumor (FWT), 174
FAMM syndrome. See Familial atypical mole melanoma syndrome

Fluorescence in situ hybridization (FISH), 215
Fluoro-2-deoxy-d-glucose positron emission tomography
        (FDG-PET), 101
Frasier syndrome, 171

G
Gamma catenin, 99
Gastrinomas, 155–156
Gastrointestinal stromal tumors (GISTs)
    c-KIT
        exon mutations, 208, 209
        imatinib inhibition, 209
    drug resistance mechanism, 209, 210
    genotypephenotype correlations, 210
    NF1-related tumors, 185
    platelet derived growth factor receptor α (PDGFR-α)
        mutations, 208, 209
        sunitinib, 209, 210
Gefitinib, 211–212
Genetic abnormalities
    cancer
        germline vs. somatic genetic alterations, 2
        oncogenes and proto-oncogenes, 2–5
        pathogenesis, 2
        techniques, 18–20
        treatment resistance, 16–18
        tumor progression, 14–16
        tumor suppressor genes, 6–13
    tumorigenesis, 1
Genetic counseling
    contracting, 24
    identification, 23
    medical information
        family history, 24–25
        individual's diagnosis, 25
        information accuracy, 25–26
    referral, 24
    risk assessment, 25–26
Genetic testing
    appropriate index testing, 27–28
    DNA banking, 28
    family members, 27
    ideal testing candidate, 26
    informed consent process, 28–29
    laboratories, 28
    psychosocial assessment and support
        post-test support, 32
        pre-test support, 31
        test results, 32
        VUS, 32
    research testing, 28
    screening process, 27–28
    test results disclosure, 28
    timing, 26–27
Genome-wide association studies (GWAS)
    breast cancer, 200, 201
    colorectal cancer, 201
    prostate cancer, 200
Genomic analysis
    cancer susceptibility, 20
    competitive genomic hybridization (CGH), 19
    gene expression profiling, 18
    GWAS studies, 20
    haplotype blocks, 19
    RNA hybridization, 18

GIST. *See* Gastrointestinal stromal tumors
GWAS. *See* Genome-wide association studies

H

Hamartomatous polyposis syndromes
   juvenile polyposis syndrome, 70–71
   Peutz-Jeghers syndrome, 69–70
   PTEN hamartoma syndrome
      BRRS and proteus syndrome, 72
      Cowden syndrome, 71
Haplotype analysis, 19
HBOC. *See* Hereditary breast and ovarian cancer
Health Insurance Portability and Accountability Act (HIPAA), 37
Helicobacter pylori infection, 97
Herediatary paraganglioma-phechromocytoma syndromes
   genetic testing, 122–124
   SDHx germline mutations, 122
   surveillance guidelines, 122
Hereditary breast and ovarian cancer (HBOC)
   bilateral prophylactic mastectomy
      bilateral salpingo-oophorectomy, 54
      BRCA gene mutation carriers, 53
      clinical characteristics, 54
   BRCA1 and BRCA2 mutations, 53
   breast cancer screening, 58
   clinical features and genetics
      anthracycline-based chemotherapy, 44
      BRCA1 and BRCA2, 42–44
      estrogen receptor (ER), 42
      founder mutations, 43, 44
      missense mutations, 43
      P-cadherin (CDH3), 42
      prophylactic oophorectomy, 44
      testing criteria, 43
   clinical management
      BRCA1 and BRCA2, 45, 46
      MRI screening, 45
      oral contraceptives, 46
      PARP inhibitors, 45
      risk-reduction mastectomy, 46
   high-risk screening *vs.* prophylactic mastectomy, 54
   lynch/HNPCC mutation, 60
   mastectomy options
      nipple-sparing mastectomy, 56–57
      skin-sparing mastectomy, 56
   patient satisfaction, 54–55
   reconstruction, 57
   sentinel lymph node biopsy, 57–58
   surgical management, BRCA1/2 carriers, 58
   technical considerations, 55
Hereditary breast cancer syndromes
   CDH1 mutation carriers, 55
   clinical testing laboratories, 42
   genetic testing, 41
   hereditary predisposition, genes, 42
   p53 mutation carriers, 55
   PTEN mutation carriers, 55
Hereditary colon cancer
   colonic polyposis syndromes
      adenomatous polyposis syndromes, 63–69
      hamartomatous polyposis syndromes, 69–72
      hyperplastic polyposis syndrome, 72–73
   Lynch syndrome, 77–86
Hereditary diffuse gastric cancer
   autosomal dominant susceptibility syndromes, 100

CDH1 gene
   cadherin–catenin complexes, 98
   hypermethylation, 99
   lobular breast cancer, 98
   somatic mutations, 98, 99
clinical criteria, 98
gastric adenocarcinomas, 98
genetic counseling and testing, 100
genotype and phenotype, 99–100
germline CDH1 mutation
   congo red-methylene blue method, 101
   signet-ring cell carcinoma, 100
   surveillance endoscopy, 101
prophylactic total gastrectomy
   gastric mucosa, 104
   germline E-cadherin mutations, 101
   intra-operative endoscopy, 103
   operative morbidity and mortality, 103
   pathological analysis, 104
   pedigree analysis, 102
   Roux-en-Y reconstruction, 104
   surgical series, 103
Hereditary diffuse gastric cancer syndrome (HDGC), 41
Hereditary leiomyomatosis with RCC (HLRCC), 118
Hereditary non-polyposis colon cancer (HNPCC) syndrome, 100.
   See also Lynch syndrome
Hereditary ovarian cancer
   bilateral prophylactic salpingo-oophrectomy, 59
   hysterectomy, 60
   risk-reducing BSO, efficacy of, 59
   risk-reducing surgery, 59–60
   surgery timing, 60
Hereditary pancreatic cancer
   breast/ovarian cancer syndrome, 91
   endocrine tumors, 90
   EUS/ERCP, 94
   exocrine neoplasms, 90
   familial atypical mole melanoma syndrome, 91
   familial cancer syndrome, 89
   genetic anticipation, 94
   genetic syndromes, 93
   high-risk patients, 93
   Lynch syndrome, 91
   MGH Screening Program, 94–95
   pancreatic ductal adenocarcinoma, 90
   Peutz–Jeghers, 90
   screening and surveillance strategies, 93
Hereditary pancreatitis and pancreatic neoplasms
   CFTR, 92
   PDAC, 91
   PRSS1, 92
   SPINK1, 91
   trypsin inhibitor, 92
Hereditary papillary RCC type 1 (HPRCC1)
   clinical presentation, 117
   molecular genetics and therapeutic implications, 117
   papillary thyroid carcinoma, 118
Hirschsprung disease (HD), 151
HPRCC1. *See* Hereditary papillary RCC type 1
Hyperplastic polyposis syndrome
   CpG island methylator phenotype (CIMP), 73
   diagnostic criteria, 72
   management, 73
   sporadic hyperplastic polyps, 72
Hypoxia inducible factor (HIF), 112

I

IHP. *See* International HapMap Project
Ileorectal anastomosis (IRA), 84
Immunohistochemistry (IHC), 28, 78
In vitro fertilization (IVF), 36
Informed consent document, 32–33
    confidentiality, 33–35
    costs and billing practices, 35
    ethical issues
        preimplantation genetic diagnosis, 36–37
        testing minors, 35–36
    genetic counselor, 37
Insulinomas, 156
International Gastric Cancer Linkage Consortium (IGCLC), 97
International HapMap Project (IHP)
    candidate gene association studies, 199
    DNA variations, 199
    haplotypes, 197, 198
    SNPs variable, 198
Iressa dose evaluation in advanced lung cancer (IDEAL), 211

J

Juvenile myelomonocytic leukemia (JMML), 185
Juvenile polyposis syndrome (JPS), 70–71

K

K-Ras oncogene, 2
Knudson hypothesis
    retinoblastoma, 165
    Wilms tumor, 171
Knudson model, 7–8

L

Leukemia, 185
Leukokoria, 163, 164
Li–Fraumeni syndrome (LFS)
    clinical features and genetics
        adrenal cortical carcinoma (ACC), 46
        classic and chompret criteria, 47
        p53 mutations, 46
    clinical management, 47
Linkage analysis, 195
Lobular breast cancer, 105
Loss of heterozygosity (LOH), 8
Low-penetrance cancer susceptibility alleles, 196, 201
Lynch syndrome
    clinical features
        extracolonic cancers, 77
        gene-specific lifetime cancer risks, 78
    diagnosis, 78
    genetic counseling, 85
    genetics and DNA microsatellite instability
        DNA mismatch repair process, 79
        germline mutation, 78
        immunohistochemical approach, 80
        polymerase chain reaction (PCR), 79
    genotype/phenotype correlations
        endometrial cancer, 84
        gastric cancer, 83
        MLH1 and MSH2 carriers, 83
        PMS2 gene defects, 84

    high-risk patients identification, 85
    hypermethylation and sporadic colon cancers, 81
    patients management
        Amsterdam criteria, 84
        chemotherapy, 85
        diagnosis, 84
        microsatellite instability, 85
        NCCN practice guidelines, 84
        sulindac, 85
    screening tests
        adenomatous polyps, 81
        MLH1/MSH2 immunohistochemistry, 80
    unselected colorectal cancer patients
        Amsterdam/Bethesda criteria, 82
        IHC, 81
        Leiden model, 82
        mismatch repair mutations, 82, 83
        molecular techniques, 81, 83
        MSI analysis, 81

M

Malignant peripheral nerve sheath tumors (MPNST), 182, 185
Mammography, 45
MAP. *See* MUTYH-associated polyposis
McCune Albright syndrome, 159
Medullary thyroid cancer (MTC)
    clinic features, 148–149
    sporadic and familial, 149
Melanocortin-1-receptor gene (MC1R), 134
MEN. *See* Multiple endocrine neoplasia
Meningiomas, 186
Microsatellite instability (MSI), 12, 78
Molecular-profiling approaches, 202
MTC. *See* Medullary thyroid cancer
Multiple endocrine neoplasia (MEN)
    medullary thyroid cancer (MTC)
        clinic features, 148–149
        sporadic and familial, 149
    type 1
        adrenal abnormalities, 157
        carcinoid tumors, 157
        clinical definition and penetrance, 154
        clinical features, 153
        CNS tumors, 157
        entero-pancreatic neuroendocrine tumors, 155
        gastrinomas, 155–156
        genetic screening, 157–158
        insulinomas, 156
        molecular genetics, 153–154
        non-functional tumors, 156
        pituitary adenomas, 156–157
        primary hyperparathyroidism, 154–155
        rare functional tumors, 156
        skin lesions, 157
    type 2
        clinical features, 145, 146
        genotype-phenotype correlations, 147–148
        molecular genetics, 145–147
    type 2A
        cutaneous lichen amyloidosis (CLA), 151
        hirschsprung disease (HD), 151
        hyperparathyroidism, 151
        pheochromocytomas, 150–151

type 2B
    clinical phenotype, 151
    screening impact, 152
    surgery timing, 152–153
Multiple endocrine neoplasia type 1 syndrome (MEN-1), 90
Multiple endocrine neoplasia type 2 (MEN 2), 121
Multiple hamartoma syndrome. *See* Cowden syndrome
Multiplex ligation-dependent probe amplification (MLPA), 80
MUTYH-associated polyposis (MAP)
    clinical features
        colorectal cancers, 67, 68
        FAP, 68
        multiple adenomatous polyps, 67
    genetic testing, 68–69
    genetics, 68
    genotype/phenotype correlation, 69
    management implications, 69
    prevention strategies, 69

N

National Comprehensive Cancer Network (NCCN), 23, 45
Neurofibroma, 184–185
Neurofibromatosis (NF)
    type 1
        clinical features and diagnostic criteria, 181–183
        genetic testing, 184
        genetics and molecular biology, 183–184
        patient management, 184
        pheochromocytoma, 185
        sporadic related tumor, 184–185
    type 2
        clinical features and diagnostic criteria, 185–186
        genetic testing, 187
        genetics and molecular biology, 186–187
        patient management, 187–188
        sporadic related tumor, 188
Neurofibromatosis type 1 (NF1), 121
Nilotinib, 207
Nonfunctional pancreatic neuroendocrine tumors (NFPNET), 156
Nonsmall cell lung cancer (NSCLC)
    EML4-ALK
        clinical outcomes, 215–216
        clinicopathologic features, 214–215
        diagnostic testing, 215
        fusion, 214
    epidermal growth factor receptor (EGFR)
        gefitinib trials, 211
        irreversible inhibitors, 213
        MET amplification, 214
        mutation, 210–211, 213
        oncogene addiction, 212
        somatic mutations, 212
        T790M mutations, 212–213
NSCLC. *See* Nonsmall cell lung cancer

O

Ocular melanoma (OM), 135
Oncogenes and proto-oncogenes activation
    gene amplifications and chromosomal translocations, 4–5
    human cancer, 3
    mechanisms, 4
Optic pathway glioma, 185

P

Pancreatic ductal adenocarcinoma (PDAC), 90
Pancreatic neuroendocrine tumors (PNETs), 111
Pediatric malignancy
    retinoblastoma
        clinical features, 163–164
        gene mutation, 165–166
        genetic diagnosis, 167–168
        management, 164
        molecular biology, 164–165
        p53, 166–167
        penetrance and mutation detection rates, 166
        pRB, 165
        RB1 gene, 165
    Wilms' tumor (WT)
        aneuploidy syndrome, 174
        clinical features, 169–171
        genetics and genotypephenotype correlations, 171–174
        management, 174–175
        Perlman syndrome, 174
        side effects, 175–176
        Simpson-Golabi-Behmel syndrome, 174
Perlman syndrome, 174
Peutz–Jeghers syndrome, 69–70
Pheochromocytoma and paraganlioma, familial
    clinical presentation, 121
    herediatary paraganglioma-phechromocytoma syndromes
        genetic testing, 122–124
        SDHx germline mutations, 121
        surveillance guidelines, 122
    VHL disease, 121
Philadelphia chromosome, 205
Phosphatase and tensin homolog (PTEN)
    Cowden's syndrome, 55
    management, 72
Phosphoinositide 3-Kinase (PI3K), 212
Platelet derived growth factor (PDGF), 2
Platelet derived growth factor receptor α (PDGFR-α)
    mutation, 208–209
    sunitinib, 209, 210
Plexiform neurofibroma, 181–182
Poly-ADP ribose polymerase (PARP), 45
Polymerase chain reaction (PCR), 79, 184
Preimplantation genetic diagnosis (PGD), 36
Primary hyperparathyroidism (PHPT), 151
Prophylactic total gastrectomy
    gastric mucosa, 104
    germline E-cadherin mutations, 101
    intra-operative endoscopy, 103
    operative morbidity and mortality, 103
    pathological analysis, 104
    pedigree analysis, 102
    Roux-en-Y reconstruction, 104
    surgical series, 103
Prostate cancer, 200
Proto-oncogenes, 4
PTEN hamartoma syndrome (PTHS)
    BRRS and Proteus syndrome, 72
    Cowden syndrome (CS), 71
PTEN. *See* Phosphatase and tensin homolog
PTHS. *See* PTEN hamartoma syndrome

R

Radiofrequency ablation (RFA)
Retinoblastoma
    chromosome 13q14 deletion syndrome, 165–166, 168
    clinical features, 163–164
    gene mutation, 165–166
    genetic counseling, 167–168
    genetic diagnosis, 167
    management, 164
    molecular biology, 164–165
    p53, 166–167
    penetrance and mutation detection rates, 166
    pRB, 165
    RB1 gene, 165
    supersellar tumor, 167, 168
Retinoblastoma tumor suppressor (RB1) pathway
    CDKN2A gene, 9
    cell cycle regulatory pathway, 8
    p16-INK4a, 10
    pRb protein, 8
Risk-reducing bilateral salpingo-oophorectomy
        (RRBSO), 46

S

Schwannomatosis
    clinical features and diagnostic criteria, 189
    genetic testing, 190
    genetics and molecular biology, 189–190
    patient management, 190
    sporadic related tumor, 190
Serous papillary ovarian carcinoma, 44
Simpson-Golabi-Behmel syndrome, 174
Single nucleotide polymorphisms (SNPs), 19
    candidate gene association studies, 199
    genomic variation, 196, 197
    microsatellite markers, 196
    The SNP Consortium (TSC), 198
Skin self-examination (SSE), 138, 139
Small cell lung carcinomas (SCLC), 2
SNPs. *See* Single nucleotide polymorphisms
Spiegelman classification system, 67
Sporadic medullary thyroid cancer (FMTC), 149
Succinate dehydrogenase B (SDHB), 117
Supernumerary nipple syndrome, 117
Suprasellar tumor, 167, 168

T

Tamoxifen, 46
Telomeres, 15
Transforming growth factor-β (TGF-β), 16, 69
Trilateral retinoblastoma, 167, 168
Tuberous sclerosis complex (TSC)
    clinical presentation, 114–115
    genetic testing, 115
    molecular genetics and therapeutic implications, 116
Tumor progression
    cell death and acquisition of immortality, 15–16
    genetic lesions
        abnormalities, 14
        epigenetic lesions and gene silencing, 14
        microRNAs, 14–15
    metastasis and angiogenesis, 16

Tumor suppressor genes
    cellular signaling and differentiation
        human cancer genes, 13
        mTORC1, 12, 13
        PTEN, 12
        TGF-b signaling pathway, 13
        TSC1/2, 12, 13
    DNA mismatch repair and microsatellite instability, 11–12
    DNA tumor viruses, 7
    genome stability and DNA repair
        ARF/MDM-2/p53 pathway, 11
        carcinogenesis, 10
        MDM-2 gene, 11
        p53 cellular stress, 10
    Knudson model
        DNA hybridization analysis, 8
        hit kinetics hypothesis, 7
        single-nucleotide polymorphisms, 8
    RB1 pathway
        CDKN2A gene, 9
        cell cycle regulatory pathway, 8
        p16-INK4a, 10
        pRb protein, 8
Tumor-specific resistance
    Bcr–Abl, 18
    DHFR gene, 17
    genetic mechanisms, 18
    multidrug resistance (mdr), 16
    therapeutic angiogenesis inhibitors, 17

V

Variant of uncertain significance (VUS), 30
Vascular endothelial growth factor (VEGF), 16
Vestibular schwannomas (VS), 186
Von Hippel Lindau (VHL) syndrome
    antiangiogenic agents, 112
    central nervous system hemangioblastomas, 110
    clinical presentation, 109–110
    germline mutations, 111
    intervention, 111
    molecular genetics, 113–114
    multiple and bilateral renal cysts, 110
    pancreatic lesions, 110–111
    papillary cystadenomas, 111
    pheochromocytoma and paraganglioma, 121
    pheochromocytomas, 110
    surveillance guidelines, 112–113
    type 1 and 2, 110

W

WAGR syndrome, 171
Wilms' tumor (WT)
    aneuploidy syndrome, 174
    clinical features
        clinical presentation, 169
        diagnosis, 169–170
        epidemiology, 169
        histology, 170
        sporadic *vs.* hereditary, 170–171
    genetics and genotypephenotype correlations
        chromosome 11p15, 171–173
        chromosome 7p, 173

chromosomes 1p and 16q, 173
    familial, 174
    WT1 gene, 171
    WTX gene, 173–174
Knudson hypothesis, 171
management, 174–175
Perlman syndrome, 174

    side effects, 175–176
    Simpson-Golabi-Behmel syndrome, 174
WTX gene, 173–174

Z

Zollinger–Ellison syndrome (ZES), 155, 156